PROMOTING

Legal and Ethical

AWARENESS

A PRIMER FOR HEALTH PROFESSIONALS AND PATIENTS

PROMOTING
Legal and Ethical
AWARENESS

A PRIMER FOR HEALTH PROFESSIONALS AND PATIENTS

Ronald Scott, PT, EdD, JD, LLM

Attorney and Physical Therapist

Cibolo, Texas

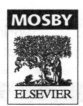

MOSBY

ELSEVIER

MOSBY
ELSEVIER

11830 Westline Industrial Drive
St. Louis, Missouri 63146

PROMOTING LEGAL AND ETHICAL AWARENESS:
A PRIMER FOR HEALTH PROFESSIONALS AND PATIENTS   ISBN: 978-0-323-03668-9
Copyright © 2009 by Mosby, Inc., an affiliate of Elsevier Inc.

Notice

Neither the Publisher nor the Author assume any responsibility for any loss or injury and/or damage to persons or property arising out of or related to any use of the material contained in this book. It is the responsibility of the treating practitioner, relying on independent expertise and knowledge of the patient, to determine the best treatment and method of application for the patient.

The Publisher

Library of Congress Control Number 2007941313

Vice President and Publisher: Linda Duncan
Senior Editor: Kathy Falk
Developmental Editor: Megan Fennell
Publishing Services Manager: Julie Eddy
Project Manager: Marquita Parker
Design Direction: Paula Catalano

Printed in the United States of America
Transferred to Digital Printing, 2011

Working together to grow
libraries in developing countries

www.elsevier.com | www.bookaid.org | www.sabre.org

ELSEVIER   BOOK AID International   Sabre Foundation

I dedicate this book with love to the love of my life, my wife Pepi.
Thanks for making my life complete over the past 35 years.

Preface

The health care system is indeed complex. From professional education to employment to clinical service delivery to reimbursement to quality management, every health care professional must be ever cognizant of existing and evolving standards.

This truism is no less applicable to ethical and legal mandates that govern health care practice. Even practicing attorneys have difficulty keeping up with a specialized area of the law in a single state system, so the task is even more challenging for health care professionals. Ethics and law modernly have often blended into a unitary standard of conduct, which must be conformed to.

This book is written with the intention of providing a roadmap to health professionals, students, and patients to the legal environment. It starts and ends with foci on professional ethics, which are inextricably intertwined with legal duties.

Chapters 1 and 2 address legal and ethical foundational principles. Chapter 2 presents a 4-quadrant legal/ethical clinical practice grid and a systems model for ethical decision making, which can be adapted for individual use by practitioners. Chapter 3 focuses on health care malpractice issues and clinical risk management. Chapter 4 addresses intentional wrongs – civil intentional torts and criminal misconduct incident to health care delivery. Chapter 5 covers ethical and legal issues in employment, and includes an alphabetized presentation of key federal employment laws and regulations, as well as detailed coverage of workplace sexual harassment.

Chapter 6 explores business law and ethics topics in alphabetical order, including, among other topics, advertising professional services, contracts, professional liability insurance, and the Sarbanes-Oxley Act of 2002. Chapter 7 examines legal and ethical issues in education, as they affect health care professionals. Chapter 8 concludes with focused ethical issues, including: informed consent, life and death decision making, nondiscrimination in health care delivery, pro bono care delivery, professional practice issues, and research considerations.

I hope that the information presented in this book helps you to better serve patients under your care, and to have greater peace of mind while doing so. Best wishes for continued practice success!

Acknowledgments

I wish to acknowledge all of the dedicated health care professionals and support professionals at all levels whose work improves the health and well-being of patients and their families and significant others. Thanks, too, to Kathy Falk, Megan Fennell, Marquita Parker, Julie Eddy, and Paula Catalano at Elsevier for their sage advice and assistance in making this book come to fruition.

About The Author

Ron Scott has been a health care professional since 1969, and an attorney since 1983. He has also been a university professor since 1985, and a writer, editor, and writers' coach since 1990.

Ron started his career as a Navy hospital corpsman and operating room technician during the Vietnam War in 1969. He subsequently attended the University of Pittsburgh's Physical Therapy Program, and graduated a McMillan Scholar and Jessie Wright awardee. He went on to earn 6 other academic degrees, including an MA in Spanish (Millersville University), MS (Samuel Merritt College), MSBA (Boston University), JD (University of San Diego), EdD (University of Texas, Austin), and LLM (Judge Advocate General's School).

Ron has been a civilian and Army physical therapist and clinical manager for 21 years. For 6 years, he was a JAG Corp attorney, specializing in criminal defense and health care malpractice claims adjudication.

After completing his military career as a Major in the Army Medical Specialist Corps, Ron became an associate professor and interim chair in physical therapy at the University of Texas Health Science Center, San Antonio. He is currently a faculty member in four programs: Husson College, Marymount University, Rocky Mountain University of Health Sciences (nursing, physical therapy, and allied health), and the University of Indianapolis.

Ron currently works full-time as an attorney-mediator, specializing in employment, family, and health law. This is Ron's twelfth book.

Contents

Chapter 4: Intentional Wrongs   89

Chapter 7: Legal and Ethical Issues in Education   203

PROMOTING
Legal and Ethical
AWARENESS

A PRIMER FOR HEALTH PROFESSIONALS AND PATIENTS

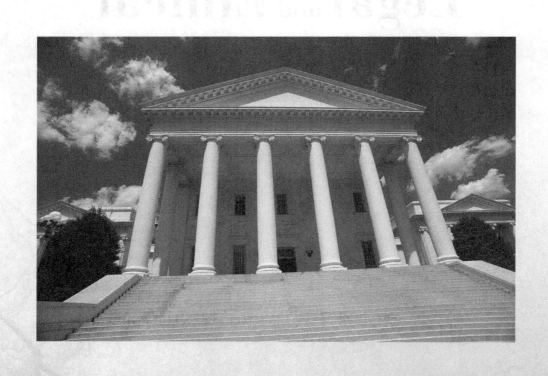

CHAPTER 1

Legal Foundations

KEY TERMS

Beyond a reasonable doubt

Case captions

Clear and convincing evidence

Clear and convincing proof

Common law

Comparative fault

Concurrent jurisdiction

Contingent fee

Contributory negligence

Declarations of rights and duties

Defendants

Diversity of citizenship jurisdiction

Due process

Exclusive jurisdiction

Expectancy

Fact finder

Fine

Frequency

Guilty

Iatrogenesis

In personam jurisdiction

In rem jurisdiction

Incarceration

Infer

Jurisdiction

Liable

Litigants

Monetary damages

Negligence

Plaintiffs

Preponderance of evidence

Presumption

Procedural due process

Public record

Punitive damages

Pure comparative fault

Remittitur

Res ipsa loquitur

Respondent

Restitution

Right of privacy

Sentenced

Severity

Special and general damages

Specific and general deterrence

Stare decisis

Statutes

Strict product liability

Subject-matter jurisdiction

Substantive due process

Tort reform

Tortious conduct

Torts

INTRODUCTION

Everyone in society—from health care professionals to ordinary citizens—must comply with established laws and regulations. Sources of legal obligations include federal and state constitutions, legislatively created statutory laws, judicial case law decisions, and administrative rules and regulations promulgated by state and federal administrative or regulatory agencies.

Legal actions against health care professionals can take place in criminal or civil courts. Criminal actions brought by the state, incident to health care delivery, are normally limited to situations in which intentional misconduct with patient injury or deaths of patients have occurred. Civil legal actions for malpractice are brought by patients against health care providers, and the burden of proof—preponderance, or greater weight, of evidence—is lower than in the criminal justice system, in which the state must prove a defendant's culpability by the standard of beyond a reasonable doubt.

Although an obvious civil litigation crisis exists in the United States, the magnitude of a specific health care malpractice crisis is less certain. Still, tort reform efforts, many designed to limit health care malpractice plaintiffs' access to courts, continue to proliferate.

THE NATURE OF THE AMERICAN LEGAL SYSTEM

The American legal system has two basic subsystems: the criminal law system and the civil law system. Each state has its own criminal and civil trial and appellate courts, as does the federal government. American criminal and civil law systems are grounded in British common (judicial) law and in the legal codes of France, Spain, and other "code" nations. Foundational British common law, the Napoleonic code, and other codes have been substantially replaced or augmented over time with American case (common) law, state and federal statutes, and laws from other sources.

Jurisdiction

State or federal courts in the criminal or civil legal system exercise **jurisdiction**, or power, over **litigants** (jurisdiction over parties, or *in personam* **jurisdiction**), over property that is the subject of litigation (*in rem* **jurisdiction**), and over specific types of cases (**subject-matter jurisdiction**). The federal courts have (or at least were expected by the founders of the United States to have) limited jurisdiction over issues involving specific federal interests, whereas state courts are courts of broad, general jurisdiction. State courts have **exclusive** (or at least primary) **jurisdiction** over purely state governmental matters, such as crimes occurring within the state (but not on federal property), domestic and family relations, establishment of private businesses (including incorporation of businesses), insurance, traffic offenses, and health care malpractice and related issues, among many other areas of interest. Federal courts have **concurrent** (shared) **jurisdiction** with states over areas such as the interpretation of state and (most) federal laws.

Federal courts also share jurisdiction with states over what would seem to be exclusively state business, including health care malpractice cases, under a concept known as **diversity of citizenship jurisdiction**. Diversity jurisdiction applies when all parties on one side of a civil case are citizens of different states than the parties on the opposing side of the case. Diversity jurisdiction was originally intended to prevent inequity, or unfairness, to an out-of-state party in a civil case that might occur in a state court. Because of the growing case burden on federal judges, however, diversity jurisdiction has been limited in recent times to cases involving a monetary amount in controversy of at least $75,000.[1]

The federal courts exercise exclusive jurisdiction over limited types of cases for which the Constitution grants the federal courts such power. These types of cases include antitrust actions; bankruptcy proceedings; federal crimes; military law and policy cases; patent, copyright, and trademark actions; and lawsuits brought against the United States.

Sources of Law and Legal Obligation

Everyone in society (with the possible exception of persons having diplomatic immunity) has an affirmative duty to comply with the administrative, civil, and criminal laws in effect in the jurisdiction. It is often said that ignorance of the law is no excuse for noncompliance. Whereas real problems exist in society regarding the selective enforcement of laws, every person—from the homeless pauper to the president of the United States—is bound by the laws of the land.

Even diplomats are not always assured immunity from answering for their conduct under the law. Consider the case of Georgy Makharadze, a Georgian diplomat who was involved in a traffic accident in Washington, D.C., in December 1996. Largely because of political pressure from the U.S. State Department, President Eduard Shevardnadze waived diplomatic immunity for Makharadze in February 1997, freeing the way for his prosecution for vehicular homicide in the case.[2]

Constitutional Law

There are four main sources of law and legal obligation (Figure 1-1). The preeminent source of legal authority is the federal Constitution, which is universally recognized as the "supreme law of the land." All other laws, regulations, and rules are subordinate in authority to the express provisions of the Constitution and to interpretations of federal constitutional law made by courts. Although there is a historical, ongoing controversy over authority to interpret the Constitution (because of the separation of powers doctrine involving the relative power of the president, Congress, and the Supreme Court), the U.S. Supreme Court is usually the final arbiter in interpreting and enforcing the Constitution.

Many cases interpreting the Constitution over the history of U.S. law have directly or indirectly affected health care delivery, including cases interpreting the meaning and scope of **due process** of law (fundamental fairness) and creating the fundamental **right of** (individual) **privacy**. The first case in which the Supreme Court established a fundamental right of privacy, *Griswold* v. *Connecticut*,[3] turned on whether a conjugate adult couple could legally purchase pharmaceutical contraceptives for birth control. The *Griswold* case is also the first and only instance in which a court created an implied federal constitutional right; and in the majority Supreme Court decision, written by Justice Douglas, one sees how this implied constitutional right of privacy was fashioned from express rights enunciated in the Bill of Rights.

Specific guarantees in the Bill of Rights have penumbras [fringe areas], formed by emanations from those guarantees that helped give them life and substance. Various guarantees create zones of privacy. The rights of association contained in the penumbra of the first amendment is one, ... the third amendment in its prohibition against

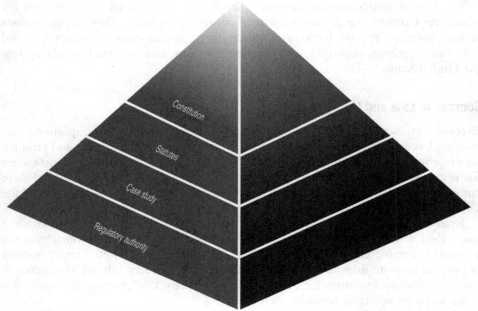

FIGURE 1-1 | Sources of law and legal authority. *(From Scott RW: Professional ethics: a guide for rehabilitation professionals, St Louis, 1998, Mosby.)*

the quartering of soldiers "in any house" in time of peace without the consent of the owner is another. ... The fourth amendment explicitly affirms the right of the people to be secure in their persons, houses, papers, and effects against unreasonable searches and seizures. The fifth amendment in its self-incrimination clause enables the citizen to create a zone of privacy which government may not force him to surrender to his detriment. The ninth amendment provides "the enumeration in the Constitution of certain rights will not be construed to deny or disparage others retained by the people."

The present case [Griswold] concerns a relationship lying within the zone of privacy created by several fundamental constitutional guarantees. ...

We deal with a right of privacy older than the Bill of Rights—older than our political parties, older than our school system. Marriage is a coming together for better or worse, hopefully enduring and intimate to the degree of being sacred. It is an association that promotes a way of life, not causes; a harmony in living, not political faith; a bilateral loyalty, not commercial or social projects. Yet it is an association for as noble a purpose as any involved in our prior decisions.[3]

Virtually all of the express provisions related to personal rights and liberties in the federal Constitution are found, not in the body of the document, but in the amendments to the Constitution. Personal rights and liberties of citizens were not written into the main Constitution by the founding fathers during the Constitutional Convention of 1787. The personal rights enunciated in the Bill of Rights—added in 1791—in large part were fashioned after the Virginia state bill of rights. The first 10 of these amendments, originally intended to protect citizens from undue interference

BILL OF RIGHTS

Amendment I: Congress shall make no law respecting an establishment of religion, or prohibiting the free exercise thereof; or abridging the freedom of speech, or of the press; or the right of the people peaceably to assemble, and to petition the Government for a redress of grievances.

Amendment II: A well regulated Militia, being necessary to the security of a free State, the right of the people to keep and bear Arms, shall not be infringed.

Amendment III: No Soldier shall, in time of peace be quartered in any house, without the consent of the Owner, nor in time of war, but in a manner to be prescribed by law.

Amendment IV: The right of the people to be secure in their persons, houses, papers, and effects, against unreasonable searches and seizures, shall not be violated, and no Warrants shall issue, but upon probable cause, supported by Oath or affirmation and particularly describing the place to be searched, and the persons or things to be seized.

Amendment V: No person shall be held to answer for a capital, or otherwise infamous crime, unless on a presentment or indictment of a Grand Jury, except in cases arising in the land or naval forces, or in the Militia, when in actual service in time of War or public danger; nor shall any person be subject for the same offense to be twice put in jeopardy of life or limb; nor shall be compelled in any criminal case to be a witness against himself, nor be deprived of life, liberty, or property, without due process of law; nor shall private property be taken for public use, without just compensation.

Amendment VI: In all criminal prosecutions, the accused shall enjoy the right to a speedy and public trial, by an impartial jury of the State and district wherein the crime shall have been committed, which district shall have been previously ascertained by law, and to be informed of the nature and cause of the accusation; to be confronted with the witnesses against him; to have compulsory process for obtaining witnesses in his favor, and to have the Assistance of Counsel for his defense.

Amendment VII: In Suits at common law, where the value in controversy shall exceed twenty dollars, the right of trial by jury shall be preserved, and no fact tried by jury, shall be otherwise reexamined in any Court of the United States, than according to the rules of the common law.

Amendment VIII: Excessive bail shall not be required, nor excessive fines imposed, nor cruel and unusual punishments inflicted.

Amendment IX: The enumeration in the Constitution, of certain rights, shall not be construed to deny or disparage others retained by the people.

Amendment X: The powers not delegated to the United States by the Constitution, nor prohibited by it to the States, are reserved to the States respectively, or to the people.[4]

with activities of daily living by the federal government (but most later applied also to state governmental intrusion), are collectively known as the Bill of Rights.

As with the federal system, laws derived from state constitutions also are "supreme" relative to other forms of state law. However, state constitutional law is subordinate to the federal Constitution. States are free to grant their citizens greater rights than are allowed by the federal Constitution but cannot take away rights, privileges, and immunities granted to citizens of the United States by the federal

Constitution. Many state constitutions afford greater rights and liberties to citizens of those states than are afforded under the federal Constitution.

Statutory Law

The second source of law is statutory law. Congress and state legislatures enact **statutes** within their scope of authority. Federal statutes, published in the United States Code (or U.S.C.), are divided by subject into "titles." Examples of important federal statutes affecting health care delivery include the Americans with Disabilities Act, the Civil Rights Acts of 1964 and 1991, the Family and Medical Leave Act, the Federal Torts Claims Act, the Health Insurance Portability and Accountability Act, Patient Self-Determination Act, the Privacy Act, and the Rehabilitation Act of 1973. State statutes enacted by state legislatures are controlling laws in areas in which the federal government does not have jurisdiction. Examples of state statutes include those creating health care professional practice acts and insurance statutes.

Common Law

The third source of law is judicial case law. These court decisions are also referred to as **common law** and encompass all judicial decisions creating legal precedent in areas in which legislatures have not enacted statutes. The earliest common law affecting the United States was English common law. Many common law legal precedents are still based on the earliest English common law. Most American civil legal authority comes from common law, including laws related to health care malpractice and business relationships involving health care professionals and others.

Although the common law is considered more flexible and quicker to adapt to societal change than the relatively rigid statutory law, common law is still characterized by relative stability. The concept of *stare decisis*, or "the decision stands," requires all lower courts in a jurisdiction to conform to prior decisions made by a higher-level court within the jurisdiction. Standing court decisions then are called precedents, and changes in existing precedents take place at the highest level courts—not at the lowest, trial courts.

Administrative Law

The final source of law derives from administrative agencies at the federal and state levels. Administrative agencies exercise delegated authority from the executive and legislative branches of government. These agencies are empowered to exercise legislative (rule-making), executive (management), and judicial (enforcement) functions. That health care professional business persons have more interface with administrative agencies than with any other legal entity is widely accepted as fact.

In their legislative role, administrative agencies promulgate everyday rules and regulations to supplement statutes and executive orders. Such administrative rules and regulations are usually previewed for public comment and debate in the Code of Federal Regulations, or CFR, before attaining the force of law. Once final, though, these rules and regulations govern business conduct in great detail. The CFR is the codification of the general and permanent rules published in the *Federal*

Register by the executive branch departments and administrative agencies of the federal government. The *Federal Register* is divided into 50 titles that represent broad areas subject to federal regulation. Each volume of the CFR is updated once each calendar year and is published quarterly.

Examples of federal administrative agencies having broad power over the business affairs of health care professionals include the Centers for Disease Control and Prevention, the Centers for Medicare and Medicaid Services, the Equal Employment Opportunity Commission, the Occupational Safety and Health Administration, the National Labor Relations Board, and the Social Security Administration. Examples of administrative agencies at the state level include health care professional licensing agencies and workers' compensation authorities.

Consider one federal agency in greater detail. The National Labor Relations Board is an independent federal agency created by Congress in 1935 to administer the National Labor Relations Act, the primary federal statute governing relations between employers and unions in the private sector. This statute guarantees the right of employees to organize and to bargain collectively through labor unions with their employers over compensation, benefits, and conditions of employment; to engage in other protected concerted activity with or without a union; and to refrain from all such activity, if desired. Health care professionals, like all other employees, have the federal statutory right to organize into labor unions to advance and protect their rights on the job. The National Labor Relations Board has broad educative, executive, investigative, judicial, and legislative roles and responsibilities.

Secondary Sources of Legal Authority

Additional (secondary) sources of law (which legislative, judicial, and executive decision makers rely on as "authorities") include professional association and institutional practice standards, protocols, and guidelines. Other secondary law sources include accreditation standards and guidelines promulgated by private accreditation agencies, such as the Joint Commission on Accreditation of Healthcare Organizations, the Commission on Accreditation of Rehabilitation Facilities, and the National Committee for Quality Assurance. (Figure 1-1).

Due Process of Law
The Fifth and Fourteenth Amendments to the Constitution require that no person be deprived of the rights to "life, liberty, and property without due process of law." Due process equates to fundamental fairness. Due process implies that all persons will be treated the same under law and will be given the opportunity to challenge legal actions against them that affect important aspects of their lives.

Substantive Due Process
The two components of due process are **substantive due process** and **procedural due process**. Substantive due process focuses on whether legal actions—particularly legislation—are substantively fair. For most actions, they must be shown to be rationally or reasonably related to a legitimate governmental purpose. For example, a state

statute requiring licensure of primary health care professionals is reasonably related to the legitimate governmental purpose of protecting the health and welfare of patients served by these professionals in the state. When legal actions adversely affect fundamental rights, such as privacy, free speech, voting, and the right to travel, substantive due process requires that such laws be narrowly written to promote a compelling or overriding governmental interest. For example, states may legally prohibit elective abortion in the third trimester, based on the state's compelling interests in protecting developing, viable fetal life.[5]

Procedural Due Process

Procedural due process focuses on administrative requirements for fairness in legal actions. Anyone whose life, liberty, or property interests—including educational degrees, employment rights, and professional licensure—would be adversely affected by such action must (1) be apprised of the nature of the action proposed and (2) be given the opportunity to respond on his or her behalf before final action is taken. An example of procedural due process is the legal requirement that, before administrative discipline of a licensed health care professional by a licensure board can take place, the **respondent** must be given adequate notice of the charge(s) against him or her and the range of potential adverse actions and must be given the opportunity to present his or her case to the decision maker.

CRIMINAL AND CIVIL LAW DEFINED AND DISTINGUISHED

Criminal law involves legal actions brought on behalf of society for violations of its criminal laws against a defendant or multiple defendants. Criminal legal actions are labeled "public" law, and their **case captions** (titles) reflect this fact. Cases may be titled *"People v. Defendant," "State v. Defendant,"* or *"United States v. Defendant."*

Civil law, however, encompasses private legal actions brought by one or more private **plaintiffs** against one or more private **defendants** (including individuals, businesses, and government agencies). All types of private actions are civil law actions, including administrative law cases; cases involving the liability of agents employed by principals; contract law cases; corporate legal actions; domestic relations cases; employment law cases; health care malpractice cases; persona and real property law cases; personal injury cases other than health care malpractice cases; and cases concerning wills, trusts, and estates. (Most private wrongs are termed *torts*, except for cases involving allegations of breach of contract. *Tort* is French for "wrong.")

Parties Bringing Actions in Civil and Criminal Cases

The party bringing criminal and civil charges against defendants differs too. In civil cases involving private wrongs, the plaintiff is always the victim of the wrong committed (or the victim's legal representative). In criminal legal actions, cases are initiated by prosecutors, who are agents of the state. Because a criminal prosecution is discretionary, the actual victim of a crime does not have an absolute right to compel the government to prosecute the offender.

Standards of Proof

Criminal Cases: Beyond a Reasonable Doubt

The standards of proof differ greatly between criminal and civil legal actions. In criminal cases—in which the stakes for the defendant are much higher than in civil cases and include the sanction of death as a punishment—the government's burden of proof is great. The government prosecutor in a criminal case must prove every element of a criminal charge by the standard of **beyond a reasonable doubt**. This standard requires that the **fact finder** (jury, or the judge, if the criminal defendant does not elect to have a jury trial) be convinced of the defendant's culpability to a moral certainty so that there can be no lingering question in the mind of ordinary, reasonable persons as to the defendant's guilt.

Civil Cases: Preponderance of the Evidence

In a civil case the plaintiff's burden of proof is much lower than in a criminal case. In civil cases, plaintiffs normally need only prove their cases by a **preponderance** (or greater weight) **of evidence**. The preponderance standard means that the plaintiff's rendition of facts is at least slightly more credible than the defendant's case presentation.

Clear and Convincing Evidence

Rarely, a civil plaintiff will be required by a court (or by legal precedent) to prove his or her case by a standard slightly higher than the preponderance standard. This intermediate standard of proof is known as proof by **clear and convincing evidence**. Clear and convincing evidence equates to "much more probable than not" that the plaintiff's version of the case is correct. *Cruzan* v. *Director, Missouri Department of Health*[6] was a case concerning whether the parents of a comatose woman in a persistent vegetative state could compel health care providers to withhold nutrition and hydration from a patient. In upholding the judgment of the Missouri (state) Supreme Court, Chief Justice Rehnquist of the U.S. Supreme Court found that the parents failed to present **clear and convincing proof** that their daughter would have desired withdrawal of such care. (Such proof was later made when the case was returned to state court, and Nancy Cruzan's food and water were taken away. She died December 26, 1990.)

Terminology for Culpability

Another difference between civil and criminal law cases is the terminology used to describe a defendant's culpability. In civil cases, defendants are found to be **liable** when the plaintiff's burden of proof is satisfied. In criminal cases, they are found **guilty**.

Comparative Remedies in Civil and Criminal Cases

The remedies afforded to plaintiffs in civil and criminal cases are also different. In tort civil cases, remedies are designed to make an injured plaintiff "whole." That is the sole purpose of tort law. In breach of contract civil cases, remedies are designed to put the parties back in the same position they would have been in had the contract never been made (**restitution**), or to award the plaintiff the "benefit of the bargain" (**expectancy**). In other types of civil legal actions, successful plaintiffs may also win awards of **monetary damages**, or they may merely be vindicated in their positions through judicial **declarations of rights and duties**.

In tort cases, successful plaintiffs may win monetary damages of two types: **special and general damages**. Special damages replace past, present, and future out-of-pocket monetary losses incurred by the plaintiff as a result of the defendant's wrongdoing, or **tortious conduct**. Included under special damages are lost wages, medical expenses incurred because of the defendant's tortious conduct, and lost future earnings capacity. General damages include monetary awards for pain and suffering and the loss of enjoyment of life resulting from the defendant's culpable conduct. Infrequently, a court will award **punitive** (punishment) **damages** against a civil defendant. Punitive damages are similar to a criminal law monetary **fine**, designed to punish a wrongdoer for egregious misconduct and to deter the offender and others from repeating the same or a similar offense.

The remedies awarded against defendants in criminal cases are more limited in type but are also more severe in effect. Criminal defendants—including health care professionals, when charged with criminal misconduct—are **sentenced** when found guilty to **incarceration** or the threat of incarceration (probation). A permanent **public record** is made of every criminal trial in which a conviction results. When criminal defendants have unjustly profited monetarily from their misconduct (such as with reimbursement fraud), a criminal court judge may impose a monetary fine on the defendant in addition to incarceration. Table 1-1 summarizes the major distinctions between civil and criminal law.

In contrast to professional ethical rules (which are introduced in the next chapter), rules of law are formal rules of conduct that govern most or all activities of all members of society—citizens and noncitizens alike. No one (except those persons possessing diplomatic immunity, for most offenses) is "above the law." Even legislators, judicial officials, and the chief executive may be sanctioned for violations of law.

The range and effect of sanctions for violations of law are much broader and potentially more severe than for pure ethics violations. Under civil law, sanctions include forfeiture of monetary resources, whereas under criminal law, the ultimate sanction is death. Under civil and criminal law, a person adjudged as culpable may lose his or her property interest in practicing a profession under license from the state after due process of law has been afforded to that person.

TABLE **1-1** ▪ Civil and Criminal Law Distinguished

Civil Law	Criminal Law
1. Private actions	1. Governmental actions
2. Plaintiff v. Defendant	2. State v. Defendant
3. Proof: Preponderance of evidence	3. Proof: Beyond a reasonable doubt
4. Liability	4. Guilt
5. Monetary damages	5. Incarceration

From Scott RW: *Promoting legal awareness in physical and occupational therapy,* St Louis, 1997, Mosby.

THE LITIGATION CRISIS

The Civil Litigation Explosion

As was mentioned in the Preface, Western nations (the United States in particular) are experiencing a civil litigation crisis that seems to be ever-expanding. In 2004, 16.5 million civil lawsuits were filed in the United States.[7] If one postulates that there are already an equal number of civil legal cases in existence in the system, then even if each case had only two litigants—one plaintiff and one defendant—then one in nine Americans may be embroiled in civil litigation at any given point in time.

Why does a litigation crisis exist? The sociologic reasons for a litigation crisis are many and are beyond the intended scope of this book. Some of the reasons relate to the nature of our legal system. The United States has 5 percent of the world's population, yet three fourths of the world's attorneys. With such a large number of attorneys, formal redress of grievances is more easily facilitated, perhaps resulting in a disproportionately high volume of litigation.[8]

In addition, the United States is the only Western nation that allows attorneys to undertake representation of personal injury clients for a **contingent fee**, in which the client contractually agrees to pay a percentage of any recovery to the attorney but is bound to pay no fee if the plaintiff does not prevail at trial. Even in the event of a loss, the client is still liable for the payment of expenses incurred by the attorney in the case, including the filing of court papers, payments to consultants and expert witnesses, and telephone and photocopying expenses.

Some authorities are critical of the role of lawyers and the law in fueling the litigation crisis. According to Leo, "[a]ll too often, litigation in America is a lucrative, lawyer-driven enterprise in which the client is not in control and is almost incidental."[9] In his book *The Death of Common Sense: How Law Is Suffocating America,* Howard[10] asserts that we have become a nation of enemies in which the rule of law is too often abused.

In cosmopolitan America, citizens may feel nameless, faceless, and relatively powerless. Litigation gives them recognition and a false sense of control. The media, schools, parents, and politicians contribute to the fervor of litigation, for everywhere one hears "I'll sue you!"

Health Care Malpractice Crisis—Fact or Myth?

Like the litigation crisis generally, the health care malpractice problem is of recent vintage. Although there has been litigation over health care delivery for many centuries, including the 1375 British case of *Stratton* v. *Cavendish* (involving failed hand surgery),[11] the floodgates of health care malpractice litigation did not open until the advent of the consumerism movement after World War II.

One of the reasons for the health care malpractice litigation crisis is related to changes in benefits for civilian workers after World War II. Employee health benefits became commonplace during and after World War II, making access to health care easy and affordable for millions of families. The benefits grew during the war, in large part, as a means of circumventing mandatory wage and price controls.[12] With enhanced access to care and increased use came greater liability risk exposure. Also, as medical and surgical technologies advanced and new drugs were discovered, the risks of patient injury, and of litigation, grew.

Media technology—especially television—became more sophisticated and widely disseminated post–World War II. After troops returned from overseas in the mid and late 1940s, baccalaureate and graduate educational opportunities were seized upon, making veterans and their families into sophisticated, demanding consumers. The consumerism movement helped spark the litigation crisis generally, and the health care malpractice crisis in particular. In recent times, readily available consumer research sites on the Internet have fueled the consumerism movement even more, perhaps offsetting diminishing governmental oversight in the area of consumer protection.

Other factors feed the health care malpractice crisis on an ongoing basis. Increasing governmental regulation of health care services, skyrocketing health care costs, and managed care initiatives designed to curb those costs have contributed to a health care environment that is ever more business-like. When patients perceive that their health care professionals are treating them in a more business-like fashion, they resent it and tend to respond in kind. So when a patient in the modern health care environment is injured by **iatrogenesis**—i.e., injury or disease caused by health care interventions—that patient is more inclined to claim against or sue his or her health care providers and the institutions vicariously responsible for them.

Tort Reform Efforts

The fundamental purpose of tort law is to award fair and reasonable compensation to persons wrongfully injured at the hands of others. The tort system strives to make victims of wrongdoing "whole" again (or as close to whole as possible through the award of monetary damages). When an imbalance is perceived in the equitable administration of justice in the tort system, adjustments are made by legislatures and/or courts to restore balance. Major adjustments to the system are labeled **tort reform**.

First Wave of Tort Reform: Expanding Litigants' Right of Access

Two eras of tort reform have actually occurred. The first era of tort reform paralleled the development of the consumerism movement post–World War II. Before and during that time, courts and legislatures began to reverse or at least relax restrictive legal rules that impeded patient-plaintiff access to the legal system and legal redress of grievances. Sweeping legislative and judicial reform took place because of the perception that injured parties were systematically impeded from receiving redress for civil wrongs. Plaintiff-oriented reforms ensued, including the relaxation of restrictive evidentiary rules, the introduction of new theories of recovery in tort, and an expansion of the classifications and amounts of monetary damages awarded to plaintiffs who prevailed in court.

Comparative Fault

One of the first important patient-oriented tort reform measures was the abolition in most states of the harsh evidentiary rule of **contributory negligence**, a rule that, with few exceptions, bars an injured party from any compensation when the injured person is at all partially responsible for his or her own injuries—even if a tortfeasor was substantially at fault. In its place a system of **comparative fault** or **negligence** was established, under which a patient's tort compensation is subject to being reduced by the degree to which the patient is at fault in contributing to his or her injuries. Although the majority of states preclude compensation altogether when a patient is found to be more than 50 percent responsible for his or her injuries, in as many as 13 states, a patient can recover tort compensation regardless of the degree of culpability attributable to the patient under a concept called **pure comparative fault**.[13]

Res Ipsa Loquitur

Another first-wave expansive tort reform measure was the easing of an injured party's burden of proof at trial, using a legal concept known as *res ipsa loquitur* (Latin for "the thing speaks for itself"). Under *res ipsa loquitur,* whenever a patient is injured as a result of the use of a treatment or modality under the exclusive control of a health care provider and the injury sustained is of the kind that normally should not occur unless the health care provider is probably negligent (e.g., a burn from a hot pack[14] or a heat-molded orthosis), the trial judge in a case may permit the jury to **infer**, or in some cases, order the jury to presume negligence against the defendant-provider. For the health care provider to escape liability for the patient's injury once *res ipsa loquitur* has been invoked, his or her attorney must dispel or rebut the inference or **presumption** of negligence through the introduction of contrary evidence.

Res ipsa loquitur is not a new concept in law. The doctrine first appeared in 1863 in an English legal case, *Byrne* v. *Boadle,*[15] in which a beer barrel "mysteriously" rolled out of a second floor window of a factory owned by the defendant. The plaintiff, a passerby below, was injured by the flying barrel. The English court held that because the victim could not prove negligence on the part of the defendant, it was sufficient to show that the incident was of a type that, in the normal course of life events, should not happen absent someone's carelessness, and that the barrel belonged to and was controlled by the defendant.

In the 1940s, courts in the United States began to allow *res ipsa loquitur* to be invoked by plaintiffs in health care malpractice lawsuits in part as a judicially imposed penalty for a perceived or factual conspiracy of silence on the part of health care professionals who refused to testify on patients' behalf against professional colleagues in court. The doctrine, however, is rarely allowed in health care malpractice cases because of the shifting of the burden of persuasion to malpractice defendants in these cases.

The three required elements for allowing a patient-plaintiff to short-circuit the normal burden of proof through invocation of *res ipsa loquitur* in health care malpractice cases are shown in Box 1-1.

Other patient-oriented tort reform measures include the development and expansion of **strict product liability**, that is, liability for injuries from dangerously defectively designed or manufactured products without regard to culpability on the part of the person held liable. In addition, there has been an increase in the frequency and amount of punitive damages imposed on health care professionals in malpractice cases, particularly where the court finds that the defendant's egregious conduct was malicious or reckless.

Punitive damages are not awarded in order to compensate an injured plaintiff. They are imposed against tortfeasors as punishment. In addition to their purpose of deterring the wrongdoer from engaging in the same or similar misconduct again,

---

BOX 1-1 ▪ **Res Ipsa Loquitur: When Does an Inference or Presumption
of Negligence Arise in a Health Care Malpractice Case?**

Critical Elements
1. The incident that led to patient injury does not commonly occur absent negligence
   on someone's part.
2. Because the health care provider exclusively controlled the instrumentality that led to
   patient injury, the party who was probably negligent is the health care provider.
3. The patient was not contributorily negligent in causing his or her own injury.

---

they also serve to deter others from following in the footsteps of the tortfeasor. These purposes are labeled **specific and general deterrence**, respectively.

In the case in which a judge believes that a jury awarded punitive damages in a civil case improperly, the judge has the power to reduce or eliminate the punitive damages award under a legal concept called **remittitur**. This occurred in the infamous case involving McDonald's restaurant in which a customer was burned by coffee supplied by the defendant that was allegedly excessively hot.[16] An award of punitive damages can also be modified or overturned on appeal.

Although the concept of punitive damages has received significant attention by federal and state legislatures under more recent, restrictive tort reform initiatives, the courts have upheld it as a legitimate element of monetary damages in malpractice and other civil cases. The U.S. Supreme Court has ruled that the imposition of punitive damages in a civil case is not unconstitutional as an "excessive penalty" under the Eighth Amendment to the Constitution.[17] The Supreme Court has also defined the requirements for courts to uphold jury awards of punitive damages, including evaluating the nature of a defendant's conduct, assessing the relationship between any harm suffered and the amount of punitive damages to be awarded, and looking at the relative amounts awarded as compensatory damages and punitive damages.[18] In *State Farm* v. *Campbell*,[19] the Supreme Court disallowed consideration by fact finders of "outside" wrongful conduct by defendants not involving plaintiffs in particular cases before courts and said that awards of punitive damages in double-digit multiples of compensatory damages are generally unconstitutionally excessive, although there may be exceptions. At the time of writing this book, the Supreme Court was considering such an exception in *Philip Morris* v. *Williams*,[20] after the Oregon Supreme Court affirmed a jury punitive damages award of $79.5 million.

A summary of first-wave tort reform initiatives appears in Box 1-2.

Prelude to the Second Wave of Tort Reform
The most significant catalyst for a second wave of health care malpractice tort reform, designed to limit the numbers of health care malpractice claims and lawsuits and reduce damages awards, was the health care professional liability insurance crisis of the 1970s and 1980s. During that time frame, the cost to providers and institutions for professional liability insurance increased dramatically, and the availability of insurance became less certain. Underwriters of health care professional liability insurance policies began to issue claims-made instead of occurrence policies to clients—and many health care

---

BOX 1-2 ■ Summary of First-Wave (Patient Advocacy) Tort Reform Initiatives

- Comparative fault: reducing tort compensation by the degree to which a patient is negligent in contributing to his or her own injuries.
- *Res ipsa loquitur* ("the thing speaks for itself"): an inference or presumption of negligence against a defendant–health care professional arising from unexplained patient injuries.
- Punitive damages: monetary damages awarded against malpractice defendants whose conduct toward injured patients was egregious and malicious. (Insurers do not normally indemnify against punitive damages, so the responsible health care professional may be personally responsible for their payment.)
- Strict product liability: liability for patient injury from dangerously defectively designed or manufactured commercial products, without consideration of culpability on the part of the commercial entity supplying the product.

Adapted from Scott RW: *Promoting legal awareness in physical and occupational therapy,* St Louis, 1997, Mosby.

organizations and physician and nonphysician providers and groups began to self-insure against liability exposure.

Although the exact number of health care malpractice legal cases in the system at any given time is uncertain, there is a significant number of cases. Malpractice lawsuit frequency rates are not universally publicized for several reasons. For cases disposed of at the claims stage of adjudication by professional liability underwriters, the data on **frequency** (numbers) and **severity** (cost) of litigation are proprietary and not normally disseminated, not even to professionals insured by these entities. Also, most health care malpractice cases that are adjudicated at trial in favor of patient-plaintiffs are settled or not appealed beyond the trial level so that case reports are nonexistent or, if they exist, are difficult to trace.

Second Wave of Tort Reform: Restricting Litigants' Right of Access

As the incidence of health care malpractice claims and lawsuits increased beginning in the 1970s and reactive defensive health care practice became commonplace, intensive pressure from medical and insurance lobbyists influenced state legislators to support restrictive malpractice reforms to limit patient-plaintiffs' access to the legal system. This counterswing of the tort reform pendulum began just as the movement toward patient-oriented tort reform was waning. By 1998, 41 of the 50 states had enacted legislative restrictive tort reform measures.[21]

Some of the second-wave tort reform measures (not all of which restrict patient-plaintiffs' rights) are as follows (Box 1-3):

1. Enacting and, after an additional 7 years' delay, implementing the Health Insurance Portability and Accountability Act of 1996.
2. Limiting time periods for validity of patient health information release authorizations, as initiated by Texas in 1998.

> ### BOX 1-3 ▪ Summary of Second-Wave Tort Reform Initiatives
>
> 1. Health Insurance Portability and Accountability Act
> 2. Limitations on time periods for valid patient release authorizations
> 3. Administrative medical (merit) review panels
> 4. Imposing caps on noneconomic monetary damages
> 5. Placing monetary limits on plaintiff attorney contingent fees
> 6. Reforming joint and several liability
> 7. Modifications to statutes of limitations and creation of statutes of repose
> 8. Relaxing the collateral source rule
> 9. Requiring periodic payment of monetary damages
> 10. Penalizing plaintiff attorneys and plaintiffs for filing frivolous lawsuits
> 11. Limiting punitive damage awards
> 12. Reforming drug label laws and drug manufacturer liability

Adapted from Scott RW: *Promoting legal awareness in physical and occupational therapy,* St Louis, 1997, Mosby.

3. Requiring that health care malpractice plaintiffs undergo administrative hearings on the merits of their cases before proceeding to trial.
4. Capping maximum noneconomic money damages for pain and suffering and loss of enjoyment of life. Although this second-wave reform has been introduced on multiple occasions since 1995 in Congress, as of November 2006, no comprehensive federal tort reform statute had been enacted by the Senate and House. Current bills would limit pain and suffering damages to $250,000 and also limit attorney contingent fees. The nonpartisan Congressional Budget Office has predicted that this law would reduce the percentage of aggregate health care expenditures attributable to malpractice from 2 to 1.5 percent.[22]
5. Limiting attorney contingent fees (fees based on percentages of money damages recovered, bargained over by attorneys and their clients as part of representation agreements). California was the first state to limit attorney contingent fees in 1975.
6. Reforming joint and several liability to prevent one defendant from being required to pay an entire judgment when that defendant is only partially responsible for a plaintiff's injuries.
7. Setting absolute time limits—based on the date of injury or manufacture of a product—within which legal action must be commenced (called statutes of repose).
8. Relaxing the collateral source rule, under which juries are prevented from learning of a plaintiff's collateral sources of compensation for injuries, including insurance coverage or partial payments by other defendants.
9. Penalizing attorneys and their clients for initiating lawsuits deemed to be frivolous, especially in the federal courts.
10. Requiring periodic payment of monetary damages, whereby future monetary damages are paid out in installments over the life of the injured plaintiff. One key purpose of this reform measure is to prevent the heirs of a plaintiff from reaping a windfall in the event that the plaintiff dies prematurely.

11. Withholding from plaintiffs (and depositing in state treasuries) a percentage of any punitive damages awarded to them in product liability cases, and deducting monies received by plaintiffs from collateral (outside) sources from final awards.
12. Reforming drug label regulations by the Food and Drug Administration, and limiting drug manufacturer liability for patient injuries resulting from medication errors.[23]

Tort Reform Outcomes

The evidence is mixed as to whether the measures undertaken in either wave of tort reform have resulted in a fair balance between patients' right of redress for injuries and cost containment in health care. Despite the need for some degree of health care malpractice reform on the part of the states and the federal government, there is also a powerful countervailing equitable consideration in favor of continued protection of patients' rights to pursue legal remedies for injuries incident to health care delivery. Patients do incur injury at the hands of health care professionals, and a small but significant percentage of injuries is the result of malpractice.

Supporting this contention are the findings of the Harvard Medical Practice Study. This interdisciplinary study involved a retrospective review of 31,429 randomly selected medical records of inpatients hospitalized in acute care, nonpsychiatric hospitals in New York State during 1984. The records were reviewed by expert panels, consisting of board-certified internists and surgeons. The panels found an adverse incident (patient iatrogenic injury) rate of 3.7 percent and attributed these injuries to probable malpractice in 27.6 percent of cases. In 15.8 percent of patient injuries, permanent disability or death ensued. The overall health care malpractice rate for iatrogenic patient injury was estimated to be approximately 1 percent.[24,25] More than 98 percent of injury cases attributed to malpractice did not result in a health care malpractice claim or lawsuit. Only about one eighth of all malpractice claims filed by injured patients studied were from patients who were deemed to have been injured as a result of health care malpractice.[26]

Several more recent studies buttress the conclusions of the Harvard Medical Practice Study. An Institute of Medicine report in 1999 concluded that as many as 99,000 inpatient deaths per year in the United States are attributable to medical mistakes.[27] Another research group, HealthGrades, found twice that number of deaths in its 2004 report.[28] The Harvard Leape study report in 2005 revalidated the 1999 conclusion of the Institute of Medicine that 100,000 patient deaths per year are the result of medical mistakes. The Leape study attributed these errors in large part to the complexity of the modern health care delivery system.[29]

Some health scholars urge that a complete restructuring of the American health care system is the only real solution to health care malpractice reform.[30] The Urban Institute, a Washington, D.C.–based research center, recommends an alternative insurance system to replace civil litigation altogether for selected medical injuries, such as severe obstetrical patient injury. Under its proposed "no fault" system, payment for specified injuries would be automatic, without resort to litigation. Such no-fault compensatory events are labeled "accelerated compensation events."[31]

In its 2005 report, *Healthcare at the Crossroads: Strategies for Improving the Medical Liability System and Preventing Patient Injury,* the Joint Commission also recommended demonstration projects for alternative no-fault health care delivery systems.

The Joint Commission report specifically recommended the establishment of special health courts of law and the use of court-appointed expert witnesses.[32]

Under President Clinton's 1993 federal Health Security Act, a demonstration project would have examined liability transfer from individual health care professionals to health alliances.[33] This proposal would have created a private-sector analog to the system already in place for federal health care professionals pursuant to the Federal Tort Claims Act,[34] under which the United States is substituted for individual provider-defendants as the party-defendant in federal sector health care malpractice lawsuits.

In a keynote address before the American Physical Therapy Association conference, Dr. Timothy Johnson aptly remarked that every component part of the American health care delivery system—care providers and their support staffs, health systems administrators, attorneys, politicians, the medical products and pharmaceutical industries, insurance carriers and underwriters, and consumers—shares blame for the current dilemma and has the fundamental responsibility to work to remedy the situation.[35]

SUMMARY

The American legal system consists of two broad component parts: the criminal justice system and the civil legal system. Cases brought by governments against private defendants are heard in the criminal system, and cases between and among private parties are adjudicated in the civil system. Allegations of health care malpractice, lodged by patients or their representatives, may give rise to civil and criminal legal actions.

A number of important differences exist between criminal and civil legal actions, most notably the burden of proof required of the plaintiff, the party initiating an action. In criminal cases the state is required to prove its case against a criminal defendant beyond a reasonable doubt, whereas in a civil case a private plaintiff must prove his or her case by a preponderance, or greater weight, of evidence—a much lower burden of proof.

Because of the growing number of civil legal cases, state legislatures and the federal Congress have initiated tort reform measures to limit the number of cases—including health care malpractice cases—heard by courts. Although a large number of health care malpractice legal cases may lack substantive merit, studies have shown that a small but significant percentage of cases involving iatrogenic injury are the result of substandard care.

CASES AND QUESTIONS

1. A patient brings a charge of "inappropriate touching of a sexual nature" against her primary care physician. In which settings can the patient initiate action?
2. You are contemplating writing a letter to your congressional representative, urging reform of the civil legal system in order to afford greater fairness to litigants, the health care delivery system, and the public at large. What original reform measures can you think of to suggest to your congressional representative?

SUGGESTED ANSWERS TO CASES AND QUESTIONS

1. At least four potential forums exist for adjudicating a case involving an allegation of intentional misconduct such as sexual assault or battery arising in the health care delivery system. The alleged victim of the misconduct may bring a civil legal action for malpractice. He or she may file a criminal complaint with the district attorney, which may lead to a felony criminal legal action against the alleged perpetrator brought on behalf of the state. The alleged victim or the district attorney may report the allegation to the regulatory agency responsible for licensing of the alleged offender. This may result in an adverse administrative action, potentially affecting the validity of the provider's professional license. Finally, any one may report the allegation of misconduct to the provider's professional association, possibly resulting in adverse action for violation of the association's professional ethics code, possibly affecting membership in the private organization. All of these potential adverse actions will have a negative impact on the personal and professional reputation of the provider, irrespective of who eventually prevails in the actions.

2. This problem optimally should be addressed by a group of students or clinicians, and suggestions for improvement in the health care litigation system should be developed through brainstorming. Remember that during a brainstorming exercise, all ideas are considered to be legitimate because to exclude ideas arbitrarily as insignificant results in a stifling of creative input.

SUGGESTED READINGS

Beck D: Is our judiciary under serious attack? Separation of powers, *Texas Bar Journal* 67(11):974, 2004.

Center for Assistive Technology and Environmental Access: *Jurisdiction of the federal courts.* Retrieved Nov 26, 2006, from www.catea.org.

The father of administrative law: remembering Kenneth Culp Davis, *University of San Diego Law Advocate* 20(2):6, 2003.

Greenberger RS: High court won't clarify 'punitive,' *Wall Street Journal* p A6, Oct 5, 2004.

Judge rules damages award in Vioxx case is excessive, *New York Times* p C11, Aug 31, 2006.

National Labor Relations Board: Retrieved Dec 1, 2006, from www.nlrb.gov.

Prosser WL: *Prosser on torts,* ed 4, St Paul, Minn, 1971, West Publishing Company.

Scott RW: *Health care malpractice: a primer on legal issues,* ed 2, New York, 1999, McGraw-Hill.

Scott RW: Legal trends: tort reform, *Clinical Management* 11(6):11-13, 1991.

REFERENCES

1. 28 United States Code Section 1332.
2. Nadien V: Shevardnadze sacrifices diplomat for $50 million, *Current Digest of the Post-Soviet Press* 49(2):24, 1997.
3. *Griswold* v. *Connecticut,* 381 U.S. 479 (1965).
3. Ibid. at 484.
4. U.S. Constitution, Amendments I-X.

5. *Roe* v. *Wade,* 410 U.S. 113 (1973).

6. *Cruzan* v. *Director, Missouri Department of Health,* 497 U.S. 261 (1990).

7. Center for Individual Freedom: *Legal Issues.* Retrieved Nov 26, 2006, from www. cfif.org.

8. Rosen B: Why are lawyers taking over the country? *New York Times* p A14, July 12, 1995.

9. Leo J: The world's most litigious nation, *U.S. News & World Report* p 24, May 22, 1995.

10. Howard PK: *The death of common sense: how law is suffocating America,* New York, 1994, Random House.

11. Furrow BR, Johnson SH, Jost TS, Schwartz RL: *Health law: cases, materials and problems,* ed 2, St Paul, Minn, 1991, West Publishing Company.

12. Cherrington DJ: *The management of human resources,* ed 4, Englewood Cliffs, NJ, 1995, Prentice Hall.

13. Matthiesen-Wickers-Lehrer website: *Contributory Negligence/Comparative Fault Laws.* Retrieved Nov 19, 2006, from www.mwl-law.com.

14. *Greater Southeast Community Hospital Foundation* v. *Walker,* 303 A.2d 105 (D.C. App. 1973).

15. *Byrne* v. *Boadle,* 159 Eng. Rep. 299 (1863).

16. Press A, Carroll G, Waldman S: Are lawyers burning America? *Newsweek* pp 32-35, March 20, 1995. In this case the trial judge reduced the jury's punitive damages award against McDonald's from $2.7 million to $440,000.

17. *BMW of North America* v. *Gore,* 517 U.S. 559 (1996).

18. Wermille S: Justices don't limit punitive damages, *Wall Street Journal* p A-2, March 5, 1991.

19. *State Farm Mutual Automobile Insurance Co.* v. *Campbell,* 538 U.S. 408 (2003).

20. *Philip Morris USA* v. *Williams,* 540 U.S. 801 (2006).

21. *Successful tort reform efforts in 1986-88,* Washington, DC, 1989, American Tort Reform Association.

22. Tokarski C: Medical liability reform stays on Bush agenda in 2005, *MedScape Today* Feb 2005. Retrieved Nov 26, 2006, from www.medscape.com.

23. Harris G: New drug label rule is intended to reduce medical errors, *New York Times* p A1, Jan 19, 2006.

24. Brennan TA, Leape LL, Laird NM et al: Incidence of adverse events and negligence in hospitalized patients: results of the Harvard Medical Practice Study I, *N Engl J Med* 324(6):370-376, 1991.

25. Leape LL, Brennan TA, Laird N et al: The nature of adverse events in hospitalized patients: results of the Harvard Medical Practice Study II, *N Engl J Med* 324(6):377-384, 1991.

26. Localio AR, Lawthers AG, Brennan TA et al: Relationship between malpractice claims and adverse events due to negligence: results of the Harvard Medical Practice Study III, *N Engl J Med* 325:245-251, 1991.

27. Institute of Medicine: *To err is Human: Building a Safer Health Care System.* Retrieved Nov 26, 2006, from www.iom.edu.

28. Health Grades: *Patient Safety in American Hospitals.* Retrieved Nov 26, 2006, from www. HealthGrades.com.

29. Leape LL, Berwick DM: Five years after *To Err Is Human, JAMA* 293:2384-2390, 2005.

30. Nutter D, Helms C, Whitcolm M, Weston W: Restructuring health care in the United States: a proposal for the 1990s, *JAMA* 265:2516-2521, 1991.

31. Bovberg R, Tancredi L, Gaylan D: Obstetrics and malpractice: evidence on the performance of a selective no-fault system, *JAMA* 265:2836-2843, 1991.

32. Modern Healthcare: *Health Care at the Crossroads.* Retrieved Feb 17, 2005, from www. jointcommission.org.
33. Reform to relieve PTs of malpractice worries, *PT Bulletin* p 6, June 2, 1993.
34. Federal Tort Claims Act, 28 United States Code Section 2674.
35. Woods E: A look at America's changing health care system, *Progress Report* 20(8):1, 1991.

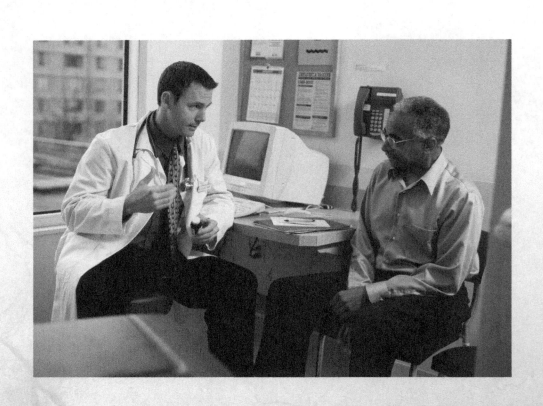

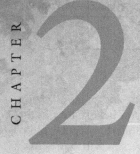

Ethical Foundations

KEY TERMS

Actor	Dilemmas	Justice
Agape	Directive	Morals
Autonomy	Distributive justice	Nonmaleficence
Beneficence	Effect	*Pro bono*
Bioethics	Ethical relativism	Problems
Categorical imperative	Ethics	Profession
Clinical ethics	*Ethikos*	Sliding scale
Code of ethics	*Ethos*	Standards of practice
Comparative justice	Fiduciaries	
Conduct	Issues	

INTRODUCTION

This chapter defines and describes morals, ethics, and law; describes the four foundational biomedical ethical principles of beneficence, nonmaleficence, justice, and autonomy; and offers a systems approach to health care professional ethical decision making. The modern "blending" of legal and professional ethical obligations is addressed, under which a substantive violation of law by a health care provider–fiduciary (person in a position of special trust) more often than not also constitutes a violation of professional ethics.

BASES FOR ETHICAL CONDUCT

Morals

Morals refer to beliefs, principles, and values about what is right and what is wrong, which are personal to each and every individual. A person's moral beliefs are often—but not always—grounded in religion. Morals may also be grounded in secular philosophical theories about right and wrong. One can be a moral person without being a religious person.

Morals, like ethics, are culture-based and culture-driven, as well as time-dependent. Only a few universal (or near-universal) morals exist, including the prohibitions against murder, rape, and incest, and the moral duty to treat others as you would like to be treated.

No one is or should feel compelled to abide by another person's morality, although individuals are clearly obliged to comply with organized ethical and legal mandates. Morals are exclusively *intra*personal. One is acting with moral virtue, or character, when he or she strives to "do the right thing."

Ethics

Ethics refers to how individuals conduct themselves in their personal and professional endeavors. The word *ethics* derives from the Greek words *ethikos,* which means character, and *ethos,* which means custom. Ethical rules of conduct are firmly grounded in moral theory.

Individuals face problems, issues, and dilemmas with ethical dimensions, which necessitate action (or nonaction) every day. **Problems** involve questions of conduct, which are relatively straightforward, temporary, and readily resolvable. **Issues** involve points of debate or controversy with strong sentiments on two (or more) sides, which are normally resolved through compromise by finding a "middle ground." **Dilemmas** entail emergent situations wherein decision makers are faced with two (or more) equally favorable or unfavorable alternative options for possible implementation. Examples of problems, issues, and dilemmas include the following:

- Clinical practice problems such as those faced by primary health care providers wrestling with patient services reimbursement policies under managed care
- Issues such as the ethics of elective abortion or whether to withdraw life support and/or nutrition for a patient in a persistent vegetative state
- Dilemmas such as deciding whether to accept or challenge a physician's invocation of therapeutic privilege (where a physician head of a health care team imposes a gag order disallowing the team to discuss a patient's diagnosis and/or prognosis with the patient)

Any ethical problem, issue, or dilemma has three fundamental elements. An agent, or **actor**, is faced with a problem, issue, or dilemma. The actor must engage in some sort of **conduct** involving action or nonaction. Further, an **effect**, or consequence, is associated with the actor's conduct related to the problem, issue, or dilemma.

Ethical theorists have analyzed these fundamental elements of actor, conduct, and effect to develop and refine their classical ethical theories. (A theory involves a set of assumptions used by theorists to explain or predict phenomena. A theory cannot be proved; it can only be disproved.) Table 2-1 lists and briefly describes the principal classical ethical theories.

HEALTH CARE PROFESSIONAL, BUSINESS, AND ORGANIZATIONAL ETHICS DEFINED AND DISTINGUISHED

Every individual comports his or her official conduct with personal or group ethical standards. These standards of conduct may differ greatly, depending on the nature of the person's occupation, profession, or position.

TABLE **2-1** ▪ **Classical Ethical Theories**

Theory	Meaning
Teleological (consequentialism ethics) From the Greek *telos,* meaning "end" or "goal"	The moral quality of conduct is assessed by focusing on its effects or consequences.
Utilitarianism	The tailoring of one's conduct so as to effect the greatest social good with a minimum of adverse consequences is one expression of consequentialism. Whether an actor effects the greatest social utility by carefully obeying established legal and ethical rules of conduct (rule utilitarianism) or by merely conducting himself or herself subjectively in such a way as to effect the greatest good, irrespective of the rules (act utilitarianism), is a matter of opinion.
Deontological (deon ethics) From the Greek *deon,* meaning "duty"	The nature of conduct is prospectively assessed, using established universal standards for behavior, including religious commandments and edicts, professional ethics codes, and rules of civil and criminal law. Under a deontological ethics approach, an actor fulfills his or her duty by following the rules, without focusing on the consequences of conduct.
Deonutility ethics[1]	This approach to ethics combines the ethical theories of teleology (consequentialism) and deontology, under which good principles and guidance are believed to bring good results.
Virtue ethics	This approach focuses on actors and their character and judgment and relations with other persons, rather than specifically on rules or consequences of conduct.

Adapted from Scott RW: *Professional ethics: a guide for rehabilitation professionals,* St Louis, 1998, Mosby.

Business ethics addresses standards of conduct for businesspersons and organizations in general. In sociocapitalist societies such as the United States, Canada, Mexico, Japan, the European community of nations, and others, the coprimary missions of private business organizations are (1) to generate monetary profits and (2) to meet express and implied social responsibilities. Social responsibility includes acts in the public interest, from affirmative action employment practices to civic charity to support for the arts to volunteerism, among a myriad of other activities.[2]

Health care professional ethical standards differ from general business ethical standards in several ways. A (declining) majority of health care entities are organized as not-for-profit businesses and therefore strive to generate net income (revenue over expenses)[3] but not profits, such as those generated in ordinary business ventures. Additionally, health care professionals treat patients who are injured or suffer from disease and are in pain and who therefore are more vulnerable to exploitation than the overwhelming majority of ordinary business clients. Health care professionals are required by law and ethical standards to maintain diagnostic, historical, and treatment-related patient information in strict confidence. Health care professionals treat patients who are injured or suffer from disease and are in pain and who therefore are more vulnerable to exploitation than the overwhelming majority of ordinary business clients. The delivery of health care to patients is often emergent, and the consequences of bad decisions are potentially dire. This is borne out by the findings of the Institute of Medicine, HealthGrades, and the Harvard University–Leape studies involving patient deaths from medical mistakes, introduced in Chapter 1. For all these reasons and more, the legal and ethical standards of conduct for health care professionals are intentionally set high—higher than for most other business pursuits.

Managed care has created a number of ethical dilemmas for health care professionals and organizations that are **fiduciaries** for their patients, meaning that they are trustees, who must place the interests of their patients above their own. From financial conflicts of interest involving provider variable or incentive pay for limiting patient care costs to "gag clauses," which inhibit free provider-patient communications, managed care has given rise to a number of significant ethical problems, issues, and dilemmas. These managed care ethical concerns are addressed in appropriate chapters throughout this text.

Jennings[4] described four situations in which a fiduciary-beneficiary relationship may exist. The first involves a classic trust relationship, in which one person gains influence or superiority over another. The second involves one person who is assigned or assumes responsibility for another person. The third involves one person who has a legal duty to act or advise another within a formal relationship. The fourth involves a specific legal duty to be recognized arising out of an interpersonal relationship. The health care professional The Hippocratic Oath–patient relationship is unique in that it encompasses all of these bases.

> The health care professional–patient fiduciary (trust) relationship is perhaps the most complete and complex of all interpersonal relationships.

What are the attributes of a **profession**? A profession has the following characteristics[5,6]:

- Defined body of accrued knowledge or expertise. The classic [original] professions—law, medicine, and the clergy—were described as having unique domains of knowledge and expertise so that no one else could carry out the professional roles of their members. Modernly, there are many more than three professions.
- **Autonomy,** or self-governance, including the establishment and enforcement of a **code of ethics** and quality standards for the professional product or service (e.g., **standards of practice** for the health care professions)
- Formal education of its members
- Research activities designed to validate and refine professional practice
- Existence of one or more professional societies or other organizations for the development of the profession and its members
- Recognition of advanced member competency through certification or other processes

PURPOSES OF PROFESSIONAL CODES OF ETHICS

Health care professional codes of ethics have four coprimary purposes.[6](p 695) First, they are **directive**; that is, they provide guidance for mandatory behavior by members of health care professional disciplines. (Professional ethics codes may also provide nondirective guidance for recommended conduct.) Second, codes must be protective of the rights of patients, clients, and research subjects and their significant others and the public at large. Third, health care professional ethics codes must be specific; that is, they must address areas of ethical problems, issues, and dilemmas particular to the disciplines governed by the various codes. Finally, health care professional ethics codes must be enforceable and enforced.

Codes of ethics may contain two general types of provisions: directive and nondirective. Directive provisions address required conduct. Nondirective provisions are of two types, addressing permissive conduct and recommended conduct. Directive provisions normally contain the words *shall, will, must, required,* or *responsible* or, in the negative, *may not, shall not,* or *will not.* Nondirective provisions addressing permissive conduct may contain the words *may* or *are not prohibited from.* Nondirective provisions addressing recommended conduct typically often contain the words *should* or *should not.*

A profession, then, has an autonomous body of accrued knowledge; it enforces a code of ethics and offers standards of practice; it provides education for its members and is involved in research activities; it promotes organizations for the development of its members; and it recognizes advanced competency.

ENFORCEMENT OF ETHICS CODES: DISCIPLINARY PROCESSES

Health care professional ethical standards are enforced by professional associations, credentialing bodies, and state licensure or regulatory administrative agencies. These ethical provisions are also indirectly enforced by the courts in civil and criminal proceedings in which violations of professional ethics also constitute violations of the law.

Readers are invited to research the ethical jurisdiction and complaint, adjudication, and appeal processes for their respective professions and to compare them with those in place for other disciplines.

Due Process and Judicial Oversight of Health Care Professional Associations

In adverse administrative disciplinary actions by state regulatory agencies against health care professionals, the federal constitutional due process clause of the Fourteenth Amendment requires that these governmental agencies afford procedural and substantive due process to respondents. State constitutions, statutes, and case law may afford additional protections to respondents in these public fora.

- Procedural due process means an adequate notice of an adverse action and a reasonable opportunity to be heard. In the case of adverse professional licensure actions, a reasonable opportunity to be heard is synonymous with the right to a hearing.
- Substantive due process means that a disciplinary procedure must be fundamentally fair, especially in light of the fact that a health care professional respondent faces potential loss of a constitutionally recognized property interest in the earned privilege of professional practice.

For disciplinary actions taken by voluntary, private (nongovernmental) professional associations, constitutional due process considerations do not apply. Instead, the internal affairs of voluntary private associations are governed by their own charters and bylaws. The private association analog of the requirement for due process is that private associations must abide by their own rules and procedures when administering discipline.

Courts always have oversight jurisdiction over state administrative agencies and their decisions, as well as over the activities of voluntary, private associations. Courts are reluctant to reverse the decisions of governmental administrative agencies, however, for several reasons. These reasons include deference to the reasonable decisions of administrative entities and considerations of time management. Reasons justifying reversal of administrative decisions include, for public agencies, the denial of due process to a respondent facing the loss of property or liberty interest, such as licensure to practice in a health care profession, and instances in which decisions are characterized as arbitrary, capricious, clearly erroneous, or the result of bias. Reasons for reversal of decisions of voluntary private associations include fraud, malice, bias, prejudicial failure to follow association rules and procedures, and instances in which decisions contravene law or public policy.

> Private associations must abide by their own rules and procedures when administering discipline.

Two other terms related to health care professional ethics warrant definition. **Bioethics** is a term used to define the identification, analysis, and resolution of ethical problems, issues, and dilemmas associated with the biological sciences, especially medicine and health care practice and research.[7] **Clinical ethics** relates specifically to ethical problems, issues, and dilemmas associated with clinical patient care activities.[8,9]

The Modern Blending of Law and Professional Ethics

Modernly, law and ethics have largely been blended into common standards of professional conduct. Often, professional conduct that constitutes a breach of ethics also constitutes a violation of law, and visa versa. Figure 2-1 illustrates the nature of the modern blending of legal and professional ethical responsibilities.

Part of the rationale for the modern blending of law and health care professional ethics is that society has become highly legalistic in recent times. U.S. citizens and residents claim against and sue one another more than anywhere else in the world. For example, in 2004, there were 16,500,000 new civil lawsuits filed nationwide.[10]

Another reason for the mixed nature of law and health care professional ethics is the fact that patients and other consumers of health care services and expertise have become more sophisticated in recent times. Patients are more aware of their rights as consumers and are more disposed to assert those rights, including through resort to the legal system.

Legal and Ethical Health Care Four-Quadrant Clinical Practice Grid

The legal and ethical health care four-quadrant clinical practice grid (Figure 2-2) illustrates acceptable and unacceptable health care clinical practice, based on compliance with or violation of legal and ethical practice rules and standards. The same model can also be applied to health care professionals in academia and research settings.

Delineation of clinical practice that clearly meets or violates legal and ethical rules and standards is relatively easy. For example, a clinician such as a certified prosthetist-orthotist who practices in compliance with applicable state and federal laws and the Canons of Ethical Conduct of the American Board for Certification is practicing in a manner that meets legal and ethical requirements. If the same provider is charged with and admits to sexual misconduct with a patient, then he or she has complied with neither legal nor ethical standards. These modes of practice can be labeled $+L/+E$ and $-L/-E$, respectively.

Professional conduct may be a violation of ethical standards but not a violation of the law, or $+L/-E$ practice. Consider the following example:

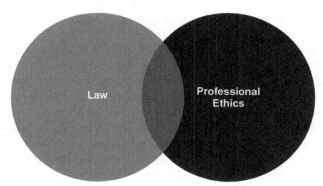

FIGURE 2-1 | Modern blending of law and professional ethics. *(From Scott RW, Petrosino C: Physical therapy management, St Louis, 2007, Mosby.)*

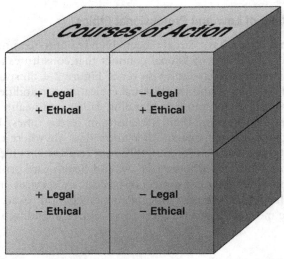

FIGURE 2-2 | Legal and ethical health care four-quadrant clinical practice grid. *(From Scott RW, Petrosino C: Physical therapy management, St Louis, 2007, Mosby.)*

> *An employment contract between a physician and a managed care organization contains a provision that prohibits the physician from discussing with patient's treatment options that are not offered by the managed care organization. (Such a contractual provision is commonly referred to as a "gag clause," which has largely been eliminated in health care professional employment contracts because of public and press pressure and resultant state and federal regulations.) Even if compliance with the "gag clause" by the physician might be upheld by a court as a legally acceptable course of action, such conduct would still constitute an actionable breach of professional ethics. Under applicable ethical standards governing patient informed consent to treatment, a competent patient must be informed by a physician of all reasonable alternatives to a proposed intervention, irrespective of whether a managed care organization elects to offer them as a matter of its business judgment. The provider in this case might face adverse administrative or American Medical Association professional association action for a breach of professional ethics, in spite of the legality of the contract.*

The most difficult mode of clinical practice to describe within the grid involves official conduct by a clinician that meets professional ethics standards but violates legal requirements, the −L/+E mode of practice. Some legal and ethics scholars might argue that a breach of professional ethics also occurs any time a health care professional's conduct violates the law. However, consider the case of a physical therapist in independent practice who treats an indigent Medicare patient in an outpatient setting. Ignorant of any possible regulatory prohibition against doing so, the physical therapist waives the patient's Medicare Part B co-payment for 20 percent of the charges but submits a bill to Medicare for its 80 percent contribution to the patient's bill.

The physical therapist, although perhaps acting ethically in providing *pro bono* services, might be in violation of federal administrative rules promulgated by the

Centers for Medicare and Medicaid Services, which generally prohibit the waiver of Part B Medicare patient co-payments.

Health care professionals should routinely evaluate their professional conduct in light of the four-quadrant grid and strive always to be clearly in compliance with legal and ethical mandates.

Despite the demise of gag clauses incident to managed care, self-imposed communications problems between primary health care providers and patients persist. In a 2003 study, Wynia and colleagues[11] reported that 31 percent of 720 physicians studied declined to offer or discuss "useful services" to patients because of the physicians' subjective judgment that the patients' health insurance would not cover those services. From an ethical standpoint, primary health care professionals must, as fiduciaries, discuss all appropriate services with their patients.

> From an ethical standpoint, primary health care professionals must, as fiduciaries, discuss all appropriate services with their patients—whether covered by patients' health insurance or not.

"Situational" Ethics

A foundational ethics question is the question of whether ethical rules and standards of conduct apply all of the time or are flexible enough to be disregarded in special situations. Situational ethics involves selective, elective noncompliance with ethics rules and standards for special circumstances.

Two general circumstances may cause a health care professional to practice situational ethics. First, a health care provider may elect not to comply with an ethical directive out of a sense of caring for a patient, colleague, or some other person. According to Fletcher,[12] this type of situational ethics occurs because of the health care professional's *agape* concern for the welfare of a patient (*agape* is Greek for love for others). Consider the following hypothetical example:

> *O, an occupational therapist employed by ABC Medical Center is treating G, a 53-year-old female patient, who is diagnosed with mild right lower limb hemiplegia incident to a left cerebrovascular accident. G is ambulatory with a standard cane and is involved in group therapy to improve performance of activities of daily living in the kitchen environment. O learned in a rehabilitation team conference that G also is diagnosed with a malignant astrocytoma of the cerebellum. G's physiatrist, P, imposed a gag order, based on therapeutic privilege, on members of the rehabilitation team—including O—that requires them to refrain from discussing G's diagnosis or prognosis with her at this time because of P's judgment that such information would harm G psychologically. During the group therapy session, G finds herself alone with O for a moment and remarks that she sometimes feels dizzy. G asks, "I don't have a brain tumor or anything like that, do I?" O answers, "Of course not! Don't worry about such a thing!"*

Has O violated professional ethics rules or standards? Does compliance with the physiatrist's invocation of therapeutic privilege supercede O's duty to comply with the Occupational Therapy Code of Ethics? That question must be answered, if it arises, by members of the Commission on Standards and Ethics of the American Occupational Therapy Association. Assume for sake of argument that the occupational therapist's conduct is deemed by the Commission on Standards and Ethics not to be violative of the Occupational Therapy Code of Ethics. Nevertheless, the conduct of the occupational therapist may still violate his or her own personal ethical standards. If, for instance, the occupational therapist believes, like deontologist Immanuel Kant,[6(note 6, p 732)] that truthfulness is a universally applicable **categorical imperative**, then the therapist has acted unethically by lying, even though the lie was occasioned by the physiatrist's order based on therapeutic privilege.

Situational ethics may also apply when a health care professional breaches professional ethics for reasons other than patient welfare, including out of malice or self-interest. Consider again the previous example (under Legal and Ethical Health Care Four-Quadrant Clinical Practice Grid) involving a physician's managed care employment gag clause provision, which disallowed the physician from discussing with patients the care options not offered by the patients' health insurance plans. Compliance with the gag clause—in violation of American Medical Association ethical standards—involves placing the physician's employment interests above patient welfare and constitutes **ethical relativism**, or **sliding scale** ethics.

Is it possible to practice situational ethics and still be an ethical person and professional? That question must be individually answered by each professional. Although every health care professional succumbs to human frailty and breaches professional ethics at some point(s) during his or her career, it may be merely rationalization to create situations under which the breach of professional ethics is routinely acceptable.

BIOMEDICAL ETHICAL PRINCIPLES

Health care professionals are guided by four foundational biomedical ethical principles in caring for patients (or conducting clinical research or educating professional students to care for patients). These four principles are beneficence, nonmaleficence, justice, and autonomy.[13]

Beneficence

Acting out of **beneficence** for a patient involves official conduct carried out in the patient's "best interests" by a health care provider. Beneficence is the manifestation of the health care professional's fiduciary duty owed to his or her patients. The Hippocratic Oath is reflective of the imperative that physicians, nurses, and allied health care professionals are bound to act in patients' best interests in clinical health care delivery. The oath reads as follows:

> *I swear ... that I will fulfill according to my ability and judgment this oath and this covenant:*
>
> *To hold him who has taught me this art as equal to my parents and to live my life in partnership with him, and if he is in need of money, to give him a share of mine, and to regard his offspring as equal to my brothers ... and to teach them this art—if they desire to learn it—without fee and covenant ...*

I will apply dietetic measures for the benefit of the sick according to my ability and judgment; I will keep them from harm and injustice.

I will neither give a deadly drug to anybody if asked for it, nor will I make a suggestion to this effect. Similarly I will not give to a woman an abortive remedy. In purity and holiness I will guard my life and my art.

I will not use the knife, not even on sufferers from stone, but will withdraw in favor of such men as are engaged in this work.

Whatever houses I may visit, I will come for the benefit of the sick [emphasis added], remaining free of all intentional injustice, of all mischief and in particular of sexual relations with both female and male persons, be they free or slaves.

What I may see or hear in the course of the treatment or even outside of the treatment in regard to the life of men, which on no account one must spread abroad, I will keep to myself, holding such things shameful to be spoken about.

If I fulfill this oath and do not violate it, may it be granted to me to enjoy life and art, being honored with fame among all men for all time to come; if I transgress it and swear falsely, may the opposite of all this be my lot.

Medical ethics and health care ethics generally have undergone a tremendous metamorphosis over time from an early deontological focus on strict compliance by physicians with the provisions of law and ethics, like the Hippocratic Oath, to a modern day period of analytical principlism,[14] under which health care professionals carefully consider the effects of their professional conduct before acting. This modern attitude is reflected in part in the Patient-Physician Covenant (Box 2-1).

Nonmaleficence

Nonmaleficence means to do no harm. Health care interventions carried out on patients' behalf, however, may cause them to suffer pain or other injury. The ethical principle of nonmaleficence requires that the health care provider not *intentionally* and *maliciously* cause harm or injury to patients under his or her care. Dr. Jack Kevorkian would assert that he did not violate the fundamental biomedical ethical principle of nonmaleficence in assisting his clients to die because his sole purpose in intervening was to alleviate the patients' suffering.

As with the other foundational biomedical ethical principles, the ethical duty of nonmaleficence applies to omissions (i.e., the failure to act when one should act) and to affirmative acts. For example, the malicious, intentional abandonment of a patient by a treating health care provider constitutes a breach of the duty not to harm the abandoned patient intentionally. An ongoing criminal investigation post–Hurricane Katrina involves a New Orleans area hospital and its staff for possible patient abandonment in the face of power outages, lack of supplies, and looting in the area.[15]

Another example of a breach of the ethical principle of nonmaleficence involves the situation in which a health care provider engages in sexual relations—nonconsensual or consensual—with a patient under his or her care. A patient may display transference emotions that are romantic toward a health care provider; however, the provider breaches the ethical duties of nonmaleficence and beneficence when he or she allows countertransference emotions to convert the professional relationship into a personal and intimate one.

BOX 2-1 ▪ Patient-Physician Covenant

Medicine is, at its center, a moral enterprise grounded in a covenant of trust. This covenant obliges physicians to be competent and to use their competence in the patient's best interests. Physicians, therefore, are both intellectually and morally obliged to act as advocates for the sick wherever their welfare is threatened and for their health at all times.

Today, this covenant of trust is significantly threatened. From within, there is growing legitimation of the physician's materialistic self-interest; from without, for-profit forces press the doctor into the role of commercial agent to enhance the profitability of health care organizations. Such distortions of the doctor's responsibility degrade the doctor/patient relationship which is the central element and structure of clinical care. To capitulate to these alterations of the trust relationship is to significantly alter the doctor's role as healer, carer, helper and advocate for the sick, and for the health of all.

By its traditions and very nature, medicine is a special kind of human activity—one which cannot be pursued effectively without the virtues of humility, honesty, intellectual integrity, compassion and effacement of excessive self-interest. These traits mark doctors as members of a moral community dedicated to something other than its own self-interest.

Our first obligation must be to serve the good of those persons who seek our help and trust us to provide it. Physicians, as physicians, are not and must never be commercial entrepreneurs, gateclosers, or agents of fiscal policy that runs counter to our trust. Any defection from primacy of the patient's well-being places the patient at risk by treatment which may compromise quality of or access to medical care.

We believe the medical profession must reaffirm the primacy of its obligation to the patient through national, state, and local professional societies, our academic, research and hospital organizations, and especially through personal behavior. As advocates for the promotion of health and support of the sick we are called upon to discuss, defend and promulgate medical care by every ethical means available. Only by caring and advocating for the patient can the integrity of our profession be affirmed. Thus we honor our covenant of trust with patients.

This covenant was produced by a group of American physicians, including Dr. David Rogers (deceased), who was former dean of medicine at Johns Hopkins University School of Medicine and former president of the Robert Wood Johnson Foundation, and Dr. Christine Cassel, who is now president and chief executive officer of the American Board of Internal Medicine. Dr. Edmund Pelligrino, senior fellow at the Center for Bioethics & Human Dignity, and Dr. George Lundberg, former editor of the *Journal of the American Medical Association,* also participated in its development. Dr. Roger Bulger, president of the Association of Academic Health Centers, and Dr. Ralph Crashaw, a practicing psychiatrist in Oregon, who has been active locally and nationally in ethical issues that pertain to physicians, were also co-authors. Finally, Dr. Lonnie Bristow, former president of the American Medical Association, and Dr. Jeremiah Barondess, president emeritus of the New York Academy of Medicine, are authors.

Justice

Justice equates to equity, or fair treatment. As it relates to the official conduct of health care professionals, justice involves comporting oneself in a way so as to maximize fairness toward all patients and potential patients requiring intervention by the provider. The concept of justice applies not only to health care professionals as individuals but to specific health care disciplines and organizations and, more broadly, to health care delivery.

Distributive justice is concerned with how equitably health care services are distributed at the macro or societal level. Distributive justice issues include political debate over universal health insurance coverage, Medicare eligibility for patients with end-stage renal disease requiring kidney dialysis, prevention and treatment of patients with acquired immunodeficiency syndrome and other catastrophic diseases, and the rationing of health care interventions near the end of life.

Comparative justice addresses how health care is delivered at the micro or individual level. Comparative justice issues include reimbursement and denial of care issues involving individual patients and the disparate treatment of patients based on age, disability, gender, race and ethnicity, or religion. The Tuskegee Syphilis Study, conducted from 1932 to 1972, is an example of a comparative justice breach of professional ethics. In this study, 400 black men with syphilis were denied lifesaving treatment (i.e., penicillin, after its discovery and release in the 1940s) so that researchers could study the effects of the disease. Publicity about this and other medical research studies led to the publication of the Belmont Report[16] and the promulgation of formal federal (and state and institutional) guidelines concerning the ethical treatment of human research subjects. On May 16, 1997, President Bill Clinton publicly apologized on behalf of the federal government in a White House ceremony to four of eight survivors of this ghoulish experiment.[17,18] Consider the following clinical practice dilemma:

> *D, a nurse practitioner, examines P, a patient who complains of severe abdominal cramping and pain. Fearing a possible bowel obstruction, D requests permission from X, a physician managed care gatekeeper, to admit P for tests. X denies the request, based on a diagnostic algorithm developed and used by the managed care organization to determine whether to admit patients with specified symptoms. D strongly believes that P should be admitted. What should D do?*

D has established a professional relationship with P and has the legal and ethical duty to take whatever action is necessary to act in the patient's best medical interests, including continuing with actions to admit him, irrespective of the reimbursement consequences of the admission. Fulfilling this duty may place D at risk of loss of employment or reinstatement with the managed care organization; however, D's higher legal and ethical duty is owed to P. To send P home might constitute a breach of professional ethics and intentional abandonment under these circumstances. Neither the law nor standards of professional ethics have changed significantly to accommodate the business of managed care.

Health practitioners are not the only professionals who face economic or other risks for "doing the right thing." Other professionals also encounter personal risks incident to fulfilling their professional duties. Consider the newspaper reporter who is jailed for refusing to violate the ethical duty not to reveal a confidential source to a judge or lawyer in a deposition, or the police, military, or fire professional who makes the ultimate sacrifice of his or her life in the line of duty. During the September 11, 2001, terrorist attack on the World Trade Center in New York City, 343 firemen and 23 policemen gave their lives in the rescue effort.[19]

A federal law related to the foundational biomedical ethical principle of individual justice is the Emergency Medical Treatment and Active Labor Act of 1986[20] (EMTALA), or the federal "antidumping law." This law was enacted largely in response to broadly publicized instances of indigent patient transfers to charity facilities by for-profit hospitals wishing to avoid a financial loss incident to their care.

EMTALA applies to all hospitals receiving federal funding for patient care. The law mandates that these facilities conduct medical screening examinations on all emergent patients and on all female patients in active labor and to stabilize bona fide emergency patients before transferring them to other (charity) facilities, without regard for the patients' ability to pay. EMTALA was intended to augment the ethical and common law duties on the part of hospitals to care for indigent emergency patients and patients in active labor and to create a uniform national standard to replace the scant number of inconsistent state laws concerning patient dumping.

Autonomy

Autonomy means self-governance. Respect for autonomy is based on respect for individual self-determination. In the health care delivery system, patients and research subjects have the right to control what is done for or to them, respectively. For patients, autonomy rights exist whether or not the patient pays for care. For research subjects, the right of control over the intervention applies irrespective of the existence or amount of compensation.

Health care professionals also exercise autonomy rights. They exercise control over physical facilities, assistants and other support personnel acting under supervision, equipment, and the examination, history taking, evaluative, diagnostic, and intervention processes within their applicable scope of professional practice.

PATIENT AUTONOMY: THE CONCEPT OF SELF-DETERMINATION

Patient autonomy rights are prominently reflected in modern-day laws and in the customary practices governing health care delivery. These laws and customs mandate, in part, strong and active patient involvement in interventional decision making. Health care organizations and professionals universally came to recognize in the twentieth century the right of patients with legal and mental capacity (or their surrogate decision makers) to be involved in, and ultimately to control, treatment decision-making processes.

This patient autonomy right of involvement and ultimate control over treatment is reflected in documents found in most or all hospitals describing patient rights and responsibilities incident to care. An excellent example of such a document is the Patients' Bill of Rights and Responsibilities of the Brooke Army Medical Center,[21] reprinted at Appendix 2-1. (The author is thankful to Brooke Army Medical Center for the use of its Bill of Rights and is grateful for its superlative and tireless medical care for returning Gulf War military servicemen and servicewomen and civilians from many nations.)

A patient's right of autonomy also includes the right to refuse treatment, after all reasonable options and the consequences of refusal of treatment have been explained to the patient. Is the patient's right to refuse intervention absolute? No. Courts have ruled on occasion that treatment may be given compulsorily to patients under special circumstances, such as when the life of a third party (e.g., fetus carried by a mother) is at risk if treatment is not provided to the patient. More and more, however, courts are ruling in ways that evince greater respect for patient autonomy, irrespective of the consequences of patient's decisions to innocent third parties.

Patients' right to choose their own health care providers is universally recognized. Laws in all states and professional ethics codes recognize this inherent patient right. Managed care and health care reform initiatives have the potential to affect patient and professional autonomy adversely in a number of ways. A draft version of the 1993 federal Clinton health reform initiative would have given regional health alliances broad authority to supervene certification and state licensure restrictions on professional practice in unspecified ways. Managed care contractual networks may create barriers to participation for providers not part of preferred provider networks. Managed care–era restrictions on provider-patient communications—such as employment contract gag clauses or limitations on parameters of practice—also derogate from the professional relationship. These restrictions must continue to be addressed by the health care professional, political, consumer, and other relevant communities.

> The four foundational biomedical ethical principles guiding the official conduct of health care professionals are beneficence, nonmaleficence, justice, and autonomy.

THE SYSTEMS APPROACH TO HEALTH CARE PROFESSIONAL ETHICAL DECISION MAKING

Health care ethical decision making, whether in clinical, educational, research, school, home, or other settings, requires careful compliance with professional and, where applicable, institutional ethical standards and with legal mandates. As with legal requirements, ignorance of ethical responsibilities is no excuse for noncompliance.

Many existing frameworks exist for ethical decision making for health care professionals. All ethical decision-making models governing patient care and health client service delivery are based on the foundational biomedical ethical principles of beneficence, nonmaleficence, autonomy, and justice and are reflective of core professional attributes and duties, including accountability, advocacy, altruism, autonomy (patient and professional), compassion, competence, confidentiality, empathy, fidelity, fiduciary status, loyalty, patience, social responsibility, team play, and truthfulness. Conducting oneself in conformity with these principles, attributes, and duties is seemingly more difficult under the current managed care paradigm, which poses significant actual and potential conflicts of interest. Most analytical ethical decision-making models have common core elements:

- Identification of a problem, issue, or dilemma having ethical implications
- Identification of relevant facts and unknowns and formulation of reasonable assumptions about the problem, issue, or dilemma
- Delineation and analysis of viable courses of action to resolve the problem, issue, or dilemma
- Selection of an option for implementation based on an appropriate ethics approach and ethical guidelines and in conformity with controlling ethical and legal directives

The systems approach augments this model with a feedback loop. Under the systems approach, a decision maker carefully monitors and obtains feedback on a chosen course of action for appropriateness, efficacy, and effectiveness—on an ongoing basis—and modifies the chosen course of action (or rejects it outright and substitutes another course of action) if, on the basis of negative feedback, it is adjudged not to be optimal. For more information on general systems theory and thinking, see von Bertalanffy's *General Systems Theory: Foundations, Development, Application.*[22]

Ignorance of one's professional ethical responsibilities is no excuse for noncompliance.

Von Bertalanffy developed systems theory in the 1920s. Today, it is widely used in engineering, the natural sciences, and business and management.

Under the systems approach to health care professional ethical decision making, a decision maker must evaluate and reevaluate a myriad of factors relevant to a problem, issue, or dilemma at all steps of the analysis. These factors include the following:

- *S*ociocultural considerations, such as gender, race and ethnicity, religion, sexual preference, and other factors, as they apply to a problem, issue, or dilemma
- *L*egal implications associated with a decision
- *E*thical imperatives (i.e., Will the decision maker's conduct conform to a governing professional code of ethics or with the decision maker's personal morals and ethical standards?)
- *E*conomic impact of a course of action on those persons affected by its implementation
- *P*olitical ramifications associated with a course of action, if any

In addition to applying these *S-L-E-E-P* factors, a decision maker should also always apply the principle of symmetry[23] to the resolution of a health care ethical problem, issue, or dilemma within the systems approach to health care professional ethical decision making. The principle of symmetry requires an actor to carry out a multidimensional analysis of a chosen course of action. The principle requires a decision maker to analyze a decision at least by assuming the opposing point of view and analyzing its implementation from that perspective.

Figure 2-3 depicts the circular flow diagram of the systems approach to health care professional ethical decision making. Primary and support health care professionals are urged to consider its implementation in their clinical decision making.

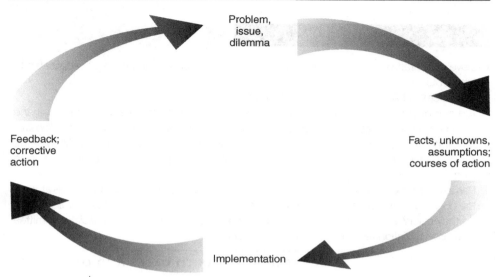

Problem,
issue,
dilemma

Feedback;
corrective
action

Facts, unknowns,
assumptions;
courses of action

Implementation

FIGURE 2-3 | The systems approach to health care professional ethical decision. *(Adapted from Scott RW: Professional ethics: a guide for rehabilitation professionals, St Louis, 1998, Mosby.)*

SUMMARY

Health care professionals must comply with their own personal moral beliefs, the civil and criminal laws of the jurisdiction in which they practice, and the professional ethics standards of their professional associations and other entities. Occasionally, these governing directives are in conflict, creating serious dilemmas for health care professionals and patients under their care.

Four foundational biomedical ethical concepts affect health care professional ethics. Beneficence involves acting in a patient's best interests. Health care professionals are their patients' fiduciaries (i.e., they stand in a position of special trust and confidence). Nonmaleficence means that health care professionals are bound not intentionally and maliciously to harm patients under their care. Justice involves equitable treatment of all patients. Autonomy evidences respect for patients' inherent right of self-determination, particularly in controlling treatment decision making. The implementation of these guiding principles has been made more difficult under managed care, in which the interests of providers and third-party payers are often in conflict with patient needs or desires.

Health care professionals must use a systematic approach to health care professional ethical decision making. The systems approach presented in this chapter shows an easy-to-follow-and-implement decision-making tool. The approach contains the following elements: (1) identification of a problem, issue, or dilemma with ethical implications; (2) identification of relevant facts and unknowns, and formulation of reasonable assumptions; (3) delineation and analysis of viable courses of action; (4) implementation of a course of action; and (5) monitoring and modification (if necessary) of an executed course of action, based on ongoing feedback.

CASES AND QUESTIONS

1. Develop a draft version of a model patient code of ethical conduct, generally applicable to inpatients.
2. Consider the following clinical practice problem:
   A group of orthotists and prosthetists in private practice in a large metropolitan area in the northeastern United States is contemplating the establishment of a *pro bono publico* (reduced or no fee) service within their practice for indigent patients needing care. Analyze the problem under the systems approach to health care professional ethical decision making.
3. Peruse your professional association code of ethics. Compare and contrast it to at least the codes of ethics of at least two other disciplines. How are the three codes similar? How do they differ? What changes, if any, might you suggest to the ethics or judicial committee of your association regarding the disciplinary code?

SUGGESTED ANSWERS TO CASES AND QUESTIONS

1. A patient code of ethics may contain the following provisions (among possible others):
   Model Patient Code of Ethics
   A patient in the inpatient setting is expected to do the following:
   I. Provide accurate and complete information to a primary health care provider relevant to a consultation or treatment.
   II. Listen carefully to information provided by your health care provider; ask relevant questions about recommended interventions; and make a definitive, intelligent, voluntary, and unequivocal decision to accept or decline a recommended intervention. Please share responsibility for your own care.
   III. Respect the rights and dignity of all other persons in the health care setting, and respect the property of others.
   IV. Cooperate with examining, evaluating, and treating health care professionals to the maximum extent feasible, and ask relevant questions throughout the process of care delivery.
   V. Conduct yourself in such a way as to maintain an optimal patient–health care professional relationship with your providers. Insist on the same level of professionalism from everyone in the process.
2. Factors for analysis under the systems approach to health care professional ethical decision making:
   • Problem: A significant number of patients require orthotist's and prosthetist's services in the community who present themselves in this clinic for care, lacking the ability to pay for those services.
   • Facts, unknowns, and assumptions: One sample factor is given for each category. Others may also apply:
     • *Sociocultural considerations:* Indigent patients presenting in this clinic for care are disproportionately working mothers and their children.
     • *Legal implications:* The assumption is that the state permits indigent patients to sign a waiver of liability for simple negligence incident to no-fee health care.
     • *Ethical imperatives: Pro bono publico* services are the epitome of ethical behavior and, in many disciplines, an expectation.

- *Economic impact:* Accepting a fixed small number of *pro bono* patients for care (e.g., three patients in the practice at any one time) is not expected to affect the profitability of the practice adversely.
- *Political ramifications:* Establishing a *pro bono publico* policy and publicizing it will enhance the business goodwill of the practice.
- Courses of action: (1) Do not accept any *pro bono* patients in the clinic, except as required by law. (2) Accept up to three *pro bono* patients (based on demonstrated need) in the clinic's practice mix at any one time.
- Option for implementation: Accept up to three *pro bono* patients (based on demonstrated need) in the clinic's practice mix at any one time.
- Feedback: Monitor the option implemented for appropriateness, efficacy, and effectiveness; modify or discontinue as necessary.

SUGGESTED READINGS

Abelson R: Medicare says bonuses can improve hospital care, *New York Times* p C3, Nov 15, 2005.

Fox W: *A theory of general ethics,* Cambridge, Mass, 2006, MIT Press.

Kirsch NR: Ethical decision making: terminology and context, *PT Magazine* pp 38-40, Feb 2006.

Patient bill of rights, Chicago, 2006, American Hospital Association.

Pear R: Medicare, in a different tack, links doctors' pay to practices, *New York Times* p A1, Dec 12, 2006.

Pear R: Nonprofit hospitals face scrutiny over practices, *New York Times* p 14, March 19, 2006.

Stern GM: Re-examining business ethics, *USA Weekend* p 12, Sept 1-3, 2006.

REFERENCES

1. Walton CC: *The moral manager,* Cambridge, Mass, 1988, Ballinger Publishing.
2. *Corporate social responsibility report,* Seattle, Wa, 2005, Starbucks Coffee Company.
3. Cleverley WO, Andrew EC: *Essentials of health care finance,* ed 6, Sudbury, Mass, 2007, Jones and Bartlett.
4. Jennings T: Fiduciary litigation in Texas, *Texas Bar Journal* pp 844-851, Oct 2006.
5. Fleming MH, Johnson JA, Marina M et al: *Occupational therapy: directions for the future,* Bethesda, Md, 1987, American Occupational Therapy Association.
6. Richardson ML, White KK: *Ethics applied,* New York, 1993, McGraw-Hill.
7. Bailey DM, Schwartzberg SL: *Ethical and legal dilemmas in occupational therapy,* Philadelphia, 1995, FA Davis.
8. Jonsen AR, Siegler M, Winslade WJ: *Clinical ethics,* ed 3, New York, 1992, McGraw-Hill.
9. La Puma J: Clinical ethics, mission, and vision: practical wisdom in health care, *Hospitals & Health Care Administration* 35(3):321, 1990.
10. Center for Individual Freedom: *The Case for Legal Reform.* Retrieved Nov 26, 2006, from www.cfif.org.
11. Wynia MK, VanGeest JB, Cummins DS, Wilson IB: Do physicians not offer useful services because of coverage restrictions? *Health Aff* 22(4):190-197, 2003.
12. Fletcher J: *Situational ethics: the new morality,* Philadelphia, 1966, Westminster Press.

13. Beauchamp TL, Childress JF: *Principles of biomedical ethics,* ed 5, New York, 2001, Oxford University Press.

14. Pellegrino ED: The metamorphosis of medical ethics: a 30-year retrospective, *JAMA* 269:1158, 1993.

15. Westen J-H: *Court documents: hospital gives lethal injections to patients during Hurricane Katrina,* Feb 22, 2006. Retrieved Dec 3, 2006, from www.lifesite.net/ldn/2006/feb/06022201.html.

16. National Commission for the Protection of Human Subjects of Biomedical and Behavioral Research: *Belmont report: ethical principles and guidelines for the protection of human subjects of research,* Washington, DC, 1978, US Government Printing Office.

17. Beck J: Apology for syphilis project overdue, *Indianapolis Star* p D2, May 18, 1997.

18. Kasindorf M: Tuskegee survivors make trek to capital for apology, *USA Today* p 6A, May 15, 1997.

19. The 9-11 Commission Report, 2004, Washington, DC, Superintendent of Documents.

20. Emergency Medical Treatment and Active Labor Act of 1986, 42 United States Code Section 1395dd.

21. *Patients' bill of rights and responsibilities,* San Antonio, Texas, 2006, Brooke Army Medical Center.

22. von Bertalanffy L: *General systems theory: foundations, development, application,* New York, 1968, George Braziller.

23. Adapted from Moore W Jr: *Ethics and values* (graduate course), EDA 388V, Austin, spring 1997, University of Texas at Austin. Used with permission.

2-1

Patient Rights and Responsibilities

BROOKE ARMY MEDICAL CENTER

Fort Sam Houston, Texas

We at Brooke Army Medical Center (BAMC) hold the welfare and safety of the patient as our highest priority. The most important person in this medical center is you, our patient. Our goal is to provide you with the best medical care available. Our success will be reflected in your satisfaction with the treatment you receive. We regard your basic human right with great importance. You have the right to freedom of expression, to make your own decisions, and to know that your human rights will be preserved and respected. The following is a list of patient rights and responsibilities.

YOUR RIGHTS AS A PATIENT

You have the right to receive respectful, considerate, and supportive treatment and service.

- We will do our best to provide you with compassionate and respectful care at all times.
- We will do everything possible to provide a safe hospital environment.
- We will be attentive to your specific needs and requests, understanding that they should not interfere with medical care for you or for others.
- We will not discriminate in providing you with care, based on race, ethnicity, national origin, religion, gender, age, mental or physical disability, genetic information, sexual orientation, or source of payment.

You have the right to be involved in all aspects of your care.

- We will make sure that you know which physician or care provider is primarily responsible for you care. We will explain the professional status and the role of persons who help in your care.
- We will keep you fully informed about your condition, the results of tests we perform, and the treatment you receive.

- We will clearly explain to you any treatments or procedures that we propose. We will request your written consent for procedures that carry more than minimal risk.
- We will make sure that you are part of the decision-making process in your care. When there are dilemmas or differences over care decisions, we will include you in resolving them.
- We will honor your right to refuse the care that we advise. (In some circumstances, especially for active duty patients, laws and regulations may override this right.)
- We will honor your Advance Directive or Medical Power of Attorney, regarding limits to the care that you wish to receive.

You have the right to receive timely and appropriate assessment and management of your pain.

- We will routinely ask if you are suffering pain. If you are, we will evaluate it further and help you get relief.

You have the right to have your personal needs respected.

- We will respect the confidentiality of your personal information throughout the institution. (For active duty persons, complete confidentiality may not be possible, based on requirements to report some conditions or findings.) We will respect your need for privacy in conversations, examinations, information sharing, and procedures. Also, you may request that a chaperone be present during an examination or procedure.
- We will communicate with you in a language that you understand.
- We will respect your need to feel safe and secure throughout the facility. Hospital employees will be identifiable with badges or nameplates.
- We will take your concerns and complaints seriously and will work hard to resolve them.
- We will respect your need for pastoral care and other spiritual services. Our Chaplain Service is on call at all times. Other spiritual support is welcome, as long as it does not interfere with patient care or hospital function.
- We will respect your need to communicate with others, both family and friends. If it is medically necessary to limit your communications with others, we will tell you and your family why.
- We will use soft fabric restraints, with close and frequent monitoring, if you become so confused that you are in danger of hurting yourself or others. We will untie the restraints as soon as we safely can do so.

You have the right to receive information on how to contact protective services.

- At your request, we will give you information on how you may contact protective services for children, adults, or the elderly. We will do this confidentially.

You have the right to participate in clinical research when it is appropriate.

- Your care provider will discuss this with you when it is appropriate. The Institutional Review Board, a committee that includes people from many parts of this community, monitors all research at BAMC. We will thoroughly explain the proposed research to you and ask your written permission to take part. If you choose not to take part in the research, it will not affect the care that we give you. Participation is completely voluntary.

You have the right to speak to a BAMC Patient Representative regarding any aspect of your care.

- We encourage patients and families to speak directly with ward of clinic personnel if there is a problem. However, if these people cannot solve it, you may contact the Patient Representative at 916-2330 (clinics) or 916-2200 (inpatient tower).

You have the right to expect that this institution will operate according to a code of ethical behavior.

- The Command at BAMC is firmly committed to managing this hospital according to the highest traditions of the military and medical professionalism and ethics. In addition, our Institutional Bioethics Committee meets regularly to review ethical topics, including organizational ethics. This committee is available to you and to our employees if a serious ethical dilemma comes up in either patient care or service.

You have a right to receive a personal copy of these patient rights.

- Copies of these patient rights are available on any ward and in any clinic at BAMC. If you cannot locate a copy for yourself, ask ward or clinic personnel. If you have any questions or comments regarding patient rights, we encourage you to contact a BAMC Patient Representative at 916-2330 or 916-2200.

YOUR RESPONSIBILITIES AS A PATIENT

- You are responsible for maximizing your own healthy behaviors.
- You are responsible for taking an active part in decisions about your health care.
- You are responsible for providing us with accurate and complete information about your health and your condition.
- You are responsible for showing courtesy and respect for other patients, families, hospital staff, and visitors. This includes personal and hospital property.
- You are responsible for keeping your scheduled appointments on time, and for giving us advance notice if you must cancel or reschedule.

- You are responsible for providing us with you current address and means of contact (such as a home phone or cell phone).
- You are responsible for providing us with current information regarding any other health insurance coverage you have.
- You are responsible for keeping yourself informed of the coverage, options, and policies of the TRICARE plan that you subscribe to as a military beneficiary. This information is available in the TRICARE Service Office. (Beneficiary Line: 1-800-406-2832).

Courtesy Brooke Army Medical Center, San Antonio, Texas.

NOTES

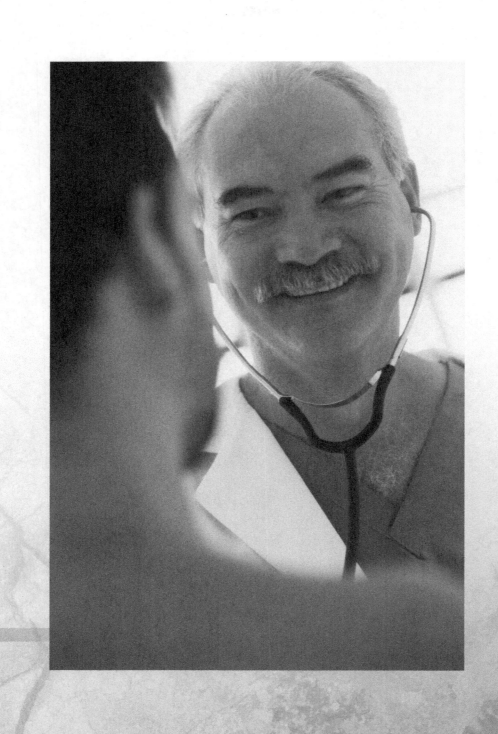

3 The Law of Health Care Malpractice

KEY TERMS

Act

Actual cause

Apparent agency

Case-in-chief

Charitable immunity

Comparative negligence

Complaint

Condition precedent

Continuous treatment
    doctrine

Corporate liability

Discovery rule

Duty of due care

Exculpatory release

Executrix

Failure to warn

Foreseeable

General damages

Health care malpractice

Impeachment

Last clear chance

Learned intermediaries

Learned treatises

Learned works

Legal causation

Legal disability

Legally competent

Loss of consortium

Malpractice

Material issue in

Medical malpractice

Omission

Ostensible agency

Past recollection recorded

Patient abandonment

Percipient

Pleading

Premises liability

Present recollection
    refreshed

Professional negligence

Proximate cause

Respondeat superior

Same or similar community
    standard

Same school doctrine

Sine qua non

Sovereign immunity

Special damages

Spoliation

Statutes of repose

Strict liability for abnormally
    dangerous activities

Strict liability for
    ultrahazardous activities

Substandard care

Substantial factor

Summary judgment

Trend

Vicarious liability

Without regard to fault

INTRODUCTION

Patient injury incident to treatment can give rise to health care malpractice liability if, in addition to patient physical or mental injury, there exists a legal basis for imposing liability. The five legal bases for liability include professional negligence, breach of a treatment-related contractual promise, intentional care-related misconduct, and strict (non–fault-based) liability for injury from dangerously defective treatment-related products or for abnormally dangerous clinical activities. Defenses to health care malpractice cases include failure to file a lawsuit within the applicable time frame, or statute of limitations, and comparative (shared) fault. Effective documentation management—including proper creation, use, and filing of incident reports—is critical to effective malpractice risk management.

Health care professionals face significant liability risk exposure primarily because they routinely interact with clients who are injured or ill and often in great physical pain and psychological distress. The concept of **malpractice**, as used in this chapter, refers to liability on the part of health care providers for patient injury. The traditional term *medical malpractice* only refers to the potential liability of physicians and surgeons for patient injury. In this book the more inclusive term *health care malpractice* is used to reflect and emphasize the fact that primary health care professionals other than physicians and surgeons are also exposed to malpractice liability incident to their professional practice. These primary health care professionals include advanced practice nurses, podiatrists, and rehabilitation professionals such as physical and occupational therapists and speech pathologists.

Health care malpractice: Liability of health care providers for patient injury.

SIGNIFICANCE OF REPORTED LEGAL CASES

What is the significance of a "reported" legal case? A reported legal case is one that was appealed by one or both sides to at least one tier of appellate review or was deemed by legal scholars to be sufficiently significant at the initial trial court level of adjudication to warrant reporting.

Just because a legal case exists, is appealed, or is reported does not in any way infer that a finding of liability resulted against a defendant–health care professional. The exclusive burden to prove liability rests with patient-plaintiffs suing defendant–health care professionals. Health care malpractice plaintiffs (i.e., injured patients or their representatives) must prove their cases to the satisfaction of a judge (acting as fact-finder in a *judge-alone* trial) or jury by a preponderance (greater weight) of evidence in order to prevail.

At the end of a trial on the merits of a health care malpractice case, a patient-plaintiff may fail to convince a jury or judge that a defendant–physical or occupational therapist committed malpractice. If such is the case, the plaintiff loses his or her case, and the defendant prevails, or wins, and is vindicated in the case.

Even before a formal trial commences, a plaintiff may lose a health care malpractice case if the presiding trial judge concludes that there is not any **material issue in** (triable) dispute. In such a case the judge will normally dismiss the case against the defendant-provider through **summary judgment**, that is, a formal finding that the plaintiff's case cannot proceed to trial because of insufficient or defective evidence.

FACTORS INCREASING HEALTH CARE PROFESSIONALS' MALPRACTICE LIABILITY EXPOSURE

External Factors

Probably the most significant external factor leading to greater health care malpractice liability exposure is the litigious nature of the American public. With 16.5 million new civil lawsuits filed in the United States in 2004 (among them, perhaps 30,000 to 50,000 new health care malpractice lawsuits), Americans are clearly overly litigious. Adding to liability risk exposure is the myriad of new and complex governmental and accreditation agency regulations. In a business environment so regulated and so scrutinized by everyone, from administrative agencies to the media, providers can ill afford not to have on retainer, and proactively seek advice regularly from, personal legal counsel.

Another liability-generating factor is the nature of the ever-changing health care delivery system. The health care milieu is moving away from what heretofore has been primarily an altruistic, patient-welfare focused, informal, and friendly system of providing health care for patients toward an arms-length, business-like, cost-containment–focused, competitive, formal, and defensive system of client management. The U.S. Supreme Court declared, in the case of *Pegram* v. *Herdrich*,[1] that the managed care health care delivery system has the blessing of the Congress and that patient care decisions made by health maintenance organization (HMO) physicians who receive variable incentive pay from their employers are not fiduciary decisions. The Supreme Court went on to rule in *Aetna Health Inc.* v. *Davila* and *CIGNA Healthcare Corp. of Texas, Inc.* v. *Calad*,[2] that health insurers and managed care organizations are not liable under state tort laws for negligent health care decisions that injure patients. The American Medical Association labeled these decisions "the demise of managed care accountability."[3]

Internal Factors

Several factors internal to specific health care disciplines predispose to greater potential malpractice liability exposure. The broadening scope of practice for many nonphysician primary health care disciplines may lead to greater liability exposure. For physical therapy, for example, the fact that 42 states permit direct access practice, that is, without physician referral, may lead to greater liability exposure as more physical therapists serve as primary care providers.[2] The trend toward clinical specialty certification in physician and nonphysician specialties may also lead to greater liability exposure—for certified specialists and nonspecialists—as the standard of care for specific practice specialties becomes more precisely articulated. Similarly, the trends toward postbaccalaureate professional-level entry to practice and advanced professional degrees and residencies may also alter the legal standard of care because more prospective expert witnesses who will establish the standard of care in court are educated beyond the baccalaureate level. Cross-training, acquisition of multiple skills, and the delegation of care (but not legal responsibility) to extenders also potentially creates greater malpractice liability exposure.

LEGAL BASES FOR IMPOSING LIABILITY FOR PATIENT INJURY

Malpractice liability occurs in the health care professional–patient relationship whenever a patient is injured during the course of care and there is a legally recognized basis for imposing malpractice liability. Health care professionals are bound to comply with the foundational ethical principle of, or "do no intentional malicious harm," when caring for patients. However, the myth that malpractice liability occurs any time that a patient is injured in the course of patient care is simply inaccurate. Judges in malpractice cases are required to practice equity, or fairness, and would not allow a jury to award a sympathy verdict in favor of a patient-plaintiff merely because the plaintiff was injured in the course of treatment. One or more of the legally recognized bases for malpractice liability must also be present.

Traditionally, medical (physicians) or health care (all disciplines) malpractice has meant liability for patient injury caused by **professional** (treatment-related) **negligence**. However, by the mid-1980s, courts and legislatures broadened the scope of potential bases for malpractice-related liability to include other legal bases for liability associated with patient injury.[4]

Under this broader definition of health care malpractice, a defendant–health care professional may face fault-based malpractice liability for patient injury caused by professional negligence, breach (violation) of a contractual promise made to a patient, and intentional conduct resulting in patient injury. A defendant—health care professional may also face malpractice liability **without regard to fault** for patient injury from dangerously defective treatment-related products and from provider-controlled abnormally dangerous treatment activities (Box 3-1).

The first three fault-based bases for health care malpractice liability—professional negligence, breach of contract, and intentional conduct—involve the delivery of care that is adjudged as being objectively substandard. **Substandard care** means care that fails to meet at least minimally acceptable practice standards for the defendant-provider's discipline.

BOX **3-1** ▪ **Health Care Malpractice**

Traditional definition: Liability of health care professionals for patient injury caused by professional negligence.

Expanded definition: Liability of health care professionals for patient injury caused by the following:

- Professional negligence
- Breach of a contractual promise regarding treatment
- Intentional conduct of the defendant–provider incident to care of a patient
- Dangerously defectively designed or manufactured treatment-related products or modalities
- Abnormally dangerous clinical activities

Adapted from Scott RW: *Promoting legal awareness in physical and occupational therapy,* St Louis, 1997, Mosby.

> **Substandard care:** Care that fails to comply with legal and ethical standards; that is, care that fails to meet at least minimally acceptable practice standards for a defendant-provider's specific discipline.

Liability for Professional Negligence

Health care professionals may be liable for malpractice when they fail to care for patients in ways that comply with legal standards of care. Negligent care may be rendered by the primary health care professional (primary liability) or by someone (an agent) under the supervision of the primary health care professional (vicarious liability). What the standard of care is, is most often established through expert testimony of health care professionals from the same discipline as a malpractice defendant by reference to authoritative texts and peer-reviewed publications or by reference to clinical practice protocols or guidelines.

The Concept of Negligence

Negligence can be considered legally actionable carelessness. The legal definition of negligence is conduct by a person who owes another a legal duty, which falls below a standard established by law for the protection of others against unreasonable risk of harm. In a health care malpractice scenario, a defendant–health care professional may be negligent in carrying out a duty owed to a patient, and the patient-plaintiff may be contributorily negligent if the patient acts in a manner that falls below a standard that the law imposes on the patient for self-protection against possible harm.[5]

"Conduct" that can form the basis for actionable negligence on the part of a health care provider may involve an **act** or an **omission** when the provider had a duty to act. An example of a negligent act might be the act of dislocating the shoulder of a patient with hemiplegia while carrying out passive mobility testing. An example of a negligent omission might be the failure to monitor a patient's intravenous line.

> **Contributory negligence:** Plaintiff-patient conduct that falls below a standard mandated by law for the patient's own protection from unreasonable harm incident to treatment.

 Conduct constituting negligence can be a positive act or an omission, or a failure to act, when a defendant had the duty to act.

Elements of Proof for Professional Negligence

A patient bringing a claim or lawsuit alleging professional negligence on the part of a treating health care professional must fulfill a litany of proof, consisting of four elements: (1) that the defendant–health care provider owed a duty of care to the plaintiff-patient; (2) that the defendant-provider violated the duty owed through conduct that constitutes professional negligence; (3) that, as a direct cause and consequence of the defendant-provider's negligent conduct, the plaintiff-patient sustained injury; and

(4) that the type of injuries that the plaintiff-patient sustained warrant the award of monetary damages.[6] The plaintiff has the legal burden to prove each of these elements to a jury or judge (acting as trier of fact) by a preponderance, or greater weight, of evidence. Before an allegation of professional negligence ever becomes a formal claim or lawsuit, the lawyer representing the plaintiff-patient evaluates the merits of the case to satisfy himself or herself that these four elements can be proved in court by a preponderance of the evidence (Box 3-2).

Duty

When does a health care professional owe a special duty of care to a patient? Possible answers include (1) whenever a patient calls for an appointment for evaluation and treatment, (2) when a patient presents himself or herself for care, (3) when a patient signs in at the reception area and is awaiting evaluation and treatment, or (4) when a health care professional accepts a patient for care. Almost always, the special duty of professional care arises only when a health care professional agrees to accept a patient for care.

Occasionally, a health care professional will not know whether a patient's diagnosis or problem falls within the professional's legal scope of practice or ambit of personal competence until after a history and physical examination are completed. It is proper, and even required by legal and ethical standards, to decline to treat a patient whose problem falls outside a health care professional's legal scope of practice or personal competence. In such instances, refusal to treat a patient does not constitute **patient abandonment**.

In the United States, unlike in some other countries, there is no general duty to help another person in need of assistance or in peril. Absent some special relationship, such as a preestablished health care provider–patient relationship, an attorney-client relationship, a minister-parishioner relationship, or a parent-child relationship, the general duty to aid another person does not apply. By way of example, consider the following hypothetical situation.

> *A man is standing on the roof of a tall building. Suddenly, a 3-year-old child walks through the door leading to the roof and ambles toward the edge of the roof, which does not have a protective fence. The toddler is walking relatively slowly, and the man has ample time to stop the toddler's movement without any danger to himself. Instead, the man silently observes as the toddler walks off the edge of the building to his death.*

BOX **3-2** ▪ **Four Required Elements of Proof in a Professional Negligence Lawsuit**

1. Duty owed by defendant
2. Duty violated by defendant
3. Causation, that is, the defendant's negligent conduct caused the patient injury
4. Monetary damages are required to be awarded to make the injured patient "whole"

Is the man legally responsible for the young child's demise? The answer depends on whether the man owed a legal duty of care to the child. Unless the man was a security guard or another type of employee of the building or somehow enticed the toddler onto the roof, he probably had no legal duty to come to the aid of the child, even though it was a clear, calm day, and he could have easily rescued the child from harm without exposing himself to any danger. Of course, it is beyond debate, under the facts of this scenario, that the man had a moral duty to help the unwitting toddler, but he probably could not be held legally accountable for his failure to act.

Under the same no-duty principle as the one presented in the hypothetical example, health care professionals generally are free to decline to accept patients for care. This commonly properly occurs, for instance, when a provider has a limited-scope practice, such as an exclusive adolescent or geriatric patient practice. In such circumstances, providers are normally free to reject patients for care who do not fall within the scope of their practice. Health care providers are not free, however, to decline to care for patients for illegal reasons, such as illegal discrimination based on a patient's race, ethnicity, religion, gender, national origin, age, or disability.

When Does "Duty" End? Issues Involving Patient Abandonment. An allegation of improper patient abandonment may arise incident to health care delivery and may be brought as a negligent or intentional abandonment charge with different legal consequences. Legally actionable patient abandonment occurs when a treating health care professional improperly unilaterally terminates the professional-patient relationship.

> **Abandonment:** Improper unilateral termination by a treating health care professional of a professional-patient relationship.

The widest imaginable range of variegated clinical treatment activities can give rise to an allegation of patient abandonment, from a clinician momentarily turning his or her back from a patient (with a resultant patient fall) to discharging a patient before the patient reaches the zenith of rehabilitative potential because of inability to continue to pay for care.

A patient is free unilaterally and summarily to terminate a health care professional–patient relationship at any time without legal consequence. The same is not true for a health care professional charged with responsibility for caring for a patient. A health care professional may unilaterally terminate a professional-patient relationship when, in the provider's professional judgment, a cure has been effected or maximal recovery or progress has been achieved. Careful documentation of the patient's status upon discharge is always required for the protection of provider and patient.

It may also be acceptable to discharge a patient for reasons unrelated to goal achievement, such as failure to pay for services or an irreconcilable personality conflict between provider and patient. In these and in similar circumstances, the freedom to discharge the patient is neither absolute nor without conditions. In the case of discharge for failure to pay for professional services, for example, a health care professional who is a preferred provider in a managed care network may have agreed contractually to treat patients for a fixed price and may not be free to discharge prematurely or to charge more than the agreed amount for whatever period treatment may entail. In the case of discharge because of an irreconcilable personality conflict, the provider must give advance notice of the intent to sever the professional-patient relationship and must also give the patient a sufficient amount of time to locate a suitable substitute, competent care provider. It is highly recommended that a provider discharging a patient under this scenario also actively assist the patient in locating a substitute provider and consult with and transfer the patient's health records expeditiously to the substitute provider to minimize the possibility of legal action by the patient for intentional abandonment.

In the case of negligent abandonment, the same four elements of proof as in any other professional negligence action must be established by the plaintiff-patient. These are (1) that the defendant–health care provider owed a duty of special care to the patient; (2) that in prematurely and improperly discharging the patient, the defendant-provider breached the legal standard of care; (3) that the breach of duty on the part of the defendant-provider caused injury to the plaintiff-patient; and (4) that the injuries that the plaintiff-patient sustained warrant the award of monetary damages in order to make the patient whole. The language used to present these four professional negligence elements is similar to language that a defendant–health care provider might see in a formal civil complaint in which the plaintiff-patient details the specifics of his or her lawsuit.

Abandonment and Substitute Care Providers. One of the special circumstances concerning patient abandonment involves whether health care professionals may temporarily transfer the care of patients to substitute health care providers of the same discipline when the primary provider is called away from the facility for additional duties, attends a continuing education course, or goes on vacation. The answer is usually yes. Just as it is legitimate to employ a substitute care provider when a primary health care professional becomes ill, it is normally acceptable to transfer a patient's care to a substitute care professional when duty (or even scheduled vacation) takes the primary provider away from the facility. In hospital and HMO settings, patients do not always have a reasonable expectation of receiving professional care from a specific provider. Instead, patients are treated by staff (in the hospital and staff HMO models) or contract (in the group or network HMO models) providers.

In private practice or preferred provider organization settings, however, patients probably do have a reasonable expectation of being treated by specific providers of choice. In such environments, providers are advised to obtain written patient informed consent for substitution of specific primary providers by other professionals. In either situation, providers should always obtain patient consent for substitution and provide a detailed care summary and instructions to the substitute professional. When applicable, referring physicians should also be notified in advance of the substitution of providers. All of these details should be succinctly but thoroughly documented in the records of affected patients.

Abandonment and the Limited-Scope Practice. Another potential problem area involves health care professionals who work only in specific, limited practice settings. What happens when a current patient asks for treatment for problems unrelated to areas in which the provider offers services? Although it would probably still be acceptable to deny care for areas outside of one's specialty practice—even for existing patients—it is recommended that specialty providers clearly delineate their scope of professional practice to patients at the outset of care so that subsequent misunderstandings (and patient dissatisfaction) do not arise.

Duties Owed to Third Parties. Although health care professionals clearly owe a special duty of care to patients under their care, an additional duty may be owed to third parties associated with patients under care. Specifically, providers may have an affirmative duty to warn third parties, law enforcement, or other authorities of specific danger incident to threats of harm made by patients. Clearly, this duty to warn others about things that patients reveal during confidential examination or treatment sessions seems to be in direct contravention of the legal and ethical duties to maintain patient diagnostic and treatment-related information in confidence.

The lead case in the area of duty to warn third parties of potential harm from patients is *Tarasoff* v. *Regents of the University of California*.[7] In that California State case, a psychotherapist employed by the University of California was treating a mentally ill patient named Poddar. During therapy sessions, Poddar threatened bodily harm to his former girlfriend. Neither the psychotherapist nor his supervisors reported the threats to the potential victim, social services, or law enforcement authorities. Poddar carried out his threat and killed his former girlfriend. Her parents sued the University of California, alleging professional negligence on the part of the psychotherapist and vicarious liability on the part of the university. In ruling in favor of the victim's parents, the California Supreme Court held that a psychotherapist owes an affirmative duty to take reasonable steps to warn identifiable third parties of foreseeable danger of serious bodily harm from patients under their care. This legal duty has been extended to physicians and other primary health care professionals by statutes or regulations in many or most states.

> A psychotherapist owes an affirmative duty to take reasonable steps to warn identifiable third parties of a foreseeable danger of serious bodily harm from patients under their care. This legal duty has been extended to physicians and other primary health care professionals.

EXERCISE

Research the practice act, code of ethics, and other practice standards of your discipline to determine whether the concept of duty to warn third parties of threats by patients of death or serious bodily harm is addressed. Share you findings with fellow students and professional colleagues.

Health care professionals may also have a duty to correct obvious errors made by other providers caring for patients.[8] A major area of concern is medication errors. Who is responsible? This multidisciplinary problem has recently resulted in Food and Drug Administration (FDA) action in the form of a new regulation designed to minimize such errors.[9] The regulation, effective June 30, 2006, requires FDA-approved patient labeling on prescription medications and preempts specific **failure to warn** lawsuits in state courts against drug manufacturers that comply with the law.[10]

DISCUSSION QUESTION

What are the relative roles and responsibilities of primary health care professionals—including physicians, pharmacists, registered nurses, occupational and physical therapists, and others—in minimizing drug administration errors? What responsibilities do patients and their significant others have in reducing such errors?

Breach of Duty

The second element that a plaintiff-patient in a professional negligence health care malpractice case must prove is that the defendant–health care professional violated a legal duty owed to the plaintiff by providing substandard care. Although every person in society owes a duty to foreseeable others to conduct himself or herself in a reasonable manner (e.g., to drive a car safely), health care professionals, because of their special knowledge, training, and experience, owe an even higher **duty of due care** to patients and others.

In establishing whether a health care professional's conduct met or violated the required professional standard of care, courts do not typically refer to a standard "cookbook" for a list of acceptable versus unacceptable procedures and interventions. Instead, courts analyze on a case-by-case basis whether what a defendant-provider did in a specific case would have been done or could have been considered acceptable by an ordinary, reasonable professional peer of the defendant acting under the same or similar circumstances.

The legal standard of care may be established in court by many sources. The most common way to establish what the standard of care is, is to ask experts from the same discipline as a defendant-provider. This usually takes place during pretrial interviews and (formal) depositions and during trial testimony. Attorneys and judges also commonly refer to official definitions of professional practice and official practice standards published by state licensure administrative agencies, professional associations, or other groups. Institutional and professional practice guidelines and protocols are also relied upon to establish the legal standard of care, as are professional journals, periodicals, and authoritative books.

Parameters of the Duty Owed. The nature of the duty owed to patients depends in part on what is permissible practice under the practice act of a profession. When a health care professional carries out treatment that is not permitted under the applicable practice act, the offender is held to the legal standard of the profession upon which the offender's practice is encroaching.

Certainly, evidence-based, peer-reviewed journals qualify as **learned works** upon which health care professional witnesses in malpractice cases may rely to formulate expert opinions on the professional standard of care. Standard textbooks for the health care professional disciplines qualify as **learned treatises**, from which opinions on the professional standard of care may also be based.

Expert Witness Testimony on the Standard of Care. Most health care malpractice legal cases are settled well before formal trials occur, through settlement, abandonment of a case, or other disposition. How and whether a case is settled often turns on the strength of expert testimony given at pretrial depositions. Health care professionals may qualify to serve as experts for a wide range of purposes, from vocational rehabilitation experts to ergonomic experts. In health care malpractice cases, however, they frequently testify as clinician-experts who establish the legal standard of care and render expert opinions on whether a defendant-provider-peer met or breached the standard of care in treating a plaintiff-patient.

Health care professional experts may serve as expert witnesses for plaintiff-patients or defendant–health care providers in malpractice cases. These experts may be asked to testify about patient care evaluation or treatment practices, the use of therapeutic equipment and modalities, informed consent practices, referral and consultation customary practice, and many other practice parameters.

In all cases in which expert witnesses are called to testify, experts establish the legal standard of care for the defendant-provider's profession and comment on whether the care rendered by the defendant met or violated legal practice standards, based on one of three geographical frames of reference:

- In the vast majority of states, what fits within acceptable legal standards is care that passes as at least minimally acceptable in the same community, or in communities similar to the area in which a defendant–health care professional practices (**same or similar community standard**, majority rule).
- In as many as 13 states, health care professionals are held to a statewide or nationwide standard of comparison, meaning that experts from anywhere within the state or from across the nation may testify on the applicable standard of care (**trend**).

The locality rule, which was the rule of law in the majority of jurisdictions earlier in this century, tended to cause unjust results in medical malpractice cases and was gradually supplanted by the same or similar community standard in a majority of states. Under the locality rule, there was often an actual or perceived conspiracy of silence in which professional colleagues in small (or even large) communities refused to come forward to testify as experts for patients against their friends and associates. This conspiracy of silence often resulted in the dismissal of clearly meritorious legal cases, which did not further the primary purpose of the tort legal system: to make whole the deserving victims injured by the negligence or misconduct of others (Box 3-3).

Irrespective of the geographical frame of reference from which an expert testifies, the expert must testify, when commenting on a defendant-provider's care, whether the defendant acted as an ordinary, reasonable professional peer would have acted under the same or similar circumstances. Experts are not allowed to testify about what they themselves would have done under circumstances similar to those at issue in a trial. The legal system is not interested in what an expert would do in practice nor in what average or best practice is among providers. What is pertinent is whether what a defendant-provider did constituted at least minimally acceptable clinical practice.

To be **legally competent** to testify as an expert, a witness must meet two basic requirements:

- Possess in-depth knowledge about the treatment procedure at issue in the trial
- Be familiar with the applicable legal standard of care in the place where the alleged professional negligence took place at the time of alleged patient injury

---

BOX **3-3** ▪ **Geographical Frames of Reference for Expert Witness Testimony on the Legal Standard of Care**

1. Majority rule: Expert practices in a similar community (or the same community) as the defendant–health care professional.
2. Minority rule and trend: Expert practices in any community, statewide or nationwide.

Because an expert's qualifications are subject to challenge through **impeachment** by opposing legal counsel, an expert must also demonstrate how he or she acquired the special knowledge that makes him or her an expert, that is, through formal or continuing education, clinical experience, or other training. When, as often is the case, a jury or judge is faced with competing expert testimony on both sides about whether a defendant-provider met or violated the standard of care, the verdict often turns on which expert is most convincing in his or her presentation.

Who may testify as an expert for or against a defendant-provider of a specific health care discipline, on the legal standard of care of that discipline? In many states, courts require that expert witnesses be of the same academic discipline as the defendant. This is often referred to as the **same school doctrine**. A number of courts, however, allow others to qualify and testify as experts in health care malpractice cases based on their personal knowledge about the procedure in issue and of the applicable standard of care for the defendant's profession obtained through formal or informal training or experience.

In one reported physical therapy malpractice case, *Novey v. Kishwaukee Community Health Services,*[11] in which a postoperative hand surgery patient sustained a tendon rupture during physical therapy care, an occupational therapist was called at trial by the plaintiff-patient as an expert witness to establish the physical therapy standard of care for postoperative hand patients. In the case, the plaintiff, who had severed his middle finger flexor tendons in an industrial accident, underwent surgical repair of the lacerations and was casted. When the cast was removed, the patient was sent to the defendant's physical therapist–employee for rehabilitation. The plaintiff alleged that his tendons were retorn during physical therapy.

At trial the patient won his case and was awarded $12,127.67 in monetary damages. On appeal, the defendant-hospital's attorney successfully argued that the occupational therapist was unqualified to testify as an expert on the physical therapist standard of care because she was not from the same "school" as the defendant's physical therapist–employee. Because of the finding by the appeals court that the occupational therapist–witness was not a proper expert in the case, the case was remanded to the trial court for reconsideration. (The case was not reported again in the legal literature, meaning that it might have been settled upon its remand.)

What is troubling about this case? The Illinois appellate court, like many other courts (and lawyers), apparently had incomplete knowledge about the professions of physical and occupational therapy. A common professional standard exists for hand therapists certified by the American Hand Society, which includes occupational and physical therapists. Physical and occupational therapists also probably share a common standard—based on similar knowledge, training, and experience—in areas such as ergonomics, functional capacity assessments, pediatrics practice, and stroke rehabilitation, among many other areas of practice.[12] Because of incomplete knowledge about these professions on the part of attorneys, primary health care professionals are urged to educate their legal counsel about their professions for any type of legal representation.

Specialty certification also has an impact on the legal standard of care. The standard used to assess board-certified clinical specialists' conduct is normally a national, rather than local or statewide, standard. Are nonspecialists permitted to testify as expert witnesses in legal cases involving defendant–clinical specialists? Yes. Just as with clinicians having different degrees, qualification as an expert witness does not turn on certification but on demonstrated knowledge about a treatment procedure in issue—whether that knowledge is derived from formal or informal training.

Direct access practice may have a profound effect on the legal standard of care for nonphysician health care professionals. For advanced practice nurses, physical therapists in independent practice, and others, an allegation that the provider in direct access practice exceeded the legal scope of practice under the state practice act may result in that professional being held to the legal standard of a professional to whom the clinician should have referred the patient for consultation—probably a physician's standard of care.

Klein[13] reported that 6 percent of professional negligence claims and lawsuits involving nurse practitioners involve issues of practice beyond scope of legal authority. According to Klein, nurse practitioners may practice independently in 14 states, through collaboration with referring entities in 23 states, and exclusively under physician supervision in 13 states.

In lawsuits involving allegations of exceeding permissible scope of primary health care practice, same-discipline expert witnesses may not be legally competent to testify about the standard of care because the medical standard of care may apply. The legal ramifications of misdiagnosis and failure to refer patients appropriately to physicians and other appropriate professionals, therefore, make it imperative to practice squarely within the boundaries of state practice acts and individual competency levels, whether physician extenders are practicing independently, with collaboration, or under supervision.

Primary health care professionals should consider it an honor to be called upon to serve as expert witnesses. Whether sought out because of professional publications, noteworthy clinical practice, or for another reason, it is a civic duty to serve as an expert witness when called upon. The duty is akin to voting and jury duty. If health care professionals do not come forward in future legal cases to establish their own standards of care, other professionals from disparate disciplines will continue to do so for these professions.

Clinical Practice Guidelines. Primary health care professionals are no doubt familiar with federal government–issued clinical practice guidelines for stroke rehabilitation, treatment of pressure ulcers, and low back pain care, published by the Agency for Healthcare Research and Quality, formerly the Agency for Health Care Policy and Research. The agency was created by Congress as part of the Omnibus Budget Reconciliation Act of 1989 and is housed within the U.S. Public Health Service.

Between 1992 and 1996, the Agency for Healthcare Research and Quality published 19 popular clinical practice guidelines for primary and support health care professionals and their patients. The agency ceased such issuance of guidelines, in part, because of their unintended use by attorneys in health care malpractice legal proceedings as evidence of the legal standard of care.

What are clinical practice guidelines, and how do they mesh into the legal standard of care? Clinical practice guidelines are different from clinical practice protocols. Protocols are relatively rigid decision matrices that call for fairly specific compliance with treatment regimens and are customarily seen in emergency and perioperative care.

Clinical practice guidelines, however, rely more on qualitative clinical reasoning and offer clinicians a number of acceptable treatment options for particular patient presentations. Valid clinical practice guidelines[14] should address all reasonable practice options and potential outcomes of these interventions (and their likelihood of occurrence). Whether or not relative values are assigned to practice options presented, the names of the authors or panels formulating the guidelines and recommendations should be delineated, and the guidelines should clearly state that the process of formulating options and assigning values has been peer reviewed. The date of publication should reflect that the guidelines are clinically current.

What, if any, legal precedent do clinical practice guidelines have in establishing the standard of care? To the extent that guidelines are inclusive of all reasonable clinical practice options, they represent the legal standard of care, although they are not pre-scriptive like protocols are. Just as with clinical protocols, however, deviation from acceptable practice standards may shift the legal burden of persuasion to a defendant–health care professional to justify why the clinician deviated from collectively established practice standards. Although the burden of proof remains with a patient-plaintiff in such cases, clearly the defendant who deviates from clinical protocols or guidelines encumbers himself or herself with a trial burden that normally a defendant does not have—the burden to justify why the clinician disregarded collective wisdom enunciated in standards or to leave it to the jury or judge to guess why.

Advantages of clinical practice guidelines include standardizing treatment pro-cesses, memorializing collective professional judgment on the validity and efficacy of treatment options, possibly reducing the number of health care malpractice claims,[15] and providing a framework for clinical decision making. Disadvantages include limit-ing available options for clinicians, creating "cookbook" health care, and causing the burden of persuasion to shift to defendant–health care clinicians in malpractice cases to justify deviation from clinical practice guidelines.

Clinicians and administrators should do everything possible to communicate that clinical practice guidelines are intended merely to guide clinical decision making and not to represent the legal standard of care. Facilities and professional associations may attempt to include a disclaimer with their clinical practice guidelines, indicating that such guidelines are not intended to represent the legal standard of care. These kinds of disclaimers may have limited effect, however, because the judges in courts of law decide what evidence is permitted at trial to represent the legal standard of care.

Causation

The third element of proof that a plaintiff-patient bears in a health care malpractice professional negligence case is to show, by a preponderance of evidence, that any breach of duty (i.e., violation of the legal standard of care) by a defendant-provider caused injury to the plaintiff-patient. The two elements of **legal causation** are **actual cause** and **proximate cause**.

Actual causation means that "but for" the defendant's substandard care delivery, the plaintiff-patient would not have sustained any injury incident to care. The "but for" desig-nation is also frequently referred to as *sine qua non* (Latin for "without which not").

For a patient-plaintiff in a health care malpractice professional negligence case to establish actual causation is fairly simple. Any direct causal link between a health care professional's conduct (action or failure to act) and a patient's alleged injuries estab-lishes actual causation. This is true even if the defendant-provider's conduct was only a **substantial factor** (along with other possible causes) in the plaintiff-patient's injuries.

Proximate causation poses a more difficult hurdle for plaintiffs in health care mal-practice litigation. Under proximate, or legal, causation a court may choose not to hold a defendant-provider liable for professional negligence, even where a breach of duty and actual causation have been established by the plaintiff.

The definition of proximate causation is elusive, even for legal scholars. In one reported physical therapy malpractice case, *Greening by Greening* v. *School District of Millard*,[16] the court described proximate causation in detail. In *Greening*, a state-employed physical therapist designed an exercise regimen for a student-patient with myelodysplasia. The program was carried out with the patient wearing leg braces, by an aide, under supervision of the physical therapist. During a treatment session the patient sustained a femoral fracture. The school district (sued by the patient's parents for vicarious liability) prevailed in the case at trial and on appeal. The appellate judge in the case described proximate cause as a natural, direct result of a breach of duty on the defendant-provider's part, with no superseding intervening act breaking the "chain" of causation.

When harm is not reasonably **foreseeable**, courts may refuse to hold health care professional–defendants liable for unforeseeable results, as a matter of fundamental fairness. Note, however, that a patient's preexisting medical conditions do not necessarily equate to superseding causes of injury that absolve a provider of liability for injuries incident to treatment, if the provider could have learned about the preexisting conditions through the taking of a thorough history or through other reasonable means, such as a thorough physical examination. Only for the reasonably unforeseeable harm may a court be willing to cut off liability under proximate causation.

Damages

The final element of proof in a professional negligence lawsuit is damages. To warrant the award of monetary damages, a plaintiff must show that he or she sustained the kinds of injuries, as a direct result of a defendant-provider's breach of duty, that require the payment of money in order to make the plaintiff "whole" again (or as whole as possible).

What kinds of losses warrant the award of monetary damages in a professional negligence health care malpractice case? Monetary outlays for additional medical care to correct or minimize the injury caused by the defendant constitute one element of damages. So do lost wages or salary (from one or more employment sources) resulting from time away from work because of rehabilitation. Economic losses, such as telephone, Internet, and traveling expenses, are also recoverable, as are (in some states) loss of a reasonable chance of recovery or survival incident to a defendant-health care professional's negligent care. These actual out-of-pocket losses specific to the plaintiff-patient are known as **special damages**.

Finally, damages may be awarded for the monetary value of pain and suffering incident to the defendant-provider's substandard care. Because of the difficulty in quantifying the monetary value of pain and suffering, a majority of states now cap pain and suffering damages at a statutory maximum amount. Pain and suffering damages and damages paid for the loss of enjoyment of life and the fear of contracting a disease related to a defendant's negligence are known as **general damages**.

Immediate family members directly and adversely affected by the plaintiff-patient's injuries may also recover monetary damages for **loss of consortium**. For spouses, loss of consortium damages include the monetary value of lost services, society, and companionship (including sexual relations) incurred over some definite period. For parents, the value of a plaintiff-child's lost economic contribution to the family unit is recoverable in some states.[5]

Other Tort Bases for Malpractice Liability

The two other tort bases for health care malpractice liability are intentional conduct causing patient injury and strict liability without regard for fault. Intentional tort liability is addressed in Chapter 4. A brief description of the two forms of strict liability in tort follows.

Strict, or absolute, liability in tort involves a socially important, but abnormally dangerous, activity that results in patient injury or patient injury from a dangerously defective commercial product. The first form of strict liability is called **strict liability for abnormally dangerous activities** (formerly called **strict liability for ultrahazardous activities**); the second is strict product liability. An issue of strict liability for abnormally dangerous activity seldom, if ever, should arise in health care clinical practice because of the emphasis on patient safety and quality management associated with health care delivery. Factors used by courts to assess whether an activity is abnormally dangerous include the following:

- Whether the activity involves a high risk of foreseeable harm
- The severity of the risk of harm
- Whether the risk of harm can be eliminated through stringent quality control or safety precautions
- Whether the activity that causes injury falls within customary practice
- The social worth or value of the activity to patients and society[5]

Hypothetical examples of activities that could be bases for strict liability for abnormally dangerous activities include high-velocity, rotary cervical manipulative thrust procedures by chiropractors, osteopaths, and physical therapists. Few cases appear in the legal literature based on strict liability for abnormally dangerous clinical activities.

EXERCISE

Brainstorm and identify at least five clinical activities from your discipline that might give rise to strict (non–fault-based) liability for abnormally dangerous clinical activities. What steps can you undertake to minimize the risk of patient harm associated with these activities?

Regarding strict product liability, courts will impose liability upon commercial distributors of unreasonably dangerously defective products that injure buyers or other foreseeable persons. According to the Restatement of Torts (Second) [a model for adoption as law by the states], Section 402A(1):

> *One who sells any product in a defective condition unreasonably dangerous to the user or consumer ... is subject to liability ... if the seller is engaged in the business of selling such a product.*[5]

Strict product liability was first imposed in the United States in California in 1944, in *Escola* v. *Coca-Cola Bottling Co.*,[17] a *res ipsa loquitur* (presumptive negligence) case involving an exploding soda bottle that injured a consumer. All other states soon followed the lead of California in establishing strict product liability as a viable cause of action in tort.

The philosophy behind strict product liability is that, between two potentially innocent parties—a commercial seller and a consumer of a dangerously defective product—the seller is the logical party to bear the risk of liability for injuries from the product because the seller is in the better position to insure against such liability and to monitor product safety. Dangerous product defects can be of three types: design defects, manufacturing defects, and inadequate warnings about potential hazards associated with a possibly dangerous product. The FDA classifies medical devices into three categories: Classes I (generally safe), II (safe with special controls; e.g., mercury thermometers), and III (necessary, but inherently unsafe, requiring premarket approval).[18]

Courts traditionally have been reluctant to impose strict product liability on health care professional–defendants because health care delivery is primarily the delivery (sale) of a professional service and not the sale of a product. This qualified immunity of health care professionals from strict product liability means that patients injured by defective medical products normally are required to claim against or sue product manufacturers.

Courts, however, will allow patients to sue health care clinicians (also classified under law as **learned intermediaries**[19] for strict product liability when health care clinicians are regularly in the business of selling products to patients, such as transcutaneous electrical nerve stimulation devices, home traction units, and exercise equipment. The professions of optometry, orthotics, and prosthetics are more vulnerable to strict product liability malpractice lawsuits because these health disciplines are coprimary service and products professions.

Primary and support health care professionals must exercise caution when asked by patients to modify care-related equipment. Product manufacturers have in place disclaimers of liability for unauthorized major modifications of equipment, which may lead to unintended strict product liability exposure for health care clinical professionals.

Ordinary Negligence Incident to Health Care Delivery

Ordinary negligence differs from professional negligence in several key respects. Any person owing a duty of due care to others may face liability for ordinary negligence. Professional negligence, however, deals with liability of members of learned (licensed or registered) professions. Professionals are rightfully held to a higher standard of care vis-à-vis their clients than are members of the public at large. The reason is that learned professionals possess superior knowledge and skills gained through advanced formal and informal education, training, and professional development. (Along the same continuum, doctoral and board-certified professional specialists may be held to even a higher standard because of their higher-level credentials.)

> **Premises liability:** Potential liability for monetary damages on the part of owners or occupiers of land for injuries incurred by patrons and others coming onto their premises.

Premises liability[20] concerns potential liability for monetary damages on the part of owners or occupiers (e.g., lessees ["tenants"]) of land for injuries incurred by patrons and others coming onto the premises. A duty of due care may be owed even to those persons entering or remaining on the premises without authorization, for example, trespassers and burglars.

In a majority of states, the law classifies the degree of duty owed to persons entering onto premises based on their status as invitees, licensees, and trespassers. For trespassers, the duty owed under this classification scheme is the lowest, often involving only the duty to post warnings about hidden constructed dangers that pose a substantial risk of serious bodily harm or death. As with most laws, there are exceptions to this barebones requirement, particularly for children (age 12 or under) who might be drawn onto hazardous premises by an "attractive nuisance," such as ladders and scaffolding.

A higher duty is normally owed to business licensees, such as delivery persons and vendors. In addition to the aforementioned duty to warn about hidden hazards, there is usually a duty owed to use all reasonable measures to protect licensees from injuries resulting from operation of the facility. For example, an occupational therapist using work simulation machinery in the clinic would be required to take reasonable steps to prevent a FedEx delivery person from being injured by that machinery while traversing the clinic on the way to the office to make a delivery.

For states using the "bright-line" duty standard based on victim status, the highest duty owed is toward invitees, including in the case of physical and occupational therapist–clinic owners the patients and their families and significant others who are allowed into the clinic. In this case the duty owed is to take all reasonable steps to protect the invitees from any foreseeable harm from their exposure to the premises. This includes an affirmative duty to undertake regular inspections of the premises to seek out potential hazards.

A minority of states have abolished the bright-line rules for duty owed to persons coming onto premises based on their status. In these states the law simply universally requires owners and occupiers of premises to act reasonably under all circumstances to protect all persons coming onto their property from foreseeable harm. The status of the entrant, then, becomes only one factor to be considered in deciding the extent of the duty owed.[21]

What is the significance of the legal distinction between ordinary and professional negligence to health care professionals? The difference is important to all parties and their attorneys. If a case is filed as an ordinary negligence case, the tort reform measures applicable only to health care malpractice legal actions do not apply. A longer statute of limitations (time line for commencing legal action) for ordinary negligence cases may exist than for professional negligence cases. In ordinary negligence cases the health care professional standard of care is not normally at issue, and often, expensive, contradictory, and confounding expert witness testimony is not needed. In some jurisdictions, such testimony is not even permitted because juries are perfectly capable of discerning common premises negligence without it. In the event of a finding of liability in an ordinary negligence case—even if it arises in a health care setting—the defendant's name is not be reportable to the National Practitioner Data Bank (which is defined and discussed later in this chapter).

So it appears that a case brought as an ordinary negligence case, rather than as a professional negligence case, can inure to the benefit of all parties. Such a case can also be of great benefit to courts because trial time may be decreased because less expert witness testimony may be required. Finally, ordinary versus professional case designation may benefit society as a whole because cases will probably cost less to bring to trial.

Vicarious Liability for Others' Conduct

The term *vicarious liability* refers to the circumstances under which an employer bears indirect legal and financial responsibility for the conduct of another person, usually of an employee. The concept of vicarious liability dates back to ancient times and in legal circles is often referred to as *respondeat superior* (Latin for "let the master answer").

> **Vicarious liability:** Indirect legal and financial responsibility for the conduct of another person, such as an employee or a clinic volunteer.

The basic rule of vicarious liability is that an employer is financially liable for the negligent conduct of an employee when that employee-wrongdoer (tortfeasor) is acting within the scope of his or her employment at the time the act or omission occurred. Therefore, when a hospital-based health care clinician is alleged to have negligently caused injury to a patient during the course of care, the hospital employing the person directly responsible for the patient's injury may be required to pay the monetary judgment if the employee's negligence is proved in court. Vicarious liability, like strict liability, is non–fault-based liability.

An employer's indirect responsibility for an employee's conduct does not in any way excuse from financial responsibility the employee who is directly responsible for negligent patient injury. A tortfeasor is always personally responsible for the consequences of his or her own conduct. Vicarious liability, however, gives a tort victim another party against which to make a claim or to sue for monetary damages incident to wrongful injury. If an employer is required to pay a settlement or judgment for the negligence of one of its employees, the employer retains the legal right to seek indemnification from the employee for this outlay.

> A tortfeasor is always personally responsible for the consequences of his or her own conduct.

Is it fair to impose liability on an employer who is innocent of any wrongdoing? In balancing the equities between an innocent victim of negligence and an innocent employer of the party directly responsible for negligence, the legal system weighs in favor of the innocent victim of negligence. Several good reasons exist for this public policy favoring victims over employers. First, it is the employer, not the patient-victim, who has the exclusive right (and duty) to control the quality of patient care rendered in the facility by all providers. Second, because the employer earns a profit from the activities of its employees, it is only fair that the employer should be held responsible for patient injuries caused by employees. Third, the employer is normally in a much better position than the patient to bear the financial risk of loss—through economic loss allocation (i.e., purchase of liability insurance)—as part of the overall cost of doing business.

An employer may be held vicariously liable for the conduct of nonemployees and for employees. In the relatively few reported cases addressing the issue, courts have universally imposed vicarious liability on hospitals for the negligence of their volunteers; in essence, equating unpaid volunteers with employees. For this reason, health care facilities using the services of volunteers should carry liability insurance for volunteers' activities.

Another area of vicarious liability involves general partnership business arrangements, wherein each general partner is considered legally to be the agent of all other general partners. Each general partner, then, is vicariously liable for negligent acts committed by other general partners when those acts are within the scope of activities of the partnership.

Several important exceptions to vicarious liability exist. Although an employer may be vicariously liable for employees' negligence, the employer typically is not liable for malicious intentional misconduct committed by employees. Such misconduct is normally unforeseeable, so it would be unfair to hold an employer financially responsible for such conduct.

Another exception to vicarious liability involves independent contractors: for example, contract nurses working in a health care facility. The legal system generally distinguishes between employees (for whom an employer is vicariously liable) and contract workers (for whom the employer generally is not vicariously liable). This distinction is based primarily on the permissible degree of control the employer may exercise over the physical details of the professional work product of these two classes of workers.

In some states, courts hold employers vicariously liable for the negligence of independent contractors under the theory of **apparent agency**, or **ostensible agency** (also called "agency by estoppel"). When a contract professional worker in a clinic setting is indistinguishable from an employee-clinician, for example, a court may hold the employer vicariously liable for contractor negligence. Therefore, it is prudent risk management for employers to take appropriate steps to ensure that patients know when they are being treated by contract workers instead of employees. Methods to accomplish this include requiring contractors to wear name tags identifying them as contractors, posting an informational memorandum about workers' status, and displaying cameo photographs of contract staff in clinic reception or waiting areas.

In some cases an employer may be not only vicariously liable for its employees' negligence but also primarily, or directly, liable for its workers' conduct under a concept known as **corporate liability**. Until the mid-twentieth century, nonprofit hospitals were virtually immune from any liability under a concept known as charitable immunity, granted in large part because of the benevolent character of these institutions. Since that time, courts in many states have imposed direct liability on hospitals and health care organizations under the theory of corporate liability.[22] In essence, courts are treating hospitals like any other ordinary business. The U.S. Supreme Court validated this status for health care organizations in its landmark managed care (non) liability case in 2000, *Pegram* v. *Herdrich*.[23]

Corporate liability may attach under at least four theories. Hospitals have been found liable for the negligent screening and hiring of professional employees, such as physicians, nurses, and allied health care professionals. Hospitals have also been held liable for the negligent credentialing and privileging of staff professionals. Hospitals have also been held directly liable for negligent failure to monitor safety adequately in their facilities. Finally, hospitals have been held liable under corporate liability for failing to establish effective quality management programs to monitor systematically the quality of health care delivered by all providers within the facility, including employees, contractors, consultants, volunteers, and others.

The 2005 Harvard University Leape study of medical mistakes[24] attributed primary culpability for patient deaths to poor leadership within complex medical systems. The study recommended a systems approach to quality management to minimize the propensity for perinatal, medication, and ventilator errors that lead to patient injuries and deaths.

Defenses to Health Care Malpractice Actions

Although a defendant in a health care malpractice case normally bears no particular burden of proof in the case, the defendant probably will put forward one or more affirmative defenses in opposition to a plaintiff-patient's **case-in-chief**. Affirmative defenses are ones that normally must be stated in the defendant's *answer,* the first responsive **pleading** to a plaintiff's **complaint**. By its apparent meaning, an affirmative defense is one in which the defendant bears the legal burden of proving the defense to the plaintiff's allegation by a preponderance of evidence.

Two key defenses available to health care malpractice defendants are expiration of the statute of limitations and comparative patient fault in causing injury. Other potential defenses include assumption on the patient's part of the attendant risks associated with a treatment and immunity and release from liability.

Statutes of Limitations

For purposes of health care malpractice litigation, the statute of limitations is a time line that begins at a point at which a patient knows (or should reasonably know) that he or she was injured at the hands of a health care provider and ends some months or years later at a time fixed by state or federal statute. The alleged victim of malpractice must file a formal civil lawsuit within the confines of that time line or be forever barred from later bringing legal action. The statute of limitations is considered a procedural, rather than a substantive, law.

> **Statute of limitations:** Period after injury during which an injured person must file a civil lawsuit or be forever barred from later initiating legal action.

The statute of limitations has several key purposes. First, the statute of limitations affords an injured person sufficient time to investigate the source and nature of an injury, consult with and retain legal counsel (if desired), file a complaint with the responsible party (and/or that party's employer and/or insurer), and attempt to settle the matter short of resorting to trial. Second, the statute of limitations creates a state of certainty (except when its exceptions apply, discussed later) and finality. Under the statute of limitations, legal cases must be commenced and brought to trial within a reasonable time frame so that witnesses to an event are still alive and available, documents and physical evidence are preserved for inspection, and parties and insurers can anticipate the resolution of pending legal disputes and their likely consequences.

A number of exceptions to the statute of limitations apply in many jurisdictions. If one of these exceptions applies, the statute of limitations is said to be *tolled*, or suspended until the exception is no longer applicable. Some exceptions concern what is termed a **legal disability** involving an alleged victim. For example, in some jurisdictions, the statute of limitations is tolled for minors and mentally incompetent victims for varying periods. Now, many jurisdictions do not suspend the statute of limitations because of a victim's minority or incompetency. This is the case in the federal civil legal system.[25]

Other exceptions that toll the statute of limitations include the **continuous treatment doctrine** and the **discovery rule**. Under the continuous treatment doctrine a court may suspend the running of the statute of limitations during the time in which the alleged victim of malpractice and the responsible health care professional maintain an active patient-professional relationship for treatment of the same condition from which injury resulted. The public policy purpose for this exception is that a tort victim should not be expected to interrupt necessary health care intervention for an active condition in order to bring legal action for malpractice.

The principle exception to the statute of limitations is the discovery rule. Under this exception, the statute of limitations may be suspended for the period during which an injured person cannot reasonably be expected to discover the injury upon which a malpractice claim may be based. The discovery rule has been invoked for conditions such as surgical sponges, needles, or instruments left inside of a surgical patient. Consider the following hypothetical example:

> *A patient is referred to physical therapy by an orthopedic surgeon with a diagnosis of cervical degenerative joint disease with mild right C5 radiculopathy. The treatment order reads, "Evaluate and treat. Consider traction and/or appropriate mobilization techniques." After taking a thorough history and conducting a comprehensive physical examination, the physical therapist makes evaluative findings and formulates a physical therapy diagnosis. The therapist then treats the patient using manual cervical distraction and manipulation techniques. The patient does not improve, and after several treatments, appears to have worsened. The physical therapist then ceases treatment, and refers the patient back to the orthopedist for reevaluation. Nine months later, it is discovered through diagnostic imaging study, that the patient sustained bony injury to the cervical spine, probably from the physical therapist's manipulation treatments. The statute of limitations would probably not begin to run until the date of discovery by the patient of the existence and source of the injury.*

Some states, pursuant to tort reform legislation, have placed absolute time limits, called **statutes of repose**, on certain types of civil actions, particularly for strict product liability actions.[26] This means that, regardless of legal disability or plaintiff inability to discover the source of an injury, the outside time limit for initiating affected legal actions covered under statutes of repose is cut off after a set statutory period. Statutes of repose are considered to be an equitable way to solve the problems of perpetual litigation involving products produced long ago and incidents resulting in injury that have become stale because of lost or destroyed evidence or unavailable witnesses.

Comparative Fault

The right of a patient to collect monetary damages for injury incident to health malpractice is not absolute. In many cases, defendant–health care professionals raise the issue of patient contributory negligence or comparative fault in cases brought against them. Just like health care professionals treating patients have a duty of due care owed to patients under their care, patients themselves have a legal duty incident to care. That duty is to conduct themselves so that their actions do not fall below a standard imposed by law for their own safety and protection. When a patient's conduct falls below the standard imposed by law for the patient's own protection, that careless conduct constitutes contributory negligence.

Courts assess plaintiff-patient conduct in two ways, depending on the state in which a health care malpractice trial takes place. Before the first era of patient-oriented tort reform earlier in the last century, most or all jurisdictions used a pure contributory negligence formula for assessing plaintiff-patient conduct. Under this formula, if a patient is at all responsible—even 1 percent or less—for his or her own injuries incident to treatment, then the patient loses a health care malpractice case brought against a defendant–health care professional or defendant-organization. This harsh rule of "all or nothing" was tempered over time with numerous exceptions that permitted meritorious lawsuits brought by plaintiffs to proceed. One of those exceptions is **last clear chance**. Under the doctrine of last clear chance, application of all-or-nothing contributory negligence is prevented when a defendant has the last clear opportunity to act reasonably to prevent plaintiff injury but negligently fails to prevent it. Consider the following hypothetical example.

> *A patient who has recently undergone lumbar laminectomy is undergoing an occupational therapy work capacity evaluation. While preparing to lift a 10-lb weight from one table to another, the patient suddenly moves toward a 75-lb weight that is on the floor and states, "Let's see how much I can lift." Even though it would otherwise be pure contributory negligence for the patient to attempt to lift the heavy weight from the floor without authorization, the patient's harm to himself might not preclude legal action for professional negligence. A legal action might be viable if the occupational therapist failed to take reasonable steps to attempt to halt the patient from attempting to lift the heavy box, under the equitable doctrine of last clear chance.*

In most states a newer method of assessing potential plaintiff fault in a malpractice case applies—**comparative negligence**. Under the doctrine of comparative negligence, plaintiff-patient contributory negligence or wrongdoing does not necessarily eliminate any possibility of a professional negligence malpractice lawsuit against a health care professional. Instead, courts assess proportional patient culpability and assign a percentage of fault to it. In most states, if the patient's percentage of fault is 50 percent or less, the patient can proceed with a lawsuit and have monetary damages reduced by the patient's proportional degree of fault. In 13 states, patients can proceed to trial and win a monetary judgment, even if plaintiff comparative fault is greater than 50 percent.[27] This subcategory of comparative negligence is called pure comparative fault. Consider the following hypothetical case.

A patient undergoing outpatient surgery for a sebaceous cyst intentionally removes an intravenous line from her arm, under a drape and out of the view of the surgeon and physician's assistant carrying out the procedure. Soon after, the patient has a mild seizure, and the physician and assistant attempt to administer medication intravenously. A 10-minute delay ensues while the assistant establishes a new intravenous line. Assuming that the state in which the patient files a health care malpractice lawsuit uses the doctrine of comparative fault to assess damages, at what level would you quantify patient comparative fault? Justify your assessment. Would the patient be permitted to proceed to trial and win any monetary damages under your assessment?

The defensive comparative fault concepts of contributory negligence and comparative negligence apply in most cases only to health care malpractice cases brought as professional negligence cases. Because, under strict liability cases, culpability on the part of a defendant is not in issue, comparative fault principles are likewise not applied in these types of cases. As always, of course, there are exceptions in the legal literature.[28] Contributory negligence and comparative fault are not valid defenses in cases involving intentional misconduct by defendants, as a matter of public policy.

Assumption of Risk

Assumption of the risk is a theoretically possible defense to a health care malpractice lawsuit. A plaintiff is considered to have assumed the risk of an activity under a defendant's control if the plaintiff (1) fully appreciates the nature and extent of the risk of injury associated with the activity, and (2) makes a knowledgeable, intelligent, voluntary, and unequivocal choice to encounter that risk.[29] Assumption of the risk applies, for instance, when a pregnant patron voluntarily elects to ride a tumultuous roller coaster at an amusement park, despite clear, posted warnings of its potential dangers.

As with comparative fault, assumption of the risk is theoretically a defense in health malpractice litigation that should be available only in professional negligence malpractice cases. Assumption of risk is not available in cases involving alleged intentional misconduct by a defendant-provider, nor can it normally be raised as a defense in cases in which a plaintiff is a member of a statutorily protected class of persons, such as those persons who are mentally incompetent or minors. Finally, no health care professional may compel a patient to waive liability (indirectly causing a patient to assume the risks of health care interventions) through a contractual **exculpatory release**.

In one reported legal case, *Schneider* v. *Revici*,[30] involving a female patient who contractually agreed with her physician to waive any liability on the physician's part for a novel form of breast cancer therapy, the federal court ruled that assumption of the risk is potentially an available defense to a health care malpractice lawsuit in which the intervention at issue is "unconventional."

The better rule to follow is that patients assume the risk of nothing in the course of health care intervention that would excuse professional negligence on the part of a health care provider owing a duty of special care toward that patient. Therefore, except theoretically, assumption of the risk is inapplicable as a defense in health care delivery.

Assumption of the risk is inapplicable as a defense in health care malpractice litigation in conventional health care delivery.

Immunity

Until recently, nonprofit religious-based health care institutions enjoyed immunity from legal actions under an equitable legal doctrine called **charitable immunity**. This immunity was granted because of the great public service rendered on behalf of the sick and dying patients who otherwise had no place of refuge in society. As health care delivery became equated with ordinary business during this century, however, the charitable immunity exception to tort liability died.

Immunity from legal actions is also a privilege enjoyed by governments under an ancient concept known as **sovereign immunity**. States and the federal government enjoy sovereign immunity from liability (i.e., cannot be sued or compelled to pay out a monetary judgment) unless they expressly waive, or give up, their sovereign immunity. The federal government, in 1946, partially relinquished its sovereign immunity from liability under a statute known as the Federal Tort Claims Act.[31] Under this statute, in the federal-sector health care setting, most patients (except active-duty military service members and their family members, when suing the federal government derivatively for wrongdoing against active-duty service members) may bring lawsuits against the federal government for professional and ordinary negligence and for a limited number of intentional wrongs. Many states have adopted waiver of sovereign immunity statutes similar to the Federal Tort Claims Act.

Under litigation brought pursuant to the Federal Tort Claims Act, individual federal health care employees are personally immune from suit under the Federal Liability Reform and Tort Compensation Act,[32] provided that their conduct falls within official federal scope of duty. State-employed health care professionals may enjoy similar personal immunity from liability under state statutes that mirror the Federal Tort Claims Act. Health care professionals engaging in *pro bono publico* (Latin for "for the public good") health care services may also enjoy limited tort immunity from liability based on state law.[33]

Releases from Liability

The release from liability is a standard legal instrument in civil law. For instance, when an insurance company settles a claim with a claimant, release from liability is used to absolve the insurance company forever of further liability resulting from the incident in question. The release from liability is also used in health care malpractice litigation to absolve a defendant or defendants of further liability exposure in exchange for a monetary settlement made to a plaintiff. These uses of a release are well-established and not generally subject to nullification, except in cases of fraud, duress, undue influence, or other overreaching by a party or by the party's agent.

The attempted prospective use of releases in the health care setting is what is legally problematic. As a general rule, an attempted exculpatory release that is made a **condition precedent** (precondition) of receiving treatment is invalid as violative of public policy. The lead reported legal case involving exculpatory releases from liability is *Tunkl* v. *Regents of the University of California*.[34] In that seminal case a terminally ill patient was admitted to a state-run charity research hospital for treatment. As a condition of admission, the hospital required the patient to sign a release from liability, which was purportedly justified because the facility was a charity hospital. The patient died and his wife, as **executrix** (personally appointed legal representative) of his estate, brought suit challenging the exculpatory release and claiming professional negligence regarding her late husband's care. In invalidating the exculpatory release, Justice Tobriner of the California Supreme Court held that California statutory law stated that "all contracts which have for their object, to exempt anyone from responsibility for his own fraud, or willful injury to the person or property of another ... whether willful or negligent, are against the policy of the law."[35] The court ruled that there could be no exception for hospitals, even charity or research hospitals, and allowed the executrix's legal action for malpractice to proceed.

In some instances a waiver of liability may be appropriate and enforceable. Consider the case in which a competent, hospitalized inpatient voluntarily elects to leave the facility midway through care "against medical advice." Before such a patient leaves the facility, a physician, nurse, or administrative official will discuss the adverse consequences of leaving against medical advice and attempt to have the patient sign a release from further liability. Such a risk management measure is appropriate. Similarly, when a patient declines what health care professionals deem to be necessary care because of religious or personal beliefs, it is appropriate to seek a limitation of liability agreement from the patient. What is repugnant to the courts are exculpatory health care releases from liability that are general. Consider the following hypothetical example.

A postoperative finger flexor tendon surgical patient is receiving outpatient rehabilitation by an occupational therapist. Suddenly one day, the patient states that she is going to quit attending rehabilitation and exercise her hand on her own. Objectively, she is still in need of professional care. As the treating therapist, explain how you would protect the patient's interests and your own interests in this situation. Answer: (1) Fully explain to the patient the consequences of discontinuing therapy prematurely. Ensure that the patient's decision to discontinue treatment is knowing, intelligent, voluntary, and unequivocal. Make sure that there is no point of dissatisfaction regarding your care that can be remedied to the patient's reasonable satisfaction. (2) Notify the referring physician of the patient's action, and carefully document the patient's statements, your counseling of the patient, and your communication with the referring physician. (3) Consult with your legal advisor, and consider asking the patient to sign a release from further liability. Be careful that the release does not attempt to absolve you of any liability incident to care because such a release would probably be unenforceable as a violation of public policy.

NATIONAL PRACTITIONER DATA BANK

The National Practitioner Data Bank was established pursuant to a federal statute, the Health Care Quality Improvement Act of 1986.[36] Congress enacted this law with several purposes in mind:

- To promote effective professional peer review by the health professions by providing "qualified immunity" from defamation or other bases of liability for statements made during these processes[37]
- To require reporting by hospitals and other health care organizations having peer review of adverse credentialing actions affecting clinical privileges involving physicians, dentists, and other licensed health care professionals
- To require the reporting of adverse licensure action against a licensed health care professional by a state licensure board
- To require the reporting of health care malpractice payments made on behalf of health care professionals to patients or their representatives by settlement or judgment[38]

Before the advent of the National Practitioner Data Bank, unscrupulous and incompetent health care providers were often able to "skip" from state to state to avoid adverse licensure disciplinary action with impunity.[39] The data bank was intended to prevent these kinds of injustices by making available to employers and licensure agencies critical information about adverse actions taken against licensed health care professionals.

The implementation of the data bank was delayed for several years after the effective date of the Health Care Quality Improvement Act, in part because of strong opposition by health care professional associations. The data bank was debated in Congress, with substantial lobbyist intervention, until its implementation on September 1, 1990. Regarding health care malpractice payments, any amount, even a nominal, so-called "nuisance" settlement amount, must be reported by payers to the data bank.

In its first year of operation (September 1, 1990, to August 31, 1991), the Data Bank recorded 15,782 malpractice payments made by insurers and health care organizations on behalf of licensed health care professionals. Of that number, 11,721 involved physician malpractice payments, 2360 involved payments made on behalf of dentists, and 1701 payments were made on behalf of other licensed health care professionals, including physical and occupational therapists. There were 2779 adverse administrative action reports for the first-year period: 2285 involving physicians, 470 involving dentists, and 24 involving other licensed health care professionals. The total number of reports made to the data bank in the first year was 18,561.[40]

Who has access to the National Practitioner Data Bank? Hospitals and other health care organizations required to query the data bank about newly licensed health care professional–employees, state licensing entities, and licensed health care professionals themselves. In limited circumstances (such as when employers fail to query the data bank as required about new health care professional–employees), plaintiff attorneys have access to information in the National Practitioner Data Bank.[41] Note that employers are also required to query the data bank for information about employed or otherwise privileged licensed health care professionals on a regularly recurring basis—every 2 years.[42] Currently, no provisions exist under the Health Care Quality Improvement Act for public access to information about health care professional adverse administrative actions or malpractice payments.

Democratic Senator Ron Wyden of Oregon, author of the legislation behind the data bank, is critical of recently publicized underreporting of health care malpractice payment data to the data bank. According to Wyden, the data bank is only as good as the information it contains.[43] Daniel Levinson, inspector general of the Department of Health and Human Services, specifically cited 474 malpractice cases from federal health agencies that went underreported to the data bank. Perhaps because of this problem, the Joint Commission has expressed a lack of confidence in the data bank and called for its redesign or replacement.[44]

PATIENT CARE DOCUMENTATION MANAGEMENT

Patient care documentation has malpractice implications just as affirmative care delivery does. Communication of pertinent information about the patient to other providers who are simultaneously treating that patient, therefore, is the principal purpose of patient care documentation. Concise, objective, timely documentation of a provider's evaluation, diagnosis, and treatment of a patient conveys to other health care professionals who treat that patient—now or in the future—insight into the patient's specific needs. Standards for formats and frequency of patient care documentation are established by statutes; licensure regulations; institution, group, or network standards; accreditation and third-party payer mandates; and professional association guidelines.

Because communication through patient care documentation is so critically important to a patient's well-being, the failure to document vital care information in the patient's record accurately, clearly, objectively, and in a timely manner constitutes professional negligence, which may be legally actionable, depending on the consequences of an omission. This type of professional negligence action for the negligent failure to communicate vital patient information to others having a need to know exists independently of any other legal action based on the quality of care rendered.

Many other legitimate purposes exist for patient care documentation, including the risk management purpose of memorializing important facts about an event for possible use in subsequent litigation. Patient care documentation is also used as a basis for planning and continuity of care, as a primary source of information for quality measurement and evaluation of patient care activities, to provide information necessary for reimbursement decisions and utilization review, to identify staff training needs, as a resource for patient care research and education, and to memorialize informed consent to treatment and patient wishes concerning advance directives, among other purposes (Box 3-4).

Documentation of patient care is as important as the rendition of patient care itself.

The patient treatment record is a legal document, referred to as a business document, which is admissible in court as evidence in health care malpractice and other civil and criminal legal proceedings. As part of the legal duty owed to a patient, a treating health care professional is responsible and accountable for accurate, clear, objective, and timely documentation of the patient's chief complaint(s), relevant history, physical examination, evaluative findings, informed consent to intervention, intervention, referral, home care instructions, and follow-up care on discharge.

Information documented about a patient serves simultaneously to protect the patient and the treating clinician. If a patient brings a malpractice lawsuit against the clinician—often years after care is rendered—what is documented in the treatment record about the patient's care may well be the best or even only objective evidence of what transpired between the patient and the health care professional at the time of

---

BOX **3-4** ■ **Purposes of Patient Care Documentation**

- Communication of critical information about a patient to other health care professionals concurrently treating the patient and having a need to know
- Basis for patient care (postdischarge) planning and continuity of care
- Primary source of information for the measurement and evaluation of patient care activities, as part of a systematic quality management (improvement) program
- Justification for reimbursement
- Source document for utilization review activities
- Identification of deficiencies in documentation and patient care performance and formulation of training needs
- Resource for patient care research and education
- Business document
- Legal document
- Provide substantive evidence on whether patient care rendered meets or breaches the legal standard of care
- Memorialize disclosure elements and patient informed consent to treatment
- Memorialize patient choices concerning life-sustaining interventions to be taken in the event of the patient's subsequent incompetence, in the form of advance directives

---

Adapted from Scott RW: *Promoting legal awareness in physical and occupational therapy,* St Louis, 1997, Mosby.

treatment. This is especially important in busy clinical practices, where because clinicians evaluate and treat hundreds or thousands of patients in a given year, memories naturally tend to fade over time.

When expert witnesses take the stand for or against defendant–health care providers to testify about whether care rendered to plaintiff-patients met or violated the legal standard of care, they rely primarily on what is documented in treatment records to formulate their professional opinions. From the standpoint of health care malpractice, documentation of patient care serves as the primary basis for expert testimony about whether the standard of care was breached or met in a given case, the standard of care being the benchmark that delineates negligent and nonnegligent care.

When a treating health care clinician is required to testify as a defendant or witness in a legal proceeding, how can the clinician recall a given patient's relevant history, evaluative findings, treatment plan, disposition, and follow-up care when the event occurred months or years earlier? Although attorneys often try to jog the memories of **percipient** (fact) or expert witnesses through leading questions (where not objected to or where allowed by judges), more often than not, reference to patient health records is often indispensable in order to refresh lapsed memories regarding past events.

When a treating health care clinician's memory (as a witness) is incomplete, patient care documentation in the treatment record can be relied upon in one of two ways during direct testimony in a legal proceeding. The preferred way is for the clinician first to review the treatment record while on the witness stand, as a stimulus to jog the witness's present memory. After reviewing the documentation, the treatment record is taken away from the witness, and the witness testifies. This form of recall is called **present recollection refreshed**.

If a clinician's present recollection cannot be refreshed by reviewing the treatment record, then the treatment record itself may have to be admitted into evidence as substantive evidence of the care rendered to the patient under an exception to the hearsay rule.[45] This exception is called **past recollection recorded**. To substitute the treatment record for live testimony, however, the clinician must swear or affirm that the treatment record was accurate at the time it was written.

A health care professional should always document in a patient's treatment record as if the entry were being prepared for court because this may in fact occur. A health care professional will be more inclined to document more carefully if he or she imagines the documentation being blown up to giant size in a courtroom. The following simple, common-sense documentation tips will help clinicians avoid legal dilemmas concerning patient care documentation:

- Always write on every line in the record (to avoid the temptation to correct an entry after the fact).
- Write with one pen, using black (or blue) ink. In the rare case in which a pen runs out of ink midway through documenting an entry, indicate in a brief parenthetical that the first pen ran out of ink and continue with a second pen.
- Correct mistaken entries by drawing a single, straight line through the error and initialing (and dating, if this is customary practice) the correction. (Do not add words such as "error" or "mistaken entry" because such words may give rise to an inference in the eyes of a jury of negligent care delivery.)
- Except when correcting contemporaneous mistakes, do not edit prior documentation entries.
- Do not back-date an omission in a patient treatment record. Once an omission is noted, document critical omitted information in a new entry with today's date.
- Write legibly. Print, type, or dictate as required to help you to communicate clearly. Remember that the failure to communicate vital patient information clearly and in a timely manner constitutes professional negligence.
- Do not express negative personal feelings about a patient in the treatment record, such as "Patient is an obvious malingerer." Lack of objectivity in documenting patient evaluation and treatment can give rise to an inference of noncompliance with the legal standard of care.
- Do not argue with or disparage other health care professionals in the treatment record. Again, such behavior gives rise to an inference of uncoordinated and negligent care.
- Avoid including in patient care documentation extraneous verbiage not related to diagnosis or treatment of patients. Information such as "Patient is a pleasant, 55-year-old Beatles record collector" probably has no place in a general patient treatment record.
- Avoid using terms and abbreviations not universally understood by all health care professionals caring for the patient. Use of cryptic, esoteric terminology constitutes a negligent failure to communicate patient information.
- Avoid documenting patient status using ambiguous terminology, such as "tolerated treatment well," without specifying the parameters of the meaning of the phrase. Health care malpractice insurers caution that such ambiguous phraseology is too vague to be useful in defending a health care malpractice charge.[46]

Even innocent corrections of prior treatment entries may be construed by courts as intentional alteration of treatment records, which can have profound adverse legal consequences for health care professionals who become defendants in malpractice cases. A court may rule that altered treatment records are inadmissible or that a jury may infer or must presume negligence against a defendant–health care provider. Intentional alteration of treatment records may also give rise to the awarding of punitive damages against a defendant-provider should be plaintiff prevail in the case. Punitive damages are not normally payable by a provider's malpractice liability insurer. The legal term for intentional treatment record loss or alteration is **spoliation**.

Although specific rules concerning the use of adverse incident reports vary from facility to facility, certain universal rules apply when documenting adverse, potentially compensable events involving patients. Potentially compensable events that warrant the generation of incident reports include patient injury or expression by a patient of serious dissatisfaction with care.

An incident report serves two purposes: (1) to alert management to possible safety hazards requiring investigation and possible correction, and (2) to memorialize important facts about an adverse event for the purpose of preventing liability on the part of the organization.

Spoliation: The intentional loss or destruction of patient treatment records.

Always document adverse patient incidents concisely and objectively. Do not assign blame or speculate as to the cause of injury in the incident report. Document as fact only those things that you personally perceive. What others related to you, as recorder, constitute hearsay and should be bracketed in quotation marks to identify the hearsay statements clearly as emanating from someone other than the recorder.

Normally, information documented in an incident report is immune from discovery by a plaintiff-patient and his or her attorney. This qualified immunity normally requires that incident reports be clearly labeled as "quality assurance/improvement/management documents" or a "report prepared at the direction of the organization's attorney for possible use in litigation."

Do not file a copy of an incident report or mention its creation in the treatment record. The information contained in its does not relate to patient evaluation or treatment. Do create a concurrent treatment entry in the record detailing patient injury and provider interventions on the patient's behalf. Consider the following hypothetical example.

> *You are a licensed practical nurse entering a patient room on a nursing unit. The patient's diagnosis is "status-post left cerebrovascular accident, with right upper limb hemiplegia." As you enter the room, you observe the patient on the floor beside his bed, in the fetal position, and moaning. You notice that the side rails are down on the side where the patient is found. The patient's wife is sitting in a chair next to the bed. She states, "The side rails were down, and he fell out of bed. The nurses always leave the damn side rails down!" You quickly come to the patient's aid, and examine and stabilize him in a supine position. There is no apparent injury. You then go to the door and call for help from other nurses and doctors on the unit.*

How do you document (1) the narrative portion of the incident report and (2) the progress note in the patient's treatment record?

1. The narrative portion of the incident report might read as follows: "Upon entering the patient's room, I observed the patient on the floor next to his bed. The
patient was in the fetal position and was moaning. The side rails were down. The
patient's wife, who was seated in a chair next to the patient's bed, stated, 'The side
rails were down, and he fell out of bed. The nurses always leave the damn side rails
down!' I examined and stabilized the patient in the supine position, after noting
no apparent injury. Nurses and physician notified."
2. The progress note might read as follows: "Upon entering the patient's room, I
observed the patient on the floor next to his bed. The patient was in the fetal
position and was moaning. Patient examined and stabilized in the supine position,
after noting no apparent injury. Nurses and physician notified."

SUMMARY

The term *health care malpractice* encompasses civil legal actions initiated by patients
or their representatives against health care providers and/or health care organizations
for patient injury incident to the delivery of professional care services. However, patient injury alone is insufficient to allow a patient to prevail against a health care
professional or organization. The injury must be coupled with a recognized legal
basis for imposing health care malpractice liability.

The legal bases for imposing health care malpractice liability consist of professional
negligence; intentional, treatment-related conduct resulting in patient injury; breach
of a treatment-related contractual promise made by a health care provider; and strict
liability (without regard to fault) for injuries from abnormally dangerous clinical procedures or from dangerously defective treatment-related products.

The overwhelming majority of health care malpractice legal cases are based on allegations of professional negligence. A plaintiff-patient alleging professional negligence by a defendant-health care professional must prove a litany of four elements,
each by a preponderance, or greater weight, of evidence at trial. These elements are
(1) that the defendant-provider owed a legal duty of special care toward the plaintiff-
patient, (2) that the provider breached the duty owed by delivering care that was
objectively substandard, (3) that the breach of duty directly caused the patient injury,
and (4) that the award of monetary damages is appropriate and necessary to make the
patient "whole."

Defenses available to defendant-health care professionals and organizations in
malpractice cases are of two general types: technical (procedural) and substantive.
Technical defenses, demonstrated in many of the reported malpractice cases lodged
against physical and occupational therapists include plaintiff-patient noncompliance
with the applicable statute of limitations, failure to comply with procedural requirements for affidavits and other pleadings and documents submitted to courts, and
personal immunity from liability (as when the federal government is responsible for
official conduct of federal workers under the Federal Tort Claims Act). Substantive
defenses include plaintiff-patient contributory negligence or comparative fault
and proof by the defendant of compliance with the legal standard of care, making
a plaintiff-patient's injuries merely an unfortunate adverse event without legal
recourse.

Health care professionals—individually and collectively, and health care organizations, systems, and networks—can and must develop and implement effective risk management strategies to minimize malpractice exposure and liability. Such measures include patient care documentation skills and management, effective communications with patients and professional colleagues, empathy and respect for patients, systematic quality and risk management, continuing and continuous professional education, training and development for staff.[47]

CASES AND QUESTIONS

1. Patient A is an outpatient in nurse practitioner B's private practice. A ambulates using a four-legged cane. On his way from the reception area to the treatment area, A trips on a frayed edge of carpeting and falls and breaks a tooth. A expresses an intention to file a claim against the clinic for malpractice. Is A's claim for malpractice valid? If so, under what theory of liability? What steps should the nurse practitioner take immediately after injury?
2. Patient C, an outpatient in a sports physical therapy clinic, is being treated for an anterior cruciate ligament deficiency with closed-chain functionally focused exercise. Z, the clinic owner and treating physical therapist, promised C that her involved (dominant) knee strength would be equal to the uninvolved leg after 6 to 8 weeks of rehabilitation. During a session, C falls, twisting and injuring her involved knee. The incident was clearly no one's fault. Does C have a valid claim for physical therapy malpractice? Under which theory or theories might she proceed?
3. D, a general practice physician in private practice, treats patient E, an outpatient with a diagnosis of mechanical low back pain, with back extension exercises. At the end of the treatment session, E suddenly complains of increased left lower limb radicular symptoms and severe low back pain. A subsequent magnetic resonance imaging study reveals an intervertebral disk herniation at L4-L5. E undergoes a surgical diskectomy the next day. On these facts alone, is D liable for malpractice? From which disciplines might health care professionals testify as experts in a subsequent health care malpractice trial?

SUGGESTED ANSWERS TO CASES AND QUESTIONS

1. Patient A's case is probably an ordinary premises negligence case and not a professional treatment-related negligence case. This is so because the source of injury was a frayed rug, causing the same kind of fall that could occur in a retail store, a private home, or anywhere else.

The main advantage for the plaintiff of the case being labeled as ordinary negligence is that the plaintiff avoids the many administrative hurdles that attach to professional negligence legal actions, such as submission of the case to an administrative merit panel and submission of expert opinions along with court pleadings. In an ordinary premises negligence case, expert testimony on the nurse practitioner standard of care is inapplicable. Experts are unnecessary because the nature of an ordinary fall is within the common knowledge of lay jurors, without the need for clarification by experts.

For the defendant, the main advantage of the case being labeled as ordinary negligence is that a finding of liability does not result in the health care professional's name being reported for inclusion in the National Practitioner Data Bank. For both parties, an ordinary negligence case should be less time-consuming, less intense, and less expensive than a health care malpractice case.

The first step that the nurse practitioner should take after injury is to ensure that the patient is safe and stable. After injuries are ascertained, emergency consultation with a physician or dentist should be accomplished, and the patient should be transferred for care by these professionals. Express empathy with the patient's situation, and show that you care.

Complete an incident report. (This applies even for private practice clinics.) In addition to accurate documentation of administrative data, such as time, place, lighting, and other relevant details about the incident, carefully complete the narrative part of the report objectively and completely. Attribute any hearsay statements made by others to their source. Do not file or mention the incident report in the patient's treatment record.

Complete an entry in the patient's treatment record regarding injuries incurred by the patient and actions taken by you and your staff on the patient's behalf. Be sure to send a copy of the patient's record with the patient for emergency medical treatment.

2. The problem states that patient C's knee injury was no one's fault. This, however, does not prevent the filing of a health care malpractice claim or lawsuit. Some persons erroneously believe that malpractice liability automatically attaches anytime a patient is injured during treatment. Such is not the case. Malpractice liability requires patient injury, plus the presence of one of the recognized legal bases for imposing liability. In this case, one of these bases for liability—breach of contract—may seem to be present because a therapeutic promise was made to the patient by the physical therapist. However, the accidental fall that caused the patient injury probably would excuse the physical therapist from the contractual promise to achieve a therapeutic result under the contractual defense of "impossibility of performance."

3. As was explained in the answer to problem 2, patient injury during treatment alone does not create health care malpractice liability. The patient must also prove, by a preponderance of evidence, the existence of one of the legal bases for imposing liability. If such a connection can be established, a malpractice case may proceed to trial.

If the case proceeds to pretrial depositions and to trial, expert witnesses for the plaintiff and defendant may be physicians, physical or occupational therapists, chiropractors, or other health care professionals from related disciplines having similar knowledge, training, and experience about low back care as the defendant, and knowledge of the applicable standard of care in effect in the community in which the defendant practices.

SUGGESTED READINGS

Bakalar N: Medical errors? Patients may be the last to know ..., *New York Times* p D7, Aug 29, 2006.

British National Institute for Health Clinical Excellence, www.nice.org.uk/

Brushwood DB: Hospital pharmacist's duty to question clear errors in prescriptions, *Am J Hosp Pharm* 51:2031-2033, 1994.

Drug Enforcement Administration: All-States Guide to Nurse Practitioner Prescriptive Authority. Retrieved March 1, 2007, from www.usdoj.gov/dea.

Freeman J: Medical negligence and the locality rule: that's how medicine is practiced here, *Iowa Med* 96(3):10, 2006.

Fusion K: 'Patient' says it all: ER waits vary widely from state to state, *USA Today* p 8D, June 1, 2006. (Low: Iowa, 138.3 minutes; high: Arizona, 297.3 minutes)

Japenga A: A little sting can become a debilitating injury, *New York Times* (online) May 30, 2006. Retrieved Feb 13, 2007, from www.nyt.com. (A 1996 study revealed that 1 in 6300 blood donors suffers a nerve injury from the large-bore needles used.)

Lieberman T: Righting wrongs: the truth about medical malpractice and the law, *AARP Bulletin* pp 10-11, April 2006.

MedicalMalpractice.com: State-by-state list of statutes of limitations. Retrieved March 3, 2007, from www.medicalmalpractice.com.

Welch HG, Schwartz L, Woloshin S: What's making us sick is an epidemic of diagnoses ..., *New York Times* p D7, Jan 2, 2007. (The "medicalization" of childhood)

REFERENCES

1. *Pegram* v. *Herdrich,* 530 U.S. 211 (2000).
2. *Aetna Health Inc.* v. *Davila, CIGNA Healthcare Corp. of Texas, Inc.* v. *Calad,* 542 U.S. 200 (2004).
3. *The demise of state managed care accountability,* Chicago, 2004, Private Sector Advocacy and Advocacy Resource Center, American Medical Association.
4. Peterson RG: Malpractice liability of allied health professionals: developments in an area of critical concern, *J Allied Health* 14:363-372, 1985.
5. Prosser WL: *Handbook of the law of torts,* ed 4, St Paul, Minn, 1971, West Publishing Company.
6. Eickhoff-Sheneck J: Exercise equipment injuries: who's at fault? *ACSM's Health and Fitness Journal* 6(1):27-30, 2002.
7. *Tarasoff* v. *Regents of the University of California,* 17 Cal. 3d 425 (1976).
8. *Gassen* v. *East Jefferson General Hospital,* 1993 Westlaw 514862 (La. App. Dec. 15, 1993).
9. Harris G: New drug label rule intends to reduce medical errors, *New York Times* p A14, Jan 19, 2006.
10. 21 C.F.R. Parts 201, 314 and 601 (Jan 24, 2006).
11. *Novey* v. *Kishwaukee Community Health Services,* 531 N.E. 2d 427 (III. App. 1988).
12. *Commonalities and differences between the professions of physical therapy and occupational therapy,* Alexandria, Va, 1994, American Physical Therapy Association.
13. Klein TA: Scope of practice and the nurse practitioner: regulation, competency, expansion and evolution, *Topics in Advanced Practice Nursing eJournal* June 15, 2006. Retrieved Dec 28, 2006, from www.medscape.com.
14. Hayward RS, Wilson MC, Tunis SR et al: How to use clinical practice guidelines: are the recommendations valid? *JAMA* 274:570-574, 1995.
15. Garnick DW, Hendricks AM, Brennan TA: Can practice guidelines reduce the number and costs of malpractice claims? *JAMA* 266:2856-2891, 1991.
16. *Greening by Greening* v. *School District of Millard,* 393 N.W. 2d 51 (Neb. 1986).
17. *Escola* v. *Coca-Cola Bottling Company,* 150 P. 2d 436 (Ca. 1944).
18. C.F.R. 880.2920 (April 1, 2006). The administrative Code of Federal Regulations (21 C.F.R. Ch. 1, Section 801.109) requires that all prescription medical devices have the statement: "Federal law restricts this device to sale by or on the order of a physician, dentist, veterinarian, or other appropriate health care professional."
19. Gerlin A: Surgeons feel trapped by implant suits, *Wall Street Journal* p B8, March 30, 1995.
20. StateLawyers.com: Premises Liability. Retrieved Aug 24, 2007, from www.statelawyers.com.
21. Keeton WP: *Prosser and Keeton on torts,* ed 5, St Paul, Minn, 1984, West Publishing Company.
22. Kearney KA, McCord EL: Hospital management faces new liabilities, *Health Lawyer* 6(3):1, 1992.

23. *Pegram* v. *Herdrich.* 530 U.S. 211 (2000). [ERISA, the Employee Retirement Income Security Act of 1974, preempts imposition of health care malpractice liability in state courts against health maintenance organizations that treat patients pursuant to employer-provided health insurance benefit plans. ERISA cases are tried exclusively in federal courts, and liability is limited to the monetary value of health benefits denied to patients. Compensatory and punitive damages are disallowed.]

24. Leape LL, Berwick DM: Five years after *To Err Is Human, JAMA* 293:2384-2390, 2005.

25. Federal Tort Claims Act, 28 U.S.C. 2401(b).

26. Center for Justice and Democracy: Jury Verdicts. Retrieved Jan 1, 2007, from www.centerjd.org.

27. Matthiesen Wickert Lehrer: Contributory Negligence/Comparative Fault Laws. Retrieved Nov 19, 2006, from www.mwl-law.com.

28. Under the Restatement (Second) of Torts, Section 524, contributory negligence is a viable defense in a strict liability case when a plaintiff knowingly and unreasonably subjects himself or herself to risk of harm. Similarly, intentional, unreasonable misuse of a product by a plaintiff may create a valid defense to a strict product liability legal action. *Daly* v. *General Motors Corp.,* 20 Cal. 3d 725 (1978).

29. *Davis* v. *Sykes,* 121 S.E. 2d 513 (Va. 1961).

30. *Schneider* v. *Revici,* 817 F. 2d 987 (2d Cir. 1987).

31. Federal Tort Claims Act, 28 United States Code Sections 1346(b) and 2671-2680.

32. Federal Employees Liability Reform and Tort Compensation Act, 28 United States Code Section 2679, reads in pertinent part:
    (b)(1) The remedy against the United States provided by Sections 1346(b) and 2672 of this title for injury or loss of property, or personal injury or death arising or resulting from the negligent or wrongful act or omission of any federal employee of the Government while acting within the scope of his office or employment is *exclusive* of any other civil action or proceeding for monetary damages by reason of the same subject matter against the employee whose act or omission gave rise to the claim or against the estate of such employee. Any other civil action or proceeding for monetary damages arising out of or relating to the same subject matter against the employee or the employee's estate is precluded without regard to when the act or omission occurred.

33. American Medical Association: *State licensing laws and volunteer physicians.* Retrieved Feb 12, 2007, from www.ama-assn.org/ama/pub/category/12455.html.

34. *Tunkl* v. *Regents of the University of California,* 383 P. 2d 441 (Ca. 1963).

35. California Civil Code Section 1668.

36. Health Care Quality Improvement Act of 1986, 42 United States Code Sections 11101 to 11152.

37. Subchapter 1—Promotion of Professional Review Activities
    (1) Limitation on damages for professional review actions
    If a professional review action ... of a professional review body meets all the standards specified ...
        (A) the professional review body,
        (B) any person acting as a member or staff to the body, and
        (C) any person who participates with or assists the body with respect to the action, shall not be liable in damages under any law of the United States (or political subdivision thereof) with respect to the action ...
    (2) Protection for those providing information to professional review bodies
    Notwithstanding any other provision of law, no person (whether as a witness or otherwise) providing information to a professional review body regarding the competency or professional conduct of a physician shall be held, by reason of having provided such information,

to be liable in damages under any law of the United States or of any State (or political subdivision) unless such information is false and the person providing it knew that such information was false.

38. Section 11131. Requiring reports on medical malpractice payments

(a) In general:

Each entity (including an insurance company) which makes payments under a policy of insurance, self-insurance, or otherwise in settlement (or partial settlement) of, or in satisfaction of a judgment in, a medical malpractice action or claim shall report ... information respecting the payment and circumstances thereof.

(b) Information to be reported

The information to be reported under subsection (a) of this section includes:

(1) the name of any physician or licensed health care practitioner for whose benefit the payment is made,

(2) the amount of the payment,

(3) the name (if known) of any hospital with which the physician or practitioner is affiliated or associated,

(4) a description of the acts or omissions and injuries or illnesses upon which the action or claim was based ...

39. Mullan F, Politzer RM, Lewis CT et al: The National Practitioner Data Bank: report from the first year, *JAMA* 268:73-79, 1992.

40. Reports to National Practitioner Data Bank, Department of Health and Human Services, September 1, 1990–August 31, 1991.

41. Using the National Practitioner Data Bank, *Medical Staff Briefing* pp 9-10, Dec 1991.

42. 42 United States Code Section 11135(a)(2).

43. Pear R: Study finds failure to file malpractice data, *New York Times* p A16, Oct 19, 2005.

44. Modern Healthcare Online: *System Failure.* Retrieved Feb 17, 2005, from modernhealthcare. com.

45. *Black's Law Dictionary,* ed 5, St Paul, Minn, 1979, West Publishing Company. Hearsay evidence includes out-of-court statements offered as evidence in legal proceedings for the truth of the matter asserted in them. The hearsay rule, in effect in every state and in the federal legal system, prevents hearsay evidence from being admitted in legal proceedings, absent a recognized exception, such as a confession (in a criminal case) or admission (in a civil case), or a dying declaration (statement made by someone near to the time of death).

46. Clifton DW: 'Tolerated treatment well' may no longer be tolerated, *PT: Magazine of Physical Therapy* 3(10):24-27, 1995.

47. Scott RW: *Legal aspects of documenting patient care,* ed 3, Sudbury, Mass, 2007, Jones and Bartlett.

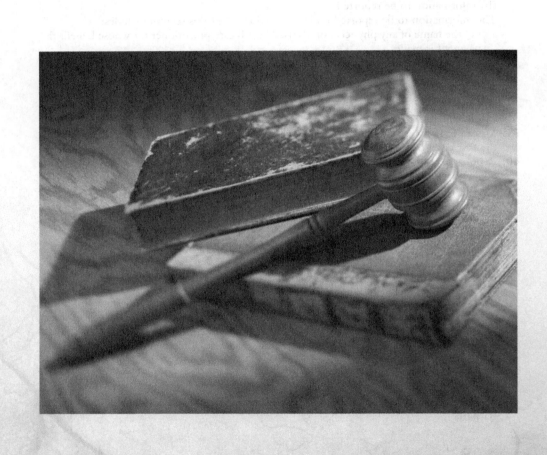

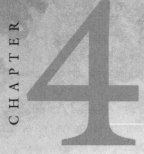

Intentional Wrongs

I N T R O D U C T I O N

This chapter introduces the concept of civil liability for intentional conduct. Legally actionable intentional conduct can consist of affirmative actions or omissions when one has the duty to act. The range of conduct that can give rise to intentional tort liability in health care settings includes assault and battery (including sexual assault and battery, a growing concern in the health care professions), defamation of character, false imprisonment, fraud, and invasion of

privacy. Recognized defenses to intentional tort legal actions include, with defamation, reporting suspected child, spousal, or elder abuse. Clinicians, managers, and administrators must
take responsibility for preventing the occurrence of intentional misconduct in health care delivery environments.

The chapter also defines basic criminal law concepts and explores offenses commonly
charged against health care professionals. Many criminal offenses bear the same names and
elements of proof as their intentional tort counterparts, including assault and battery, sexual
assault and battery, and fraud. Crimes by and against health care professionals are on the rise
and are highlighted in the concluding section of the chapter.

The successful prosecution of most crimes by the state requires proof of two elements:
culpable conduct (*actus reus*) and a culpable state of mind (*mens rea*). The burden of
proof on the state in a criminal case is proof of guilt beyond a reasonable doubt.

> Defenses to most crimes include consent by the victim (not normally applicable in
> the health care setting), defense of others and self-defense, infancy, insanity, in-
> toxication, and the statute of limitations. Avoidance of allegations of health care
> clinical misconduct that can give rise to criminal and civil liability is the formidable
> responsibility of all health care practitioners and administrators.

INTENTIONAL TORTS

Intentional wrongs committed against individuals or property are referred to as **intentional torts.** As the phrase implies, legally actionable intentional conduct requires
some kind of injury to a person or to a person's property. The "injury" can be something as seemingly innocuous as interfering with a person's right to exclusive use of
his or her tangible property or touching someone in such a way that may reasonably
be construed as offensive.

> **Intentional tort:** Conduct in which a person intends that the resulting conse-
> quences of the act or omission occur or in which the person
> engaging in the conduct knows with substantial certainty
> that the occurrence of certain results are probable, with
> resultant injury to a person or to a person's property.

The word *wrong* associated with "intentional wrong" may be a bit misleading as
used in this context, in that the person committing an intentional tort need not have
any specific intent to injure a victim (or the victim's property). The tortfeasor merely
has to act with intent, or volition, to effect a desired or probable result through his
or her conduct. When that conduct results in injury to a person or to a person's
property, an intentional tort action may arise.

A legally actionable intentional tort may exist even where the party whose conduct
is in question did not intend to do an act that results in personal injury. That the

person intentionally engaging in some type of conduct knew that the conduct was substantially certain to cause a legally actionable result is often sufficient.

Normally, no intentional tort occurs when a person engaging in conduct is unconscious or acts reflexively. For example, consider the following hypothetical case examples:

> *A physical therapist assistant, acting under proper supervision of a licensed physical therapist and in compliance with the applicable state practice act, applies electrode pads from a neuromuscular stimulation device to a patient's lateral forearm musculature to effect extensor muscle reeducation. As the assistant activates the device, it malfunctions, sending a surge of electrical current into the control box of the device. In a purely reflexive act, the assistant flails her arm into the air. Her moving arm strikes the patient in the left side of the face, resulting in a deep scratch to the patient's cheek, and a corneal abrasion to the patient's left eye. Does the physical therapist assistant's "harmful and offensive" touching of the patient constitute the intentional tort of battery?*

Answer: Probably not. Although the physical therapist assistant would be legally responsible for unintended patient injury if she had been flailing her arms in response to being told about a pay raise, for example, in this case her conduct was unintentional. It also cannot be said that she knew with substantial certainty that, by turning on the neuromuscular stimulator device, it would surge and her arm would flail into the air, striking and injuring the patient. It would be a different case if the stimulator device had failed in a similar manner in the recent past and the physical therapist assistant was using it anyway, knowing with substantial certainty that a surge of electricity would probably cause her to flinch reflexively. The law will not impose intentional tort liability for a nonvolitional act, unless it was reasonable to assume that the nonvolitional act would take place.

> *X, a registered nurse employed by ABC Community Hospital, enters the break room and observes Y, an aide, sleeping in a chair. X applies a hand to Y's shoulder, gently shaking Y awake. Startled by being awakened suddenly, Y lashes out a fist, striking X in the face, knocking off X's glasses. Has either X or Y committed an intentional tort, that is, battery? (Battery, as discussed later in this chapter, involves the intentional harmful, offensive, or otherwise impermissible touching of another person.)*

Answer: Probably neither X nor Y committed the tort of battery upon one another. X presumably acted reasonably as a representative of management in awakening Y during working hours. A certain amount of physical contact between persons—even in the "intimate zone"[1] of contact—is a reasonable consequence of normal social relations. A different conclusion would result if X's touching of Y was unreasonable, either by applying excessive force to Y's shoulder or by touching Y in a private zone of contact. Y's act of striking X is considered legally to be an unconscious act, for which Y normally is not legally responsible.

In a legally actionable intentional tort action, then, there is no requirement for the injured party-plaintiff to prove **malicious intent.** That is, there is no requirement that a defendant's intention was to commit wrongdoing. It is sufficient that the defendant's conduct was volitional and intended (or substantially certain) to cause some even innocent result that causes injury to another person. If a defendant is proved to have had malicious intent incident to an intentional tort, then a court is more likely to permit the award of punitive damages against the wrongdoer.

One legal concept related to intent is the transferred intent doctrine. Under **transferred intent,** a defendant intends to direct conduct toward one person but unintentionally affects another person. For example, consider the following hypothetical scenario:

> *During a staff Christmas party in the cafeteria at Anywhere Medical Center, a food fight spontaneously erupts involving several employees. Within seconds, the food fight escalates to the point where one of the participants reaches into a punch bowl and retrieves a small piece of ice. The employee, C, throws the ice cube at D, who is engaged in the fray. D ducks, and the ice cube strikes E, another employee who is just entering the cafeteria to attend the party, in the right eye. Even though C had no intent to strike E, C is liable under the concept of transferred intent for injuries sustained by E because C acted with intent toward D.*

Why would a patient allegedly injured by a health care professional in the course of a professional-patient relationship bring a civil legal action for an intentional tort versus ordinary or professional negligence? In labeling a malpractice case as an intentional wrong case instead of as a negligence case, the patient has several advantages. In proving an intentional wrong case (as with an ordinary negligence case), the patient normally does not have to introduce (expensive) expert testimony about the professional standard of care because a lay jury or a judge normally can discern the nature and consequences of intentional conduct without the need for expert witness assistance. Also, if the court finds the defendant's conduct to have been egregious, it may allow for the award of punitive (or punishment) damages in the case. Punitive damages are over and above the normal compensatory monetary damages designed to make a tort plaintiff "whole."

The main disadvantage to a plaintiff in bringing a health care malpractice lawsuit as an intentional tort case is that a defendant–health care professional's liability insurer may not be legally obligated to indemnify the insured for liability for malicious intentional torts or for punitive damages, necessitating **execution of the judgment** (collection of monetary damages) from the defendant personally, a prospect that is less certain than collecting the award from the defendant's professional liability insurer.

Acts Versus Omissions

The kinds of conduct that can give rise to intentional tort liability—in the health care delivery setting (or any other setting)—are affirmative **acts** and legally actionable omissions. Acts involve affirmative, volitional, intended conduct in furtherance of a specific result. For example, the application of nontherapeutic touch during a massage is an example of an affirmative act giving rise to potential intentional tort liability. So is striking a person without legal justification or excuse (i.e., committing battery). By definition, affirmative acts of battery designed to arouse or gratify the sexual desires of the aggressor or of the victim constitute sexual battery. Sexual battery, a subset of the tort of battery, is discussed later in this chapter.

Legally actionable omissions involve the intentional and wrongful failure to act when one has the legal duty to act. Once a health care professional has assumed a legal duty of care for a patient, the provider is obligated by law to act reasonably toward the patient until the professional-patient relationship is properly terminated. When a provider leaves a patient under care without supervision or improperly refuses to treat a patient, the intentional tort of patient **abandonment** becomes an issue. Similarly, when a health care professional intentionally fails to communicate critical patient information to others having an official need to know, an intentional tort issue arises. Consider the following hypothetical example:

> *A surgical nurse is assisting an operating room technician in setting up a surgical suite for an orthopedic case. In the course of depositing sterile instruments onto the sterile back table, the nurse, in haste, knowingly drops an unsterile electrocautery cable onto the field, contaminating the sterile field and the "scrub" technician, who begins to touch instruments on the field. The orthopedic surgeon and the anesthesiologist are already visibly furious about routine delays in starting the case and would be incensed if the nurse revealed that the sterile field was contaminated. The field would have to be broken down to start over again. The nurse elects not to admit that the cable that was placed on the table was unsterile. If the surgical patient becomes infected as a result of the nurse's intentional (mis)conduct, then the patient will have an actionable claim for battery. (In this case, the harmful touching would be indirect, involving the unsterile electrocautery device that infects the patient.)*

Assault and Battery

Assault and **battery** are terms that, although used interchangeably by laypersons, really define two separate torts. The torts of assault and battery often go hand in hand in a real-life case; however, it is possible to have one tort occur without its complementary intentional wrong. These torts are discussed separately.

Assault

Assault involves a situation in which a victim reasonably anticipates, or has apprehension or fear about, an impending battery. Although apprehension and fear are possible elements of the tort of assault, they are really two different concepts. A victim can apprehend (or sense) that harmful, offensive, or otherwise impermissible physical contact (i.e., battery) is imminent, yet not be in fear of it. Such might be the case when a patient knows that a health care provider is about to kiss the patient without permission. But assault may also involve a fear of a touch, such as when a person flinches or winces in anticipation of an impending blow by another. In either case the victim is displaying a normal reaction to an unwanted wrongful touch.

Another excellent example of assault is represented by a scene in the feature film, *The Hand That Rocks the Cradle*,[2] in which the female protagonist finds herself at the beginning of the film in her gynecologist's examining room with her legs placed in stirrups. Sensing that the gynecologist's imminent touch is improper, the protagonist flinches in disgust. This conduct alone on the part of the gynecologist gives rise to a legally actionable assault. The patient would have a cause of action, or case, even if the gynecologist had noticed that the patient was aware of his malicious intent and arrested his movement toward her without ever touching the patient.

In making the tort of assault legally actionable, the legal system serves to protect a person's privacy right to carry out activities of daily living free of the fear or anticipation of a battery at the hands of another. Considering the large number of reported assault and battery cases in society,[3] one may wonder how effective the legal system really is in protecting the rights of citizens to be free from the threat of violence. Because of the availability and threat of legal redress, every act of assault and battery carries with it a potentially high cost in terms of civil and criminal liability and adverse administrative consequences for the offender.

Assault: Reasonable anticipation or fear by a person of an impending battery.

Battery

Battery involves unjustified and unexcused harmful, offensive, or otherwise impermissible intentional contact by a tortfeasor with another person. Harmful contact includes volitional actions by the offender that cause pain, impairment, or disfigurement of a victim. Offensive contact includes direct and indirect acts of touching that offend a person's sense of dignity, such as when a health care profession inappropriately touches a patient's breasts or genitals.

A victim may be the subject of a battery without experiencing a prior assault. In the hypothetical example involving the nurse who contaminated a sterile surgical field, the patient, who was the victim of a battery, could not have apprehended the harmful touch (by the unsterile instruments) because the patient was sedated and the patient's view was obscured by a drape sheet. Similarly, when a patient is asleep, the patient cannot sense an impending battery (e.g., from a kiss or from touching of a sexual nature), so the patient becomes the victim of a battery without an assault.

Several recognized **complete defenses** to the torts of assault and battery exist. The first recognized defense is consent. If a person who otherwise would be a victim of assault and/or battery knowingly and voluntarily consents to harmful or offensive contact, then there is no legally actionable assault or battery. For example, a customer of a prostitute solicits sadomasochistic sex with the prostitute, and the prostitute complies, tying and beating the customer. Even if the customer is injured, there may be no actionable assault or battery claim against the prostitute or the prostitute's employer if the customer consented to the beating.

In health care delivery, public policy considerations normally preclude consent by a patient or client to an assault or battery. So, even if a patient nominally consents to some socially impermissible contact such as sexual relations with the patient's health care provider, an action for assault and battery may be viable on the grounds that the patient's "consent" is invalid as a matter of law. A patient cannot consent to sexual contact incident to routine health care delivery (with limited exceptions for situations such as legitimate sexual therapy) because the patient's consent would violate public policy.

Another legitimate defense to assault and battery is self-defense. Even in the health care treatment setting, a provider has the legal right to defend himself or herself from harmful or offensive contact by another person, including a patient. A health care provider may be privileged to use whatever physical force (or threat of force) is necessary to repel an attack, even to the point of meeting deadly force with deadly force.

The same legal rules apply for legitimate defense of others. Consider the following hypothetical example (based on a real case):

> *A patient with a diagnosis of bipolar manic-depressive psychosis suddenly attacks a neurosurgical resident who is examining the patient at bedside. The patient begins to choke the resident, and the resident cries for help. Two licensed practical nurses and one patient come to the resident's aid and attempt in vain to pry the psychotic patient's fingers from the resident's neck. As the resident begins to lose consciousness, one of the nurses and the good Samaritan patient begin to strike the aggressor hard in the face. The other nurse draws and administers an ampule of chlorpromazine (Thorazine) intramuscularly into the aggressor's arm. After a few seconds, the psychotic patient releases his grip on the resident's neck and falls to the ground, unconscious. Did the nurse and patient who struck the aggressive patient commit battery?*

Answer: No. The nurse and patient had the legal right to use reasonable force to protect the neurosurgical resident, who was in real danger of losing his life.

Defamation

Definition

Defamation includes legally actionable untrue communication(s) of purported fact about a person that harm the victim's positive personal reputation in the eyes of a significant number of other persons in the victim's community. Defamatory communications cause other persons to hold the target of the defamation up to ridicule, disgust, or scorn. **Business disparagement** (also called **trade libel**) involves verbal or other communications that harm a target person's business, rather than exclusively personal, reputation in the relevant community.

Two primary classifications of defamation are slander and libel. **Slander** is a defamatory communication that is transmitted orally or through signing. **Libel** includes defamatory communications transmitted by all other means, including writings, film, videotape and audiotape, and computer transmissions. Slanderous communications are transitory, whereas libelous communications are considered to be of a more permanent nature.

> **Defamation:** False communication(s) of purported fact about a person that harm the victim's positive personal reputation in the eyes of a significant number of other persons in the victim's community.
>
> **Slander:** A defamatory communication transmitted orally or through signing.
>
> **Libel:** A defamatory communication transmitted by all other means including writings, film, videotape and audiotape, and computer transmissions.
>
> **Business disparagement** (also called trade libel): Verbal or other communications that harm a target person's business reputation in the community.

A special category of defamation is **defamation** *per quod.* Under this concept, a communication made to others is not, on its face, defamatory. The communication may even appear to be complimentary of the target person. However, a defamation results once the negative implication of the primary communication (called the **innuendo**) is realized, after the communication is coupled with extrinsic facts (called the **inducement**) that make the communication defamatory. Consider the following hypothetical example:

> *A, a physical therapist working in a comprehensive outpatient rehabilitation facility, announces to the assembled rehabilitation team at a weekly meeting that B, an occupational therapist (who is not present at the meeting), became "certified" today in psychiatric therapy. Later that day, it is discovered that B was hospitalized for a nervous breakdown. Everyone then realizes that A meant to ridicule B by inferring that B's certification was as a psychiatric patient. The original statement—seemingly innocent—then becomes a legally actionable defamation under defamation per quod.*

To win a defamation lawsuit, a target person of a defamatory communication must normally prove special damages specific to the victim, not just generalized pain and suffering damages. One exception involves communications that constitute **defamation** *per se.* Under defamation *per se,* certain comments about persons are actionable without proof of any damages, such as statements ascribing a loathsome, communicable disease—such as venereal disease—falsely to another person.

Several complete defenses to a legal action for defamation exist. The first is the defense of truth, that is, that what was said or otherwise communicated about a defamation plaintiff was, in fact, true. Although proof of the truth of a purportedly defamatory communication brings an end to a defamation legal action, it may give rise to another intentional tort action for wrongful **invasion of privacy.** (Invasion of privacy is discussed subsequently.)

Another defense to defamation is **privilege.** Certain members of society—rightfully or not—are afforded by law an absolute (or complete) privilege to make defamatory statements about others. These include sitting judges in legal proceedings from the bench, congresspersons, and high-level executive officials acting in their official capacities.

Health care professionals, like prosecutors and defense attorneys in legal proceedings, have a qualified privilege under certain circumstances to make statements believed in good faith to be true about others but that in fact are false and therefore defamatory. For health care professionals, for example, there is a qualified privilege under federal statute to give good-faith testimony in credentialing administrative actions about the competency of a physician under inquiry, without fear of defamation liability.[4] Health care professionals also are normally immune from defamation liability incident to good-faith official reporting of suspected child, spousal, or elder abuse (discussed subsequently).

Constitutionally Protected Speech

One other defense to defamation related to privilege involves communications that are protected from suppression under the federal Constitution. Since the landmark U.S. Supreme Court decision in *New York Times* v. *Sullivan*[5] in 1964, it may be permissible for one person (particularly if that person is from the media) to "publish" (i.e., communicate to others) defamatory information about a target person who is a public official or a public figure. To enjoy constitutional immunity from defamation liability, the person making a false statement about a public official or public figure must prove that he or she acted without actual knowledge of the falsity of the statement and did not communicate the defamatory information in reckless disregard of the truth.

Public officials, although not encompassing all public employees, includes policy-making governmental officials at all levels—federal, state, and local—and from all three branches—executive, legislative, and judicial. Examples of public officials also include persons who are political appointees to policy-making positions, such as heads of governmental task forces. As has become evident in recent political campaigns and appointment hearings, seemingly every aspect of these public officials' public and private lives is open to investigation and dissemination.

Public figures are not subject to the same degree of permissible scrutiny under law as public officials. Public figures are those persons who have achieved some degree of public fame or recognition incident to some pursuit or who have voluntarily injected themselves into the public eye regarding some subject of public interest. Only areas related to their fame or reputation are permissible areas of scrutiny, not their entire lives or life histories. Examples of public figures include the leaders of major health care professional associations.

Why should the legal system shield from defamation liability false communications made about public officials or public figures? The stated rationale for this constitutional privilege to defame is that the press's and public's right to know important information about public officials and public figures outweighs the privacy rights of those who have voluntarily placed themselves in the public eye.

Reporting Statutes and Requirements

As mandatory reporters, health care professionals in most or all states are required by statute to report certain findings incident to patient care activities. Included among these reportable findings is objective, credible evidence of possible child, spousal, and elder abuse.

Child Abuse

All states mandate reporting of actual or suspected child abuse and/or neglect. State statutes must require such reporting in order to qualify for federal funds under the Child Abuse Prevention and Treatment Act.[6] A Rand Corporation survey found that as many as 40 percent of health care professionals and educational professionals admit to not reporting suspected child abuse.[7] The primary stated rationale given for failing to report child abuse as required by law was that professionals were disillusioned with what they perceived as overtaxed and understaffed child protection service agencies. Another rationale for not reporting was that professionals stated that they were uncertain about the nature of their legal duty to report suspected child abuse.

Perhaps an unstated reason for failing to report suspected child abuse is the fear of liability exposure. Health care and other professionals have been subjected to liability exposure for reporting and failing to report suspected child abuse.[8,9] Even when a health care or other professional is vindicated in a defamation lawsuit involving a report of suspected child abuse, the cost in terms of stress, injury to personal and professional reputation, and monetary outlays may be very high.

Domestic (Spousal) Abuse

Each year, as many as 4 million women (accounting for 90 to 95 percent of total domestic abuse cases) may be victims of domestic violence at the hands of their partners.[10] The continuum of types of spousal abuse range from battering with or without weaponry to sexual assault and battery to prolonged torture and murder. Health care professionals in all but five states are required by law to report suspected acts of spousal abuse to law enforcement authorities.[11]

The duty incumbent on health care professional clinicians is formidable. Providers are expected to be able to identify indices of possible abuse. Providers also routinely and expressly make inquiries of patients about possible domestic abuse, make reports when indicated to appropriate agencies, and provide professional support and empathy. Imparting information about options to affected patients, addressing immediate safety concerns of patients and their children, properly documenting suspected abuse, and making appropriate client referrals to support agencies and other providers is part of the duty indicated.

The reporting of spousal or other abuse in the face of client resistance to reporting creates an ethical dilemma, with the ethical principles of confidentiality and compliance with legal mandates in opposition. The reluctance to report is even stronger when the provider knows or reasonably believes that law enforcement or social service agencies will not protect the patient, exposing him or her to further violence.

In 2002, 247,730 rapes and sexual assaults were reported in the United States.[12] Health care providers must be cognizant of overt and even subtle signs of sexual abuse in patients, including among other considerations, reticence, lack of eye contact, reluctance to shake hands or allow other physical contact, inappropriate dress, unexplained injuries, panic attacks during examination or conversation, and crying.

Elder Abuse

The phenomenon of elder abuse is less well recognized than child abuse or spousal domestic violence. Yet elder abuse is a massive social problem in the United States, Great Britain, and other countries and is a problem that health care clinicians may fail to recognize and address.[13]

Health care providers should screen for elder abuse just as they should for child or spousal abuse. The health care professional should watch for notable physical findings and behavioral characteristics of elder abuse that are identifiable in the client and the elder's caregiver.

Physical warning signs of possible abuse in the elder abuse or neglect victim may include the following:

- Untreated injury
- Unexplained injury
- Pain or withdrawal from touch
- Seemingly minor skin bruising, lacerations, and/or burns
- Malnutrition and/or dehydration
- Unexplained weight loss

- Pallor, sunken eyes and/or cheeks
- Poor personal hygiene
- Soiled clothing; clothing inappropriate for the season

The following are commonly noted behavioral characteristics of patients who are victims of elder abuse or neglect:

- Anxiety, nervousness, apparent fear
- Reticence, failure to make eye contact, withdrawal
- Allowing a caregiver to answer when questioned about health-related complaints
- Refusal of treatment intervention
- Depression
- Anger, hostility, belligerence
- Inappropriate apparent euphoria
- Lethargy

The abused elder patient's caregiver may display the following behavioral characteristics:

- Intoxication, drug use
- Aggression and/or history of violence
- Indifference to caregiver education efforts
- Verbal abuse of the patient
- Answering questions for the elderly patient
- Verbal and physical cues of a sexual nature that may indicate sexual abuse of the elderly patient, such as inappropriate touching of the patient and inappropriate patient dress for the clinical environment

Health care professionals are urged to educate themselves about the common and subtle indices of possible elder abuse and to take appropriate action to prevent further abuse, including client and family/significant other education and reporting suspected abuse to social service entities or law enforcement authorities as required by law. Failure to recognize and act on obvious signs of likely abuse, on the part of health care providers, constitutes professional negligence, for which liability may attach.

Other Reporting Requirements

Other forms of mandatory reporting requirements include the reporting to appropriate state health agencies of suspected or known infectious diseases[14] and enumerated occupational diseases[15] under state statutes. Nonphysician health care professionals who evaluate and treat patients without physician referral have the same duty to recognize and report disease, injury, and abuse as physicians have.

False Imprisonment

False imprisonment, as it applies in the health care delivery environment, involves an allegation that a health care professional or someone employed by the provider acted intentionally to restrict a patient's movement unlawfully. False imprisonment allegations can arise from actions such as the involuntary commitment to hospitals of a patient with a psychiatric diagnosis and the unjustified physical restraint of a patient.

False imprisonment: An intentional act to restrict a patient's movement unlawfully.

Another basis for false imprisonment liability exposure involves a situation in which a health care professional is alleged to have compelled a patient to remain in a specific location to undergo treatment against the patient's will. Cases also have been reported in the legal literature involving allegations of false imprisonment involving health care professionals attempting to stop, or actually prohibiting, patients from leaving the clinic area pending resolution of outstanding billing charges.

Certain nuances and qualifiers to false imprisonment liability warrant elaboration. False imprisonment is an intentional tort; therefore, any allegedly wrongful act on the part of a defendant–health care provider would have to have been done with the specific intent to confine a plaintiff-patient's free movement. Negligent, or careless, action that results in the confinement of a patient would not normally be sufficient to give rise to false imprisonment liability. Consider the following hypothetical scenario:

A certified occupational therapy assistant is treating a hospital patient in the patient's room on a ward. The patient requires a chair or her walker at one side of her bed in order to rise and ambulate to the bathroom. The patient's chair and walker are moved away from bedside during the activities of daily living treatment session. Despite the patient having told the occupational therapy assistant of this fact and the assistant promising to reposition the chair and walker after treatment, the assistant forgets to do so and leaves the room. Because of this oversight, the patient cannot get up to use the toilet. The patient calls in vain for nursing assistance to help her get up and finally urinates in bed, soiling her clothing and the bed linen.

Is the certified occupational therapy assistant liable for false imprisonment? No. Although the intentional actions of the certified occupational therapy assistant resulted in the confinement of the patient to a limited area, that is, the patient's bed, the certified occupational therapy assistant did not act with the specific intent to confine the patient. The assistant's actions constituted negligence, at worst.

Another nuance to false imprisonment liability is that verbal threats of physical force directed at a patient or threats of harm to a patient's property, resulting in a patient electing to limit volitional movement, may also constitute wrongful false imprisonment. False imprisonment liability, unlike most other torts, normally does not require proof of special damages, such as incurring additional medical expenses or resultant lost wages, in order for a plaintiff-patient to prevail.

One qualifier to false imprisonment liability is that a victim must be conscious of the fact that he or she is being confined or threatened with force if he or she moves. Therefore, legally, comatose or perhaps even disoriented patients cannot be "falsely imprisoned" by restraint, threats, or involuntary hospitalization.

Often, an act that constitutes false imprisonment (or assault or battery) also gives rise to another tort action—**intentional infliction of emotional distress.** Intentional infliction of emotional distress occurs when a defendant intentionally engages in extreme, outrageous conduct (such as unlawful false imprisonment of a patient) that results in severe emotional distress to a plaintiff.

Fraud

Black's Law Dictionary defines **fraud,** in part, as "an intentional perversion of the truth."[16] The intentional tort of fraud may be defined as the intentional false representation or concealment of a material fact designed to deceive another person, which causes that person to act (or not act) in some manner to the victim's legal detriment. Fraud is often thought of as being synonymous with "misrepresentation"; however, the latter term is used exclusively to describe fraudulent conduct that involves affirmative action by a wrongdoer.

> **Fraud:** The intentional false representation or concealment of a material fact designed to deceive another person, which causes that person to act (or not act) in some manner to the victim's legal detriment.

Fraud in health care reportedly accounts for 10 percent of all health care expenditures.[17] Defraudation primarily takes place as a result of fraudulent billing for services, the receipt of bribes and kickbacks for patient referrals, and self-referral. Self-referral has decreased dramatically as a result of enactment and implementation by Congress of *Stark I* and *II*,[18] which prohibit physician self-referral of Medicare and Medicaid patients for the following types of services, among others, in which the physician has a financial interest:

- Clinical laboratory services
- Diagnostic imaging services
- Durable medical equipment and supplies
- Home health services
- Inpatient and outpatient hospital services
- Occupational therapy
- Orthotics
- Parenteral and enteral nutrients
- Physical therapy
- Prosthetics

The Stark law regulations took substantial time to come to finality. First published in 1995, Stark I did not take final effect until January 4, 2002, and Stark II until July 26, 2004.[19]

Federal anti–health care fraud statutes and regulations are intended to prohibit the offer or receipt of payment of bribes, kickbacks, and rebates in exchange for Medicare or Medicaid patient referrals. A limited number of regulatory exceptions to Stark exist under which providers may be immune from prosecution or civil liability for health care activities such as in-office ancillary services, rural practices, and certain personal services arrangements with independent contractors. The existence of such safe harbors from prosecution and liability are particularly important to providers in managed care environments, who must have a certain degree of practice flexibility.

Civil legal action against health care professionals for defraudation of federal health care programs can take place under a federal statute titled the False Claims Act of 1863.[20] Under that Civil War–era statute, the intentional submission of a false claim to the federal government, which results in reimbursement by the federal government, may subject an offender to mandatory civil money penalties of between $5500 and

$11,000 for every false claim submitted, plus treble (triple) damages, based on the amount that the government was defrauded. The federal government or a private citizen (under the *qui tam* [Latin for "who as well"] provisions of the statute) may initiate civil legal action against an alleged offender. If a private citizen initiates a *qui tam* action for fraud against an offender and the action is successful, the private citizen receives between 10 and 30 percent of the government's recovery, plus the award of reasonable legal expenses.[21]

The federal government is making significant headway in battling health care fraud. In 2005 the Department of Justice recovered $1.47 billion in judgments and settlements against providers and others in health care fraud legal actions.[22] The Health Care Fraud and Abuse Control Program, enacted pursuant to HIPAA, the Healthcare Insurance Portability and Accountability Act of 1996, is a coordinated program managed by the attorney general and Department of Health and Human Services and designed to prevent and prosecute health care fraud. Monies collected by the program are transferred to the Medicare Trust Fund.[23]

Invasion of Privacy

In perhaps no environment (except for military service) is individual privacy sacrificed to so great a degree as in health care delivery settings. As part of their fiduciary duty owed to patients under their care, health care professionals are obligated by law and ethics to jealously safeguard patient confidences, except where they are required by law to disclose them or when disclosure is made to other health care professionals having a need to know the information disclosed. Occasionally, health care providers, administrators, and support personnel unlawfully fail to respect patient privacy, resulting in the intentional tort of invasion of privacy.

As in defamation cases, invasion of privacy legal actions are premised on an allegation of wrongful disclosure of information to third parties. The four principal forms of legally actionable invasion of privacy in the health care delivery environment are the following:

- Intrusion upon a patient's seclusion or solitude
- "False light" publicity about a patient
- Misappropriation of a patient's name or likeness
- Public disclosure of private facts about a patient

Unreasonable Intrusion Upon Patient Solitude

To be liable for invasion of privacy under the **unreasonable intrusion** prong of this tort, a defendant must intentionally intrude; (1) physically or otherwise, upon the seclusion or solitude of another person; (2) in such a way that is deemed highly offensive to an ordinary, reasonable person (i.e., the fact finder in litigation). Everyone—even patients—have the right to reasonable privacy or seclusion. Of course, for patients—especially inpatients—there are few areas where seclusion can be experienced.

Many scenarios involving intrusion on a patient's solitude take place in the health care setting. One involves the opening of a patient's mail or a private drawer of a nightstand in order to peruse a patient's private property. Another is the unauthorized photographing of a sleeping or comatose patient—even if the photograph is never shown to anyone. Consider this hypothetical example:

X is a male medical photographer employed at HMO Health Care Center. Y is a female outpatient under care in the gynecology clinic. During one treatment session, X suddenly opens the curtain to Y's cubicle while Y is undressing, in order to see her in a state of partial undress. Does X's act constitute a tort? Yes. X is liable for invasion of Y's privacy by intruding on her reasonable seclusion. (Note that X might also be liable for other torts, such as intentional infliction of emotional distress and sexual misconduct. X's conduct might be legally excused, however, if exigent, or emergency, circumstances (such as a fire in the clinic) existed that required X to enter the cubicle where Y was undressing.)

False-Light Publicity

False-light invasion of privacy, like the remaining two prongs of the intentional tort of invasion of privacy, involve situations in which a defendant violates a plaintiff's privacy rights in some way and disseminates private information about the plaintiff to third parties who do not have a right to know, or legitimate need for, the information. The three classic elements to actionable false-light invasion of privacy are as follows:

- The defendant disseminates private information to others about a plaintiff and somehow casts the information conveyed in such a way as to place the plaintiff in a false public light.
- The defendant's actions are objectively unreasonable and highly offensive.
- The information disclosure is done with **malice** (knowledge of the fact that the disclosure would place the plaintiff in a false public light or reckless disregard for the consequences of the act).

Consider the following hypothetical example:

F is a 44-year-old male orthopedic patient in a physical therapy clinic and a prominent physical therapy professor in the city's only health care professions university. F sustained an open right femoral fracture and a right distal radial fracture when he fell from his roof while inspecting the structure for hail damage. F is required to wear a bulky right long-leg cast and a right forearm cast. He has been fitted by his physical therapist, G, with axillary crutches with a right forearm support device. With F's written consent, G takes a photograph of F ambulating in the clinic with his crutches for the stated purpose of using the photograph in a viewbook of the clinic to show the range of services that it offers. Sometime after F's discharge from the clinic, G has the photograph enlarged to poster size and displays it in the clinic with the caption, "This could be you, so BE CAREFUL!" Has G committed the tort of false-light invasion of privacy? Maybe. G had consent to use F's photograph for the limited purpose of including it in a clinic viewbook. In this case, G exceeded the scope of F's authorization for permissible use of the photograph. The photograph may be construed to paint F in a false public light, that is, to make him look clumsy and unintelligent. Whether this misuse of F's photograph constitutes false-light invasion of privacy becomes a question for the fact finder (jury or judge) at trial in a civil legal case. (Even if G's conduct is not adjudged to be false-light invasion of privacy, it may constitute unlawful misappropriation, discussed next.)

Misappropriation

Misappropriation invasion of privacy involves the unauthorized use of a plaintiff's name and/or likeness, usually but not always, for a defendant's commercial gain. Unapproved use of a plaintiff's name or likeness for noncommercial purposes is also legally actionable as misappropriation.

This branch of invasion of privacy is particularly applicable to health care delivery because health care professionals are frequently asked by commercial product manufacturers and others to involve patients in research studies. In addition to the ethical considerations surrounding the use of patients in clinical research, clinicians are urged to remember that misuse, or "overuse," of patient information may give rise to misappropriation liability.

Public Disclosure of Private Patient Facts

The three elements to the tort of **public disclosure of private facts** invasion of privacy are as follows:

- The defendant publicizes information about a person that is of a personal nature.
- The disclosure is highly offensive from the viewpoint of an ordinary, reasonable person.
- The subject matter of the disclosure is not legitimately in the public interest.

Every person has constitutional (federal and state), statutory, and common law rights to legitimate privacy and intimacy. These rights are perhaps the most fundamental in American society, a nation which prides itself on respect for individual rights and freedom. The constitutional right of privacy is the only judicially recognized personal freedom that is not enumerated in the Constitution. This implied right was added to those enumerated in the Constitution by the U.S. Supreme Court in 1965[24] and was based on language from multiple enumerated rights in the Bill of Rights. HIPAA, enacted in 1996 and implemented in 2003 (discussed in greater detail in Chapter 8), adds high-profile, albeit limited, protection for patient information privacy.

Examples of actionable public disclosure invasion of privacy abound in the health care setting. Health care attorneys frequently say at continuing education courses that any lawyer could discover almost any private fact about a patient just by walking through the corridors of a hospital and listening to what others say. Hopefully, this assertion is not factual. However, actions such as the release of patient information from medical records without patient authorization, revelation of a patient's human immunodeficiency virus status or sexual preferences, and disclosure of other private facts about a patient, among other actions, may give rise to public disclosure invasion of privacy litigation. Consider the following hypothetical example:

B is a 32-year-old female patient with a diagnosis of hemorrhoids. B is being evaluated for treatment by C, a physician's assistant. During the course of evaluation, C notices that B has significant prominent stretch marks on her abdomen from her two previous pregnancies, a fact that B struggles to keep private. After B's initial treatment session, she leaves the hospital and is scheduled to return the next day for follow-up. While in the cafeteria with fellow staff professionals later that day, C reveals, in the course of a conversation about pregnancy, that B has prominent stretch marks on her abdomen. This revelation—even though factual and even if considered trivial by those who hear it—constitutes actionable public disclosure invasion of privacy.

Sexual Misconduct

The incidence of allegations of sexual misconduct involving professionals is disproportionately high in the health care environment. The fact that sexual misconduct involving health care professionals and patients occurs at alarmingly high rates tarnishes the reputation of all health care disciplines. This section describes sexual misconduct that constitutes sexual assault and battery and other impermissible forms of sexual contact, such as meretricious consensual sexual relations between providers and patients. The discussion in this section does not extensively address the topic of employment-related sexual harassment. Sexual harassment is discussed in greater detail in Chapter 5.

Clinical health care professions are, of necessity, hands-on professions. Health care professionals at all levels spend substantial time in close physical contact with patients during their care.

Health care professionals elicit and assess a great deal of personal information about patients during the course of patient history taking and examination and assimilate this information into care plans. In the ensuing professional relationships, health care professionals become privy to many intimate details about patients' private lives. Just as in psychotherapy, law, and religion, patients who share their intimate thoughts may experience **transference** with their health care providers, within the therapeutic relationships.

A patient may be vulnerable to abuse because of the trust that the patient places in his or her health care professional. The patient may develop intense affection for his or her treating clinician and may sense an urgent need for approval, creating a kind of parent-child relationship. Romantic feelings may develop as well. These transference emotions are normal phenomenon in a patient and must not be exploited by health care professionals responsible for the patient's care.

A health care professional serves as a fiduciary to his or her patient, meaning that the provider has a legal and ethical duty to act principally in the patient's best interests. Therefore, one of the highest duties incumbent upon a health care professional is to ensure that the professional-patient relationship does not turn into an intimate, personal, or sexual relationship. Any reciprocal countertransference of feelings that arise in the clinician must be sublimated in order to prevent the sexual abuse of the patient. Even when not prohibited by law, sexual relations with patients during the pendancy of the provider-patient professional relationship are always wrong.

From a legal perspective, there are two possible classifications of sexual abuse involving health care professionals and patients. The first type of health care–related sexual abuse is **sexual assault** or battery, which can be defined as any nonconsensual touching of a patient's or health care provider's sexual or other body parts (or clothing) by the other party, for the purpose of arousing or gratifying the sexual desires of either party to the relationship, or for the purpose of sexually abusing a patient.[25]

Commission, by a health care professional, of sexual assault or battery upon a patient can give rise to civil liability, not only for the tort of malicious intentional sexual assault or battery but also for intentional infliction of emotional distress and professional negligence. Concomitant legal and adverse administrative actions may also ensue in criminal court, before state licensing and board certification entities, before judicial committees of professional associations of which the offender is a member, and before credentials committees at institutions where the offender holds clinical privileges.

A finding of civil liability against a health care professional for sexual assault or battery may result in a civil court award of punitive (punishment) damages against the wrongdoer and in favor of the patient-victim in addition to the normal compensatory damages for lost wages, medical expenses, and pain and suffering incurred by the victim. A finding of liability for a malicious intentional tort and the award of punitive damages may mean that the defendant-provider's professional liability insurer is relieved of the legal responsibility for indemnifying the provider for the judgment, making the provider personally liable for the monetary judgment rendered against him or her.

The second type of health care–related sexual abuse involves meretricious and specious provider-patient intimate relationships labeled **consensual.** In such relationships a patient falls in love with his or her health care provider and the provider reciprocates. Because of transference of emotions, the inherent vulnerability of patients dependent upon their providers for care and support, and providers' fiduciary duty of good faith and trust toward their patients, the concept of "consent" on the part of patients to sexually intimate meretricious relationships with health care professionals responsible for their care has no real meaning. The health care professional is always singularly responsible for the creation of such a relationship. Patients, however, are not bound by professional ethical or legal standards for their behavior in provider-patient intimate relationships.

> The concept of "consent" on the part of patients to sexually intimate meretricious relationships with health care professionals responsible for their care has no real meaning.

In the legal profession, the ethical rules prohibiting sex between attorneys and clients are not as clear or comprehensive as they are for most health care professionals. Rule 1.8j of the American Bar Association's Model Rules of Professional Conduct reads, "A lawyer shall not have sexual relations with a client unless a consensual sexual relationship existed between them when the client-lawyer relationship commenced." Only 19 states have adopted this or similar rules of conduct governing attorney-client sexual relations.[26] The Disciplinary Rule 5-111 of New York only prohibits sexual relations that are coercive with most law clients, except for domestic relations cases, where such relations are prohibited altogether.

From the viewpoint of many legal commentators, these approaches fail to recognize the fact that any sexual relationship between a professional and client is inherently potentially exploitative and therefore to be avoided at all costs. A more reasoned approach to nonconsensual and putative "consensual" sexual relationships between professionals and their clients or patients is one that, considering the fragile psychological and emotional status of patients (and legal and other clients) and the actual impropriety or appearance of impropriety of such relationships, prohibits them altogether.

EXERCISE

Access the professional code of ethics of your discipline. Find the provision, if any, addressing sexual relations between members of your profession and patients or clients. Conduct a comparative search of the professional codes of ethics of at least two other health disciplines.

What should a health care professional do when an intimate relationship with a patient cannot be avoided? Because most health care professional ethics codes prohibit an intimate relationship simultaneously with a professional-patient relationship, a provider who is about to enter into an intimate relationship with a patient, despite this prohibition, must expeditiously disengage from further care of the patient and take appropriate steps to transfer the patient, with appropriate coordination, to another competent health care professional. Some authorities have suggested a minimum 6-month waiting period before commencing any intimate relations.[27]

Health care clinical professionals and managers and administrators have the legal and ethical duty to take all appropriate measures to prevent allegations of sexual abuse and actual sexual abuse of patients in the health care delivery environment. Simple risk-management measures that can be implemented include the following:

- Provide a same-sex chaperone for observation of patient evaluation and treatment, available upon patient request or when a health care provider believes that the chaperone's presence is required.
- Implement a "knock-and-enter" clinic policy, under which any staff member having a need to open a closed door to a room in which a patient and provider are located may do so after giving due warning by knocking.
- Establish an informed consent policy that ensures that patients understand the nature of all questions asked during patient history taking and of all therapeutic procedures—especially those that are intensively hands-on—and always obtain informed consent before initiating them.
- Provide ongoing continuing education to professional and support staff on how to prevent sexual abuse and harassment.

Sexual Abuse

The incidence of sexual abuse of patients is well documented and publicized in the professional and popular literature. Sexual abuse is estimated to occur in 7 to 11 percent of encounters between patients and psychotherapists, family practice physicians, gynecologists, internists, and surgeons. A similar prevalence is estimated for attorneys, clergy, educators, and social workers. Sexual abuse of these patients ranges from verbal abuse to sexual intimacies (including kissing and fondling) to sexual intercourse. Of the total number of reported cases of sexual abuse involving psychiatrists and patients, 80 percent are estimated to involve male therapists and female patients; 13 percent, female therapists and female patients; 5 percent, male therapists and male patients; and 2 percent, female therapists and male patients.[28]

CRIMINAL LAW

A licensed or certified health care provider confronted with an allegation of professional misconduct may face legal action in one or more of the following venues based on a single incident: (1) in civil court, for health care malpractice; (2) in adverse administrative proceedings affecting one's professional license and/or certification; (3) before a judicial committee of a professional association of which the respondent is a member, for a violation of professional ethics; and (4) in criminal court. All of these judicial and administrative legal actions may take place simultaneously, but more probably will be conducted at different times because of docketing, evidentiary, and other considerations.

Health care professionals, like other business professionals and citizens in general, are directly affected as potential victims by the rampant violent crime wave sweeping the United States and by so-called nonviolent, "white-collar" crime while at work,[29] home, or elsewhere. Reported criminal legal case files also reveal that health care professionals are no less subject to being charged as perpetrators of crime than other similarly situated professionals. The primary purpose for the material presented in this chapter is to familiarize health care professionals with basic criminal law and procedure so that they understand it better and have a healthy respect for its power.

Classifications and Types of Criminal Actions

Unlike morals and ethics, which govern the conduct of select individuals or groups of persons, the law compels all persons within its reach (jurisdiction) to comply with its mandates. The purpose of law, then, is to delineate what constitutes socially unacceptable conduct and to impose sanctions for noncompliance. A crime may be generally defined as conduct that violates a recognized duty owed to society as a whole, for which society will demand satisfaction.[30]

With few exceptions,[31] conviction for all crimes requires a bifurcated form of proof of culpability: (1) proof of commission of a criminal act (the *actus reus*, Latin for "guilty act"); and (2) proof of a wrongful state of mind *(mens rea)*. Criminal law recognizes varying degrees of *mens rea* along a continuum, ranging from **specific,** malicious criminal intent at one extreme to **criminal negligence** (gross negligence or recklessness) at the other extreme.

There are many ways to classify crimes. For instance, crimes are classified according to whether they affect persons or property interests and whether they involve, or do not involve, allegations of **moral turpitude.**[32] As alluded to previously, crimes may also be classified as violent or nonviolent offenses.

Criminal activity is also classified as *mala in se* (Latin for "wrongs in themselves") or *mala prohibita* (Latin for "prohibited acts"). *Mala in se* crimes include wrongful acts that are clearly criminal, such as the wrongful use of violence against another person (e.g., robbery) and fraud offenses. *Mala in se* crimes are often also labeled as "substantive" offenses.

Mala prohibita crimes, however, consist of "petty" offenses that are only criminal law violations because society says that they are so. *Mala prohibita* crimes are not inherently wrongful. Offenses such as speeding while driving a motor vehicle, minor building code violations, and failure to maintain a current vehicle registration are examples of *mala prohibita* "criminal" offenses.[33]

The two basic types of crimes are misdemeanor offenses and felony crimes. **Misdemeanor** offenses include crimes of relatively minor importance, such as moving traffic violations, which generally are punishable by incarceration for less than 1 year and/or fines of less than $1000. Jurisdictions may subdivide misdemeanor offenses into categories, or classes, ranging from A (most serious) to C (least serious).

Crime: Any social harm defined and made punishable by law.

Felony crimes include all of the classic serious offenses, such as felonious homicide, robbery, burglary, rape, and fraud. Felonies are generally punishable by imprisonment for greater than 1 year and in some cases even by death. Like misdemeanors, felonies are often subdivided into categories, or degrees, ranging from capital offenses (punishable by death) to third-degree offenses (punishable by a maximum of 5 years' imprisonment).[34]

Public Interest

Unlike tort (civil) legal actions, which involve disputes between private parties over "private wrongs," criminal legal actions involve disputes between the state and a private defendant over "public wrongs." The term *the state* is intended to be inclusive of all governmental prosecutorial entities, at the city, county or parish, state, and federal levels.

Crimes, then, are wrongs against society and social order. Society exclusively circumscribes what conduct is and is not criminal (by statute), and societal interests are satisfied through sentencing when an alleged criminal offender is convicted of a crime. An individual crime victim does not have an absolute right to have a criminal case prosecuted. Criminal prosecution is largely discretionary to public prosecutors.

Criminal legal cases differ, then, in many respects from civil (tort) cases that may emanate from the same wrongful conduct. Criminal wrongs are public wrongs against society as a whole, whereas torts (e.g., health care professional intentional [mis]conduct malpractice) are private wrongs against the personal interests of private victims. Criminal cases are prosecuted at the discretion of public officials, whereas private parties prosecute civil tort cases. Also, criminal law is largely statutory law, whereas tort law may be statute-based but largely is common (judicial) law.

Parties

In tort cases and other forms of civil litigation, the parties to the cases are private parties—individuals, business entities, and even governmental entities. Civil cases are captioned ("titled") with the private litigants' names. For example, a physical therapy malpractice case might be captioned, *Smith by Smith*[35] *v. Doe, R.N.*

In criminal cases, however, cases are captioned with the title of the governmental entity as plaintiff and the name of the private defendant. A criminal case against a physical therapist might be captioned, *People* (or State, Commonwealth, or United States) v. *Doe, R.N.* The victim of a crime is not a party in a criminal case.

> The victim of a crime is not a party in a criminal case.

Elements and Burdens of Proof in Criminal Cases

In tort cases, civil plaintiffs must fulfill their evidentiary burden of proving specific elements of the torts in issue in order to prevail. For example, in a health care (professional negligence) malpractice case brought by a patient against a health acre professional, the patient must specifically prove each of the following elements:

1. The defendant–health care professional owed a duty of special care to the plaintiff-patient
2. The defendant-provider somehow breached or violated the duty owed in the course of professional care delivery
3. The defendant's breach of professional duty caused the patient to sustain injury
4. The injuries sustained by the patient warrant the payment of monetary damages in order to make the patient "whole"

The civil plaintiff must prove all of the required elements of his or her case by a preponderance (or greater weight) of evidence to the satisfaction of a civil jury or a judge.

In a criminal prosecution, the state's attorney-plaintiff also bears the entire legal burden to prove the state's case against a criminal defendant. Each and every statutory element of a crime must be proved in order to prevail. Failure of proof of any material element of a criminal case results in acquittal (a finding of "not guilty").

In part because of the relative potential severity of criminal sanctions (compared with civil sanctions) and in part because of constitutional, statutory, and judicially imposed safeguards designed to protect the rights of criminal defendants, the quantum of proof required for a criminal conviction is much greater than that required to prevail in a civil case. The state's representative in a criminal case must convince a trier of fact of a criminal defendant's culpability beyond a reasonable doubt in order to merit a guilty verdict. This lofty standard of proof requires that the criminal defendant's guilt be proved to a "moral certainty" so that there is no legitimate, lingering question concerning the defendant's culpability in the minds of any jurors or in that of the judge.

Why is such a high burden of proof required of government prosecutors in criminal cases? The adage goes, "Society would rather free a truly guilty defendant than to wrongfully convict an innocent one." The adverse consequences to a criminal defendant's life, liberty, and property interests are potentially so severe that the strongest proof of culpability under the law is required for a conviction.

A verdict of "not guilty" in a criminal case does not equate to a lack of culpability on the part of the defendant. The verdict simply stands for the proposition that a unanimous finding of guilty beyond a reasonable doubt could not legitimately be reached by the fact finders in the case. As O.J. Simpson (and interested parties following his very public legal cases) discovered in 1995, a finding of not guilty in a criminal case does not preclude the institution of a civil case based on the exact same facts that formed the basis for criminal prosecution. The "not guilty" finding in the criminal case only precludes retrial in the same jurisdiction (i.e., state or federal system) of the defendant for the same offense. This Fifth Amendment constitutional protection against criminal retrial is called double jeopardy.

Defenses to Criminal Actions

Like the civil law system, the criminal legal system recognizes a number of defenses to criminal charges that defendants can attempt to take advantage of in order to escape liability. Some of these defenses operate as complete defenses to exonerate defendants from any criminal liability, whereas others are incomplete defenses that may serve to exonerate criminal defendants of some, but not all, offenses. Normally, the burden of establishing (proving) affirmative defenses is incumbent upon criminal defendants, not the state.

Examples of legitimate defenses to criminal charges include alibi, automatism (a state of unconsciousness), coercion, consent (of the victim), defense of others, duress, entrapment, immunity from prosecution, infancy, intoxication, insanity, mistake of fact or (sometimes) of law, self-defense, and expiration of the statute of limitations. The following comments are intended only to introduce some key concepts about selected defenses to criminal liability, not to be an exhaustive overview of this area of law.

In the health care delivery setting, public policy considerations do not permit the use of the defense of patient consent (in civil or criminal litigation) to wrongful conduct on the part of a defendant–health care provider. Self-defense and defense of others (including of staff, patients, and visitors in health care environments) do allow for the use of anticipatory or reciprocal force to prevent or to repel the imminent application of criminal force. The objective entrapment defense normally requires that a criminal defendant not be predisposed to commit a crime in the absence of an unlawful inducement by law enforcement officials or agents. Mistake of law is normally a tenuous defense, unless a criminal defendant can prove justifiable reliance on an official, erroneous pronouncement of law. Generally, though, the adage, "ignorance of the law is no excuse" applies.

The fact that a criminal defendant is a minor may operate as a defense to successful prosecution. This defense is known as the "infancy" defense. At early common law, minors 7 years of age or younger could not be held to account for criminal conduct at all. For minors between the ages of 7 and 14, there was at common law a rebuttable presumption that the minor was incapable of forming the *mens rea* to commit a criminal act, which the state could try to rebut in order to try the minor as an adult for the offense. Between ages 14 and the age of legal majority, the rebuttable presumption at common law was that the minor could form the requisite criminal intent to commit any crime, and the legal burden to rebut that presumption rested with the minor's criminal defense attorney. Most states have retained this approach to holding minors responsible for criminal acts, whereas other states have enacted other systems for liability determination.

The defense of intoxication may relieve a criminal defendant of legal responsibility for criminal conduct, particularly if the actor's intoxication was involuntary, that is, he or she was drugged or forced to imbibe alcohol. Even voluntary intoxication may operate as a complete defense to crimes that require a specific criminal intent, such as murder, sexual battery, and fraud. Voluntary intoxication cannot successfully be proffered as a defense to crimes where the required culpable mental state is recklessness or criminal negligence, as in most crimes arising from driving while intoxicated or, in the case of health care providers, treating patients while impaired.

Courts use several tests to adjudge whether a criminal defendant is insane. The federal system uses a standard developed after President Reagan was shot by John Hinckley. Under this standard, a defendant must prove the following by clear and convincing evidence:

> As a result of severe mental disease or defect, the defendant was unable to appreciate nature and quality or the wrongfulness of his or her act(s).[36]

Other jurisdictions use a more traditional rule of decision, the M'Naghten test, which excuses criminal behavior under the defense of insanity if the defendant is incapable, because of a substantial mental defect, from distinguishing right from wrong.[37] Courts differ on whether a criminal defendant bears the burden of proving insanity (by a preponderance of, or clear and convincing, evidence) or whether the state bears the legal burden of establishing a criminal defendant's sanity (beyond a reasonable doubt).

Anticipatory or reciprocal deadly force may legitimately be used to prevent or repel deadly force (i.e., force reasonably likely to cause imminent serious bodily harm or death). The statute of limitations defense is similar to the civil health care malpractice statute of limitations defense. The statute of limitations is a time bar to initiation of legal action. Although some defenses, such as the failure of police to comply with Miranda rights warnings,[38] are Constitution-based, the defense of statute of limitations is purely a technical defense. This means that a criminal defendant who successfully invokes it literally "gets off on a technicality." The statute of limitations does not apply to two criminal offenses: murder and treason.

Criminal Procedure

Unlike the civil legal system, in which both parties to a lawsuit are simultaneously aided and impeded by the same procedural rules regarding evidence, testimony, and burdens of proof, in criminal procedure, a criminal defendant enjoys substantially greater protection than the state. This is so primarily because of the dire potential consequences to the defendant of a conviction, including imprisonment, loss of reputation and citizen privileges, and even imposition of the death penalty.

Special federal constitutional rights operate in favor of criminal defendants. These rights include the following:

- Fourth Amendment protection against (most) warrantless searches and seizures of property and against unreasonable searches and seizures of property and the person of the defendant

- Fifth Amendment requirement for fundamental fairness in judicial proceedings: "due process of law," prevention of involuntary self-incrimination by the defendant, and protection against retrial, after acquittal, for the same charges (double jeopardy)
- Sixth Amendment rights to have the assistance of personal legal counsel, to have a speedy and public trial, to confront adverse witnesses before and at trial, and to have one's criminal action heard before a jury of one's peers (i.e., citizens drawn from the local community)
- Eighth Amendment rights not to be subjected to cruel or unusual punishment or to have excessive bail or criminal fines imposed before or at trial

Statutes, case law, and state constitutions may afford criminal defendants even greater rights than those enumerated in the federal Constitution. These sources of law, however, may not limit or take away the basic federal constitutional rights of criminal defendants. The following section describes basic criminal procedures common to all jurisdictions: arrest, indictment or information, arraignment, pre-trial (discovery) processes, trial, and appeal.

Arrest

In the United States, unlike in many other countries, individuals generally enjoy the right to be free from unreasonable intrusion on their privacy and freedom of movement from the police and the state. Although police may temporarily detain anyone based on reasonable suspicion of criminal activity, they may not arrest a person without probable cause, that is, evidence of a substantial likelihood that (1) a crime has been committed and (2) the person to be arrested committed the crime.

Before questioning an arrestee about criminal activity, police officials must apprise the person being subjected to custodial interrogation of his or her Miranda rights, which are based on the Fifth Amendment right against self-incrimination. The Miranda warnings consist of the following points:

- The right not to speak to police about any offense
- The fact that anything said might be used by police and, by the state, against the person
- The right to have an attorney present during questioning and to have the government provide an attorney, if the arrestee cannot afford to retain one[39]

Without proof that these rights were explained to a criminal defendant and proof that the defendant waived, or gave up, the right to not to speak, evidence obtained from any subsequent interrogation (directly or indirectly) may normally not be used against the defendant in a criminal trial.

Indictment or Information

After arrest and processing, a grand jury, a magistrate, or another judicial official determines anew whether probable cause exists to bind the suspect over for criminal trial. The formal complaint that results is called an indictment (if issued by a grand jury) or an information (if issued by a public official).

Arraignment

After the issuance of a formal indictment or information, the criminal suspect is arraigned, that is, brought before a trial judge to be apprised of the formal charges against him or her and to be required to enter a plea (answer) to the charges. Most criminal cases are disposed of without resort to a full trial by plea bargaining, in which criminal defendants and prosecutors bargain over specific offenses to be pleaded guilty to, sentencing limitations, and conditions to be imposed on the parties. Conditions include cooperation and assistance by the defendant in other prosecutions and recommendations of the prosecutor regarding sentencing, among others. A plea bargain is an express business contract between a criminal defendant and a criminal prosecutor and a necessary instrument for any semblance of efficiency in the operation of a very busy legal system.

Pre-trial (Discovery) Processes

Pre-trial discovery in criminal cases is similar to discovery processes in civil cases. During this period, the prosecution and the defense interview witnesses and prospective witnesses, locate and examine evidence, and formulate trial strategies and tactics. Plea bargaining often continues during pre-trial discovery. The state has the affirmative legal duty to turn over expeditiously to the defense any exonerative and exculpatory evidence. Judges order the parties to appear in court for pre-trial conferences and hearings (especially in the federal court system) to monitor processes and to narrow issues.

Trial

As described before in this chapter, at trial a criminal defendant nominally has no legal burdens. He or she is presumed innocent until proved guilty by the state, beyond any legitimate, reasonable doubt. Even in the face of seemingly overwhelming physical and testimonial evidence against a criminal defendant, a "not guilty" verdict can result. This is what happened in 1995 in the celebrated California case of *People v. O.J. Simpson*. Despite substantial public dissatisfaction with the decision, it must fairly be conceded that the jury could have legitimately found reasonable doubt, based on alleged racism and evidence tampering on the part of former Los Angeles Police Detective Mark Fuhrman.

Appeal

Whenever a guilty verdict results in a criminal case, the defendant has an absolute right to appeal the case for a review of legal and factual issues by an appellate court. At the appellate level, the case is largely a "paper case," without live witnesses or the presence of another jury.

Although it is often said that a defendant enjoys the right to appeal his or her case to the U.S. Supreme Court, such is not the case. The U.S. Supreme Court reviews selected criminal cases as a matter of judicial discretion and normally hears only those cases presenting important constitutional issues.

State and Federal Jurisdiction and Interests

The overwhelming majority of criminal cases are tried in state courts because such cases exclusively affect intrastate interests. The Tenth Amendment to the U.S. Constitution reserves the general "police power" to the states as follows:

> The powers not delegated to the United States by the Constitution, nor prohibited by it to the States, are reserved to the States respectively, or to the people.[40]

Federal criminal courts try cases involving criminal activity having interstate, national, or international effects, such as drug and mail fraud cases, crimes committed on federal installations and against federal officials, and immigration cases. Federal criminal and civil procedure may differ greatly from that of state court systems.

Remedies and Sentencing Principles

In civil tort legal system the principal purpose of a liability award in a given case is to make a tort victim "whole." Remedies in tort are flexible and are largely based on judicial precedent guided by the principle of *stare decisis*.[41] In the criminal legal system, however, remedies are primarily based on statute and are more formalized for specific offenses. Criminal court judges may be required to comply with relatively rigid sentencing guidelines (as in the federal system) when sentencing criminal defendants.

In a criminal case the remedy awarded reflects societal needs and concerns, as well as any impact on individual victims of crime. The criminal law equivalent to the civil remedy of monetary damages is incarceration or the threat of incarceration (probation) of a criminal defendant. A criminal sentence serves to make society whole, in a sense, by punishing the criminal wrongdoer.

The factors that are considered in arriving at a criminal sentence, referred to as sentencing principles, reflect societal needs for the following:

- Retribution, or punishment of an offender, that is, "just desserts"
- Isolation of a dangerous offender from members of society
- Specific deterrence of further criminal activity by a convicted criminal
- General deterrence of others who know of a criminal's conduct and might otherwise be tempted to emulate it
- Rehabilitation of an offender to make him or her a productive member of society

A specific sentence in a given case reflects how a sentencing authority (judge or jury) weighs and prioritizes these sentencing principles. In addition to incarceration or probation, a criminal defendant may be ordered to make monetary restitution to a crime victim or to multiple victims. A convicted criminal may also face a criminal monetary fine as part of sentencing and risk the forfeiture of personal property and assets, either those used in the commission of a crime or those obtained with illicit assets as "fruits" of the crime.

Crimes in the Health Care Environment

Crimes of Violence

Health care-related crimes have the same elements of proof as general crimes of violence. However, the additional consideration is patient-victims are particularly vulnerable to exploitation because health professional-perpetrators are fiduciaries, owing special duties of trust and fidelity to their patients.

Assault and Battery

Criminal assault and battery are essentially the same under criminal law as under civil law. Assault involves the apprehension or fear, on the part of a victim, of impending unlawful harmful or offensive contact. Battery involves the unlawful application of harmful or offensive force, by a perpetrator, to the person of a victim.

A subclassification of criminal battery that too frequently arises as an allegation in the health care environment is criminal sexual battery. Such battery involves any nonconsensual touching of a patient's or a health care provider's sexual or other body parts (or clothing) by the other party, for the purpose of arousing or gratifying the sexual desires of either party, or for the purpose of sexually abusing a patient.

A health care provider facing an allegation, or multiple allegations, of sexual assault or battery incident to patient care may be required to defend himself or herself in criminal court and in civil court and before licensure boards and professional association ethics committees. Conviction of a health care professional of sexual assault or battery of a patient in a criminal trial provides overwhelming evidence in the form of a public record that can be readily obtained and used against the provider in civil, administrative, and professional association proceedings.

Robbery

Robbery may be defined as the unlawful, forcible taking of a victim's property from the person of the victim. Robbery is distinguished from other unlawful seizures of property, such as larceny and burglary, in that (1) the property seized is taken directly from the person of the victim (as in a mugging) and (2) there is involved the use or threat of force. Thus theft of property that occurs while a victim is asleep—a hospital patient, for example—would not constitute robbery because no force was used or threatened. Similarly, when a pickpocket lifts a victim's wallet—in the hospital or in any other setting—the crime committed is larceny, but not robbery. A criminal charge of robbery may be elevated from simple to aggravated robbery if a deadly weapon is brandished during the crime or if the victim suffers serious injury during the unlawful taking of the victim's property.

Homicide

Homicide literally means the killing of one human being by another. Many patient deaths occur in health care settings. Most patient deaths, however, do not give rise to criminal charges against health care professionals. Some patient deaths facilitated by health care professionals, however, such as through the unlawful practice of

active euthanasia, may give rise to criminal prosecution. A few criminal cases against physicians and other providers have been publicized in recent years, the most notorious being the Michigan state court prosecutions against Dr. Jack Kevorkian, a former pathologist, for alleged physician-assisted suicide. Kevorkian was convicted of second-degree murder on April 13, 1999, for assisting amyotrophic lateral sclerosis patient Thomas Youk to end his life with a lethal injection that was recorded by Kevorkian on videotape. In all, Kevorkian reportedly assisted 130 persons to commit suicide.[42]

Health care providers responsible for the deaths of patients under their care may be charged criminally with any of the following homicide offenses.

Criminal homicide constitutes murder when (a) it is committed purposely or knowingly or (b) it is committed recklessly under circumstances manifesting extreme indifference to the value of human life. Such recklessness and indifference are presumed if the actor is engaged or is an accomplice in the commission of, or is attempting to commit robbery, rape or deviate sexual intercourse by force or threat of force, arson, burglary, kidnapping, or felonious escape.[43]

In addition to a specific intent to murder, the state of mind of extreme criminal negligence constituting a "depraved heart" can be a basis for conviction for murder.

Manslaughter

Manslaughter involves a less culpable state of mind than murder and can be defined as an unlawful homicide without malice, or the specific intent to kill the victim. This crime can be subdivided into voluntary and involuntary manslaughter.

Voluntary. **Voluntary manslaughter** involves a victim's death that occurs during the commission of some unlawful act, such as during a fight arising from the "heat of passion."[44] The death of a patient during an illegal abortion would probably give rise to a charge of voluntary manslaughter against a physician performing the abortion.

Involuntary. Involuntary manslaughter occurs when a victim dies during the (reckless) commission of a lawful act.[45] Consider the following hypothetical example:

> *A patient with extensive third-degree burns is being treated by a physical therapist in a whirlpool tub. A radio is positioned by the therapist on the edge of the tub to distract the patient's attention during débridement. If the radio falls into the water, causing the electrocution death of the patient, the most likely unlawful homicide charge against the physical therapist would be involuntary manslaughter because the patient's death arguably occurred during the (reckless) commission of an otherwise lawful act.*

Negligent Homicide

Negligent homicide involves the death of a victim caused by another person, where the latter's conduct constitutes gross negligence. Gross negligence is conduct that falls well below the standards established by law for the reasonable protection of others. As with involuntary manslaughter, in criminally negligent homicide, the perpetrator displays neither wanton depravity nor any specific intent to kill another human being. Most homicide charges lodged against health care professionals for patient deaths are labeled as criminally negligent homicide.

Nonviolent Crimes

Fortunately for patient safety and the safety of others, most criminal activity that occurs in health care settings involves the commission of nonviolent, or so-called "white-collar" offenses. However, nonviolent crime arguably has an equally devastating impact as violent crime does on society in general and on business in particular. The following are selected examples of nonviolent crimes that affect business (including the business of health care delivery).

Burglary

Burglary is now defined as the unlawful breaking and entry (trespass) onto another person's property with the specific intent to commit a felony crime on the victim's premises. Although the felony crime intended to be committed may be a violent offense, most often the intended felony is larceny. An example of burglary is when a thief breaks into a health care clinic at night to steal a computer that is visible through a closed window. As with robbery, a burglary charge can be elevated to **aggravated burglary** if a deadly weapon is used in commission of the crime.

Larceny

Larceny is defined as the unlawful taking of another person's property with the intent to deprive the true owner of its use permanently. Threshold amounts for the value of property taken determine whether the crime to be charged is a misdemeanor (**petit larceny**) or a felony (**grand larceny**). Shoplifting is a form of larceny, as is stealing a vehicle (grand theft auto).

Embezzlement

Embezzlement is theft of money or other property by someone in a fiduciary (special trust) relationship with the victim. Unlike in larceny, the embezzler is in lawful possession or engaged in lawful use of the victim's property at some point. Although the eventual return of the victim's property may operate in **extenuation and mitigation** to reduce the severity of a criminal sentence, the crime of embezzlement is complete once the wrongful misappropriation occurs.

Employment and Reimbursement Fraud

Fraud in any setting involves the unlawful misrepresentation of a material fact, specifically intended to deceive a victim and cause him or her to act to the victim's detriment. The U.S. Government Accountability Office estimated that for fiscal year 2004, $20 billion of $297 billion in total Medicare and Medicaid expenditures were lost to fraud.[46] HIPAA provides funding for federal anti–health care fraud law enforcement activities. In 2001 the Department of Justice successfully prosecuted 465 defendants in health fraud cases.[47]

Although most health care fraud involves active misrepresentation to third-party payers of health care (non)delivery, passive fraud is of growing concern, especially under managed care models. Passive managed care health fraud (more accurately "abuse") involves deliberate underprovision of health care to plan beneficiaries to prop up profits. This area of fraud and abuse is more difficult to investigate, ferret out, and eliminate. However, state and federal agencies are making slow, incremental progress against it.

An interesting example of (pre)employment fraud involved Eugene Roscoe, who purportedly was a physical therapist. Roscoe reportedly "earned" more than $100,000 per year from job interviews. He allegedly undertook job interviews in 38 states before his arrest in Houston, Texas. Reportedly, Roscoe was never licensed.[48]

Corporate Crime

Perhaps the fiercest weapon that federal law enforcement authorities have in the fight against corporate crime—violent and nonviolent—is RICO, or the Racketeer Influenced and Corrupt Organizations Act,[49] which Congress enacted as part of the Organized Crime Control Act of 1970. Although authorities reasonably debate the intended scope for RICO, it has been used successfully to curb the encroachment of organized crime into legitimate business—including health care delivery. RICO makes interstate racketeering activity a federal felony crime that may be prosecuted anyplace along the trail of criminal activity. Racketeering includes the unlawful commission of (or **conspiracy** [unlawful agreement] **to commit**) two or more of 26 enumerated federal felonies or 9 specified state law offenses.[50] In addition to criminal prosecution under RICO, the government and private individuals may sue defendants civilly for monetary damages.

The USA Patriot Act[51] was modeled after RICO. The Patriot Act was enacted post–September 11, 2001, to give the federal government new tools to fight domestic and international terrorism. The controversial Patriot Act, reauthorized by Congress on March 2, 2006, expands surveillance, wiretapping, detention, and expulsion powers of law enforcement authorities. Many persons believe that the Patriot Act unduly encroaches on civil liberties. Under the current president's interpretation of the law, all international phone calls are subject to interception and eavesdropping, with or without court order.

One of the most publicized health care corporate fraud legal cases involved Richard Scrushy, the former CEO of HealthSouth. The federal government charged Scrushy with conspiracy, false reporting, fraud, money laundering, and violating Sarbanes-Oxley (a federal statute discussed in detail in Chapter 6.) Scrushy faced life in prison and several millions of dollars in fines. He did not take the stand in his own defense. The jury in Birmingham, Alabama, acquitted him of all charges on June 28, 2005. Scrushy was found guilty of bribery in a subsequent federal case on June 29, 2006, along with former Alabama governor Don Siegelman.[52]

SUMMARY

Liability for intentional conduct may have more seriously adverse consequences for health care professionals than does liability for professional or ordinary negligence. For intentional acts that are found to be malicious, such as sexual battery, health care professionals may face loss of licensure and professional association membership, as well as personal monetary liability for an adverse judgment because insurers are generally not legally obligated to indemnify their insured against such losses.

The types of tortious conduct that can give rise to intentional tort liability range from assault and battery to defamation of character to fraud, among other volitional conduct. Allegations and the commission of sexual assault and battery by health care providers against patients pose a serious threat to the professional reputations of all hands-on health care disciplines. Health care clinicians, managers, and administrators must work together, proactively and aggressively, to prevent such allegations from arising in all health care practice settings.

Regarding defamation of character, one important exception to intentional tort liability involves compliance with statutory reporting requirements, under which health care professionals are obligated to report to authorities suspected child, domestic (spousal), and elder abuse. A good faith report by a health care professional, grounded in reasonable suspicion, will not result in defamation liability, even if the report is unsubstantiated by authorities.

Because one must act consciously and deliberately in order to be held liable for intentional conduct, careful thought before taking any official action incident to patient care delivery is perhaps the best, as well as the simplest, risk management measure that health care professionals can undertake to dampen intentional tort liability.

The application of criminal law to health care has received ever-increasing attention in recent years. Out of a single act or omission—such as the wrongful injury to or death of a patient—a health care professional can face legal action in civil and criminal court, as well as adverse administrative action before licensure boards and professional associations.

A criminal act almost always requires culpable conduct *(actus reus)* and a culpable state of mind *(mens rea)* to subject a defendant to possible criminal liability. Violent (e.g., sexual battery) and nonviolent (e.g., reimbursement fraud) criminal offenses are on the rise in the health care environment, as are federal and state investigatory and prosecutorial efforts. RICO has given criminal prosecutors a most formidable weapon to brandish and use in the fight against health care fraud and other related racketeering activities.

CASES AND QUESTIONS

1. A nurse practitioner attending a risk management seminar inquires about risk management measures that should be taken to prevent misunderstandings about the nature of therapeutic touch in an intensively hands-on gynecological practice. What would you advise the audience to do?
2. You are an occupational therapist in a multispecialty outpatient rehabilitation clinic. The clinic's manager and co-owner of the private group practice directs you to bill Medicare for patient no-shows at one half the billing rate of normal clinic visits. Can you legally and ethically comply with the manager's order?

SUGGESTED ANSWERS TO CASES AND QUESTIONS

1. In all settings, patients should clearly understand the nature of therapeutic touch. Thorough education about procedures to be used and relevant anatomical structures, including the use of anatomical models, should help patients understand parameters of examination and recommended treatments. Patients must be given legally sufficient disclosure information

about recommended treatments so that they can make valid, voluntary, and intelligent elections of treatment. Considerations of modesty, privacy, and common sense require that health care clinicians adequately drape patients undergoing examination and treatment. Patients have the absolute right to request and have present a same-gender chaperone during evaluation and treatment. Clinics that cannot comply with these requirements must take immediate steps to rectify their noncompliant practices.

2. No. Billing for care that is not delivered under false pretenses constitutes actionable intentional fraud. A finding of defraudment against Medicare or Medicaid, known as "program-related misconduct," results in automatic exclusion from participation in these programs for a minimum of 5 years. Additional adverse action in federal (criminal) court and before licensure boards and professional associations may also result. Commission of an illegal and unethical act is not legally justified because a superior orders an employee to carry it out.

SUGGESTED READINGS

Bloom JD, Nadelson CC, Notman MT, editors: *Physician sexual misconduct,* Washington, DC, 1999, American Psychiatric Press.

Child Welfare Information Gateway: *Mandatory reporters of child abuse.* Retrieved Feb 17, 2007, from www.childwelfare.gov.

Model penal code, Philadelphia, 1981, American Law Institute (originally published in 1962).

Oslund v. *United States,* Civ. No. 4-88-323 (U.S. Dist. Court, District of Minnesota, Oct. 23, 1989); Federal Tort Claims Act lawsuit by Veterans Administration hospital patient against an occupational therapy intern.

Robinson DJ, O'Neill D: Access to health records after death: balancing confidentiality with appropriate disclosure, *JAMA* 297:634-636, 2007.

Rodriguez MA, McLoughlin E, Nah G, Campbell JC: Mandatory reporting of domestic violence injuries to the police, *JAMA* 286:580-583, 2001.

Scott RW: Sexual misconduct, *PT Magazine* 1(10):78-79, 1993.

US Constitution.

Walters R, Marin M, Curriden M: Are we getting a jury of our peers? *Texas Bar Journal* 68(2):144-146, 2005.

Williams BA: Sex, lies and bar complaints, *Virginia Lawyer Register,* pp 1-2, Nov 2001.

REFERENCES

1. There are four potential physical areas of social interaction between individuals. The public zone includes distances where physical contact is unlikely, such as in a concert hall or across a public street. The social zone includes distances of between about 4 and 12 feet and encompasses normal business relations between colleagues in an office or university environment. The personal zone involves arms-length business transactions between two or more persons and includes encounters such as an interview between a health care clinic's receptionist or provider and a patient. The intimate zone involves hands-on or skin-to-skin contact between persons. Certain health care professionals are privileged as part of their professional licensure to enter patients' intimate zones for legitimate professional purposes. For more on social distances, see Purtilo R: *Health professional and patient interaction,* ed 4, Philadelphia, 1990, WB Saunders (p 149).

2. *The hand that rocks the cradle,* Hollywood Pictures, Nov 1992.

3. In 2005, 1,390,695 violent crimes were committed in the United States. Of that number, there were 862,947 aggravated assault cases. Retrieved Feb 13, 2007, from www.fbi.gov.

4. 42 United States Code Section 11111(a)(2).

5. *New York Times* v. *Sullivan,* 376 U.S. 254 (1964).

6. 42 United States Code Section 5101 et seq.

7. 40% of health professionals admit not reporting abuse, *PT Bulletin* pp 6, 40, Feb 21, 1990.

8. *Landeros* v. *Flood,* 551 P.2d 389 (Cal. 1976); addresses potential physician liability for failure to diagnose and report battered child syndrome.

9. *Kempster* v. *Child Protective Services,* 515 N.Y.S. 2d 807 (App. Div. 1987); addresses potential liability on the part of health care professionals for making reports of suspected child abuse.

10. National Organization for Women: *Violence against women in the United States.* Retrieved Feb 13, 2007, from www.now.org .

11. Hyman A, Schillinger D, Lo B: Laws mandating reporting of domestic violence, *JAMA* 273:1781-1787, 1995.

12. Bureau of Justice Statistics: *Violent Crime.* Washington DC, 2003 US Department of Justice.

13. Kingston P, Penhale B: Elder abuse and neglect: issues in the accident and emergency department, *Accid Emerg Nurs* 3:122-128, 1995.

14. Chorba TL, Berkelman RL, Safford SK et al: Mandatory Reporting of infectious diseases by clinicians, *JAMA* 262:3018-3026, 1989.

15. Freund E, Seligman PJ, Chorba TL et al: *Mandatory reporting of occupational diseases by clinicians, JAMA* 262:3041-3044, 1989.

16. *Black's law dictionary,* ed 5, St Paul, Minn, 1979, West Publishing Company.

17. Department of Health and Human Services, Department of Justice: *Health care fraud and abuse control program annual report for FY 2005.* Retrieved Feb 14, 2007, www.usdoj. gov/dag/pubdoc/hcfacreport2005.pdf.

18. Section 1877 of the Social Security Act, 42 United States Code Section 1395nn.

19. *With Stark II Rules, CMS has tried to respond positively to industry requests for greater clarity,* Austin, Texas, April 15, 2004, Vinson & Elkins LLP.

20. 31 United States Code Section 3729 et seq.

21. Ibid. at Section 3730(d).

22. Annual Report, note 17.

23. MEDICARE: *HCFA'S USE OF ANTIFRAUD AND ABUSE FUNDING, June, 1998.* Retrieved at www.gao.gov. on Sept. 6, 2007.

24. *Griswold* v. *Connecticut,* 381 U.S. 479 (1965).

25. Adapted as a composite definition of sexual assault and battery from the following criminal law codes: *The model penal code,* Section 213.4, American Law Institute, Proposed Official Draft, 1962, and Colorado Revised Statutes, Section 18-3-401(4).

26. Brock RH: *Sex, clients, and legal ethics,* March 2001. Retrieved Feb 17, 2007, from www. texasbar.com.

27. Stromber CD, Haggarty DJ, Leibenluft RF et al: Physical contact and sexual relations with patients. In *The psychologist's legal handbook,* Washington, DC, 1988, Council for the National Register of Health Service Providers in Psychology.

28. Sherman C: Behind closed doors: therapist-client sex, *Psychology Today* 26(3):67, 1993.

29. Violence in the American workplace is a most serious human resources management problem. Between 1993 and 1999, 900 persons per year were victims of homicide in work settings, and workplace violence accounted for 18 percent of violent crimes. Mental health custodians (69/1000) and professionals (68.2/1000), nurses (21.9/1000), and physicians (16.2/1000) led health care professionals as victims of violent crimes. Bureau of Justice Statistics, US Department of Justice, Dec 20, 2001. Retrieved Feb 18, 2007, from www. ojp.usdoj.gov.

30. Adapted from *Black's law dictionary,* ed 5, St Paul, Minn, 1979, West Publishing Company.
31. For example, the crime of statutory rape, or carnal knowledge of a (usually female) child (consensual sex with a legal minor) is punishable (in most states) even if the adult party made a legitimate and reasonable mistake as to the minor's status as a minor. Valid and reasonable mistake of age eliminates *mens rea.* However, conviction under such circumstances is justified by basing it on social policy disfavoring sexual relations between adults and minors.
32. Moral turpitude describes intentionally wrongful *mala in se* criminal conduct that violates public standards of moral decency. Crimes of moral turpitude evince heinousness, vileness, and depravity. These crimes include offenses such as nonconsensual sexual relations (ranging from intercourse to lewd and lascivious behavior) between health care professionals and patients and consensual or nonconsensual sexual activity between adults and young children. Traditionally, conviction of crimes of moral turpitude was alone a legitimate basis for adverse action affecting professional licensing, certification, and health professional association membership. Now, though, the precise definition of "moral turpitude" is so difficult to articulate that it may be successfully challenged as unconstitutionally "vague" when it is invoked as a basis for adverse professional actions.
33. Perkins R: *Perkins on criminal law,* ed 2, Mineola, NY, 1969, Foundation Press.
34. See generally *Model penal code,* Philadelphia, 1981, American Law Institute (originally published in 1962).
35. The malpractice plaintiff's name in the case caption, *Smith by Smith,* indicates that Smith, a legal representative (e.g., parent or guardian), is bringing suit on behalf of Smith, the real party in interest.
36. Insanity Defense Reform Act of 1984, 18 United States Code Section 17.
37. See M'Naghten's Case, 8 Eng. Rep. 718(1843).
38. See *Miranda* v. *Arizona,* 384 U.S. 436 (U.S. Supreme Court, Chief Justice Earl Warren, 1966).
39. Baird PD: Critics must confess, Miranda was the right decision, *Wall Street Journal* p A19, June 13, 1991.
40. U.S. Constitution, Tenth Amendment, 1791.
41. *Stare decisis* is Latin for "the decision stands" and, as a legal principle, requires lower courts within a jurisdiction to abide by the prior judicial pronouncements of higher-level courts within the jurisdiction, applicable to the same or similar facts. Only when constitutional or statutory law or public policy considerations require it will case precedent normally be overturned.
42. Courttv.com: *Dr. Jack Kevorkian.* Retrieved Feb 19, 2007, from www.courttv.com/trials/famous.
43. *Model penal code,* Philadelphia, 1981, American Law Institute, Section 210.2.
44. *Model penal code,* Philadelphia, 1981, American Law Institute, Section 210.3(1)(b).
45. *Model penal code,* Philadelphia, 1981, American Law Institute, Section 210.3(1)(a).
46. US Government Accountability Office: *Medicare Fraud and Abuse.* Retrieved Feb 17, 2007, from www.gao.gov.
47. Guiney MA: *Health Insurance Portability and Accountability Act.* Retrieved Feb 17, 2007, from www.usd.edu.
48. Harlan C: He apparently succeeded better than most of us at avoiding work, *Wall Street Journal* p B1, March 14, 1991.
49. See Title 18, United States Code Sections 1961 et. seq.
50. Ibid. at Section (1)(A).
51. 18 United States Code Section 2331 et al.
52. Scrushy, former Alabama governor found guilty. Retrieved Sept 6, 2007, from www.money.cnn.com.

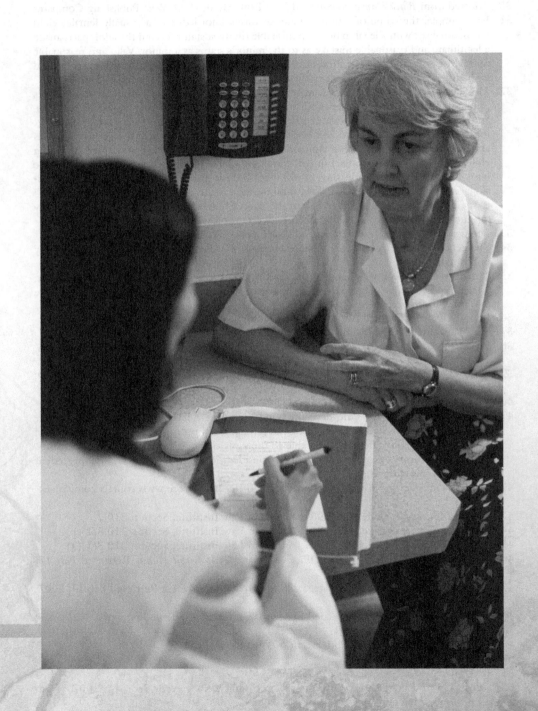

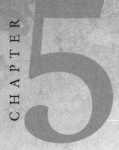
Ethical and Legal Issues in Employment

KEY TERMS

Ab initio

Defamation of character

Disability

Exculpatory drug testing

Negligent hiring

Periodic drug testing

Preemployment drug screening

Postaccident drug testing

Quid pro quo

Random drug testing

Reasonable suspicion drug testing

Restrictive covenants

Undue hardship

Whistle-blowing

Wrongful discharge

INTRODUCTION

This chapter overviews key ethical and legal employment-related issues. The principal federal statute governing employment discrimination is Title VII of the Civil Rights Act of 1964, which prohibits discrimination in all aspects of employment based on race/ethnicity, gender, religion, and national origin. Augmenting Title VII are the Americans with Disabilities Act of 1990 and the Age Discrimination in Employment Act of 1967, which prohibit employment discrimination against disabled and older workers, respectively. The vast majority of employment in the United States is "at will," meaning that the employee or employer can terminate the relationship without notice or penalty. Employment at will creates a significant job-security problem for health care professionals under managed care.

The chapter addresses in detail the ethical and legal issues surrounding sexual harassment and patient-initiated sexual behaviors. The presentation includes a detailed examination of quid pro quo and hostile work environment sexual harassment and concludes with a discussion of special duties and problems involving health care academicians, clinical faculty, and health care professional students.

EMPLOYMENT AT WILL VERSUS EMPLOYMENT UNDER CONTRACT

Traditionally, all employees were employed "at will." The vast majority of employees are still employed at will. Under the common law concept of employment at will, an employee is free at any time to terminate his or her employment with an employer, with or without justification. The reciprocal right rests also with the employer under employment at will. Absent some legally recognized exceptions, an employer is free, under employment at will, to discharge an employee at any time, with or without just cause.

Employment at will is generally mutually advantageous to employees and employers. Whenever a better employment opportunity arises, an employee knows that under employment at will he or she can terminate an existing employment relationship (with reasonable advance notice) and take advantage of the new opportunity without stigma. Similarly, in a time of corporate downsizing, employers can generally adjust the size and composition of their workforces without adverse legal consequences (with due regard to their social responsibility[1]).

Several recognized exceptions to the concept of employment at will exist. Obviously, a valid employment contract for a specific term of days, weeks, months, or years is an exception to employment at will. Such a contract must comply with all of the legal requisites for a valid contract, including a valid offer and acceptance (mutuality of assent), consideration (mutuality of obligation), legal capacity of the parties to contract, legality of the subject matter, and compliance with the statute of frauds, as applicable.

Some courts have found language in employee handbooks, such as a promise not to discharge an employee except for just cause or the promise of "steady employment" to be implied contractual promises that modify the common law doctrine of employment at will. An employer may be able to disclaim an implied employment contract in an employee handbook by prominently featuring the express disclaimer in the handbook and phrasing it clearly in simple English.[2] Many other employers have chosen to do away with employee handbooks to avoid altogether the possible declaration of an implied employment contract incident to language in the handbook.

Courts have also declared illegal employee discharges based on protected conduct under federal or state statutes. Examples of such wrongful discharges include discharges for **whistle-blowing** (making a good faith report of a suspected violation of law to appropriate authorities); union activities permitted by law; illegal discrimination against racial and ethnic minorities, women, and disabled workers; and the proper filing of workers' compensation and disability claims. Rarely, courts have also declared illegal, as violative of public policy, employee discharges that are deemed fraudulent, malicious, or abusive, such as when a supervisor conspires with co-workers to create a case for discharge against an employee.

Similarly, it would constitute **wrongful discharge** for an employer to fire an employee who refuses to commit an illegal act. In physical and occupational therapy, an example of such a wrongful discharge might be the situation in a managed care setting in which a clinical therapist is fired for refusing to allow unlicensed support personnel to carry out clinical duties that cannot legally be delegated to them.

LABOR-MANAGEMENT RELATIONS

Before 1926, organized labor activity in the United States was significantly impeded by industry, state and federal government, and public opinion. At various points in time, organized labor was viewed as a criminal or communist conspiracy or both. As a result of this unfair and distorted view of organized labor, ordinary employees existed largely at the mercy of their employers, and arbitrary wage cuts and terminations without cause were commonplace.

In 1926, Congress enacted the Railway Labor Act,[3] which for the first time permitted collective bargaining over compensation, benefits, and conditions of employment between railroad (and later airline) employees and their employers. In 1935, Congress expanded the scope of workers' rights granted under the Railway Labor Act to nearly all of the private sector when it enacted the National Labor Relations Act (NLRA), or Wagner Act.[4] The NLRA specifically sanctioned as legitimate organized union activity on behalf of private sector employees and bargaining units and declared collective bargaining to be public policy. The NLRA also defined certain employer misconduct as "unfair labor practices" and created the administrative agency, the National Labor Relations Board, to oversee collective bargaining activities in the private sector.

Unfair labor practices were later extended to unions by the Labor-Management Relations Act of 1947,[5] or Taft-Hartley Act. Federal public sector employees were first given the right to organize and bargain collectively over conditions of employment by an executive order signed by President Kennedy in 1962.[6]

It was not until 1974 that Congress authorized employees of nonprofit hospitals to engage in union activity by amending the NLRA. Health care unions are required by statute to give advance notice of an impending strike to the Federal Mediation and Conciliation Service, which then will attempt to avert the strike through mediation.[7] Except where restricted by law (e.g., by federal employees or during a national emergency), the exercise by unionized employees of the strike option is recognized by law as a legitimate, last-resort option under collective bargaining, just as the lock out is for employers.

Under administrative rules established by the National Labor Relations Board, hospital-based employees can only form into eight bargaining units (with a minimum of six employees in each) representing physicians, registered nurses, other health care professionals, technicians, skilled maintenance workers, other non–health care professional employees, clerical employees, and guards. Implementation of the NLRB's plan was delayed until the U.S. Supreme Court approved it in a case decision in 1991, after it was challenged in the courts by the American Hospital Association.[8]

For a variety of reasons, the percentage of the total workforce represented by unions has decreased dramatically since its high point of about one third of the workforce in the mid-1950s.[9] In 2006, 12 percent of the workforce was unionized, down from 12.5 percent in 2005. In that same year, 7.4 percent of private sector employees were members of unions, whereas among government employees, 36.2 percent were union members. With the ongoing drastic restructuring of health care delivery under managed care and the actual and threatened reimbursement cuts by the federal government, unions may attract health care professional members in larger numbers if they carefully analyze and target this population and meet its special needs.

SELECTED FEDERAL AND STATE LAWS AND AGENCIES

Age Discrimination in Employment Act of 1967; Older Workers Benefit Protection Act of 1990

The Age Discrimination in Employment Act of 1967 (ADEA),[11] as amended, prohibits employment-related discrimination by private and public sector employers of workers age 40 or older (except executives and top policy-making officials). The legal analysis used to process and adjudicate age discrimination cases under federal law parallels that used in Title VII, Civil Rights Act of 1964 cases. Therefore, employment discrimination against older workers is prohibited in recruitment, selection, job assignment, compensation, training, promotion, layoff, discharge, and conditions of employment.

The ADEA was augmented in 1990 by the Older Workers Benefit Protection Act,[12] which clarified the intent of Congress that benefits protection was included in age-related federal antidiscrimination statutory law. The amendment also permits employers to ask dismissed older workers to waive their rights to sue for age discrimination under the ADEA in exchange for compensation. Affected employees have 21 days to sign such waivers and 7 days thereafter to revoke their decisions.

The Equal Employment Opportunity Commission (EEOC) is the federal agency that administers and enforces the ADEA (and several other federal antidiscrimination laws). State statutes and judicial law may afford additional protection to older workers. In 2006, the EEOC processed 13,569 age discrimination complaints, down from 16,585 in 2005.[13]

Americans with Disabilities Act of 1990

The Americans with Disabilities Act of 1990 (ADA)[14] was enacted by Congress on July 26, 1990, for the express purpose of "establish[ing] a clear and comprehensive prohibition of discrimination on the basis of disability."[15] This federal statute completed the decades-long effort of Congress, under the Fourteenth Amendment (due process and equal protection) and under its plenary power to regulate interstate commerce, to prohibit employment discrimination in the public and private sectors. For the approximately 43 million Americans with physical or mental disabilities, the ADA ensures equal access to public accommodations and services and equal opportunities in employment.

Before the ADA was signed into law, 34 states had already enacted legislation protecting disabled workers against employment-related discrimination. The ADA was modeled after the Rehabilitation Act of 1973,[16] which prohibits disability-related employment discrimination in federal executive agencies and by the approximately 50 percent of private sector businesses that contract with the federal government.

The ADA has five sections, or "titles," that protect the rights of persons with disabilities. Title I protects against disability-related employment discrimination. Title II ensures equal access for the disabled to public services (i.e., all activities of state and local governments), including public transportation services. Title III ensures equal access for the disabled to public accommodations, including all private businesses and services (except for some private clubs and all religious organizations and places of worship[17]). This title includes private sector health care facilities under its jurisdiction. Title IV provides for equal access by disabled patrons to telecommunications services. Title V is a miscellaneous section addressing, among other considerations, the relationship of the ADA to other federal statutes, key definitions, and an affirmation that the states cannot claim immunity (Eleventh Amendment) from the requirements of the ADA.

Title I became effective for businesses employing 25 or more persons on July 26, 1992, and for businesses with 15 or more employees on July 26, 1994. Title I covers private and public employers, employment agencies, and labor union organizations.

Title I of the ADA prohibits employment discrimination by employers against employees and job applicants who are qualified to perform the essential functions of their jobs. This prohibition against employment discrimination is all-encompassing, applying to recruitment, selection, training, benefits, promotion, discipline, and retention. The ADA does not, however, establish a quota system for hiring or retaining disabled workers.

If a job candidate with a disability is legitimately found to be unable to perform the essential functions of a position, then that person may be rejected as a candidate for employment for that position. The legal burden of challenging such a decision rests with the rejected candidate, who must prove that he or she is the best qualified person for the position. Qualification standards also require that a candidate not pose a "direct threat" to others in the workplace, that is, "a significant risk to the health or safety of others that cannot be eliminated by reasonable accommodation."[18]

Title I includes several key definitions. **Disability** is defined in one of three ways.[19] An employee or job applicant has a disability if one or more of the following is true:

- The person has a physical or mental impairment that substantially limits one or more major life activities.
- The person has a record of such an impairment.
- The person is regarded as having such an impairment.

"Major life activities" include all of the important activities of daily living well known to health care professionals, including the ability to see, hear, and communicate, as well as cardiorespiratory function, ambulation, self-care, the performance of manual tasks, and formal and informal learning activities, for example.[19]

Precisely which functions are "essential" for any given job is a matter of business judgment for employers.[20] Prudent liability risk management and fundamental fairness require, however, that standards in job descriptions and delineation of essential functions for positions be clear, ethically and legally justifiable, and in writing. Business decisions regarding the labeling of job tasks as essential functions should be reviewed by a legal counsel of a practice before implementation.

A "qualified individual with a disability" means a job applicant or employee who can perform essential job functions, with or without reasonable accommodation. "Reasonable accommodation" is defined by the EEOC as follows[21]:

Any change or adjustment to a job or work environment that permits a qualified applicant or employee with a disability to participate in the job application process, to perform the essential functions of a job, or to enjoy benefits and privileges of employment equal to those enjoyed by employees without disabilities ... and may include:

Acquiring or modifying equipment or devices
Job restructuring
Reassignment to a vacant position
Adjusting or modifying examinations, training materials, or policies
Providing qualified readers and interpreters, and
Making the workplace readily accessible to and usable by people with disabilities.

Reasonable accommodation must be carried out upon request of an applicant or employee (or if a disability is obvious to the employer), unless the employer can prove that to do so would amount to an "undue hardship." **Undue hardship** is defined as a situation in which accommodation is excused because to do so would be unduly burdensome (excessively disruptive, costly, or difficult to implement in light of an employer's size and financial situation) or would fundamentally alter the very nature of the employer's business operations.[22] The accommodation provided need not be one specifically requested by a disabled applicant or employee, just one that enables the applicant or employee to perform the essential functions of his or her job. The applicant or employee can be asked to contribute to funding the accommodation if its cost amounts to an undue hardship for the employer.[23]

The ADA does not require that employers hire or promote anyone but the "best qualified"; however, the law mandates that disabled applicants and employees be afforded equal consideration in the selection process. Excluded from the statutory definition of "disabled" are the following:

• Current illegal drug users and abusers of alcohol
• Compulsive gamblers, kleptomaniacs, and pyromaniacs
• Pedophiles, exhibitionists, and voyeurs
• Homosexuals and bisexuals
• Persons with gender identification and miscellaneous sexual behavior disorders (including transsexualism and transvestism)[24]

Employers must continuously review their hiring, promotion, training, and benefits programs to ensure compliance with the ADA. Employers must especially ensure that, during the hiring process, prospective employees are judged on their abilities, not disabilities, and that candidates and current employees are made aware of their ADA rights (through posting of federal antiemployment discrimination requirements in a prominent place[25]).

Regarding preemployment inquiries and screening tests, the following rules apply. It is unlawful to inquire about applicants' disabilities and to require preoffer medical examinations. Preoffer drug screening tests, however, are permissible by management.

Once a conditional offer has been extended to an applicant, it is permissible to carry out a job-related medical examination, if such an examination is universally given to all similarly situated conditional offerees. A final offer of employment may lawfully be conditioned on the results of such an examination.

According to final EEOC regulations on preemployment questions released in October 1995, it is permissible for an employer to inquire about an applicant's ability to perform specific tasks, including requiring a demonstration of job skills, as long as such an inquiry is made of all applicants. Although it is generally unlawful to inquire about reasonable accommodation(s) during preoffer interviews, the EEOC sanctions such inquiries when one or more of the following occurs:

• The employer reasonably believes that reasonable accommodation might be required for a job because the applicant displays an obvious disability, such as blindness or paralysis.
• The applicant voluntarily discloses an unidentified disability, and the employer reasonably believes that accommodation might be required.
• The applicant requests accommodation.

The EEOC establishes rules and regulations interpreting and enforcing the ADA. In 2005 the EEOC received 14,893 charges of disability discrimination. The EEOC resolved 15,357 disability discrimination charges in fiscal year 2005 (October 1, 2004 to September 30, 2005) and recovered $44.8 million in monetary benefits for charging parties and other aggrieved individuals (not including monetary benefits obtained through litigation).[26]

Litigation over the scope of duty on the part of employers to provide reasonable accommodation to disabled workers has helped to clarify the mandates of the ADA. In cases decided soon after the implementation of the ADA, some court decisions that favored employees included requiring a teacher's aide for a teacher with physical and mental limitations after an automobile accident,[27] ordering reasonable alternatives for an employee unable to drive (an "essential function") because of terminal cancer,[28] mandating lifting restrictions for a nurse with low back dysfunction,[29] and requiring home-based work for a clerical employee with multiple sclerosis.[30] Courts have also ruled in favor of employers, for example, holding that extensive workplace redesign required to accommodate a paraplegic employee constitutes excessive cost and therefore undue hardship[31] and accommodation short of a total workplace smoking ban for an asthmatic employee is acceptable.[32]

Courts are divided, in reasonable accommodation ADA litigation cases, over whether the employee or the employer bears the legal burden of proof in the case. Some courts take a middle ground, first requiring a disabled employee to establish that he or she can perform the essential functions of a particular job (with or without accommodation) and then shifting the burden of proof to the employer to establish why the employer should be excused from providing accommodation.[33]

The following represent a sampling of more recent ADA cases decided by the U.S. Supreme Court and federal courts of appeal. In *Barnett*,[34] the court ruled that no change in an existing seniority system is required in order to accommodate an ADA-covered disabled employee, absent a showing by the employee of special circumstances. In *Chevron*,[35] the court held that an employer may refuse to hire and accommodate a disabled worker with a serious medical condition that might worsen on the job (e.g., liver diseased worker in a toxic environment). The *Garrett*[36] case ruled that, because of state immunity under the Eleventh Amendment to the Constitution, state employees cannot win monetary damages against their state employers under Title I of the ADA, only equity remedies. *Gorman*[37] held that neither can plaintiffs win punitive or punishment damages under Title II of the ADA (lawsuits against public agencies). *Karracker*[38] held that the Minnesota Multiphasic Personality Index is a mental examination subject to ADA restrictions (that is, no preoffer testing is permitted). In *Kirkenburg*[39] the court ruled that certain correctable conditions (e.g., eye disorders corrected with glasses) are not covered disabilities under the ADA. *Martin*,[40] a Title III public accommodation case, declared that a professional golfer with chronic severe low back pain has the right under the ADA to use a golf cart in lieu of walking during tournaments. Finally, *Williams*[41] held that an ADA-covered disability is only one that severely restricts life activities of central importance, not ambiguous impairments like "living with pain."

Consider the following case:

> *Misty is a personal trainer in private practice. Her three metro offices employ 15 staff members. Puchi is a highly qualified applicant for a massage therapist position. During the interview, Misty observes that Puchi is blind. How should Misty proceed?*

Despite the substantial number of administrative and litigation cases involving the ADA, employers should not be fearful of the ADA. In addition to reinforcing the social responsibility of a business to recruit, hire, train and develop, retain, and promote workers with disabilities, the ADA makes good business sense. The cost of total public support of a person who has a disability averages $1 million over the person's lifetime, whereas employment of that person results in a net gain to public coffers of $65,000 in taxes paid. Studies and experience show that persons with disabilities want to work and perform their work very well, relative to the total workforce. Even persons with severe physical or mental disabilities or both can be highly successful in the workplace through supported employment.[42]

Employers who are strongly committed to the principles of the ADA also benefit from an enhanced public image and increased goodwill. Employers should not take a defensive approach to compliance with the ADA because, as has been the case with health care malpractice prevention, a defensive posture only serves to increase the likelihood of litigation.

Despite the call from some legislators in Congress for ADA reform,[43] based in part on the perceived financial burden of compliance for business, the ADA remains a linchpin for employment and civil rights, crucial to the prestige and maintenance of the United States as a world leader. Health care professionals—especially those in rehabilitation—have a unique opportunity to serve as consultants to employers (to meet their legal responsibilities) and to employees (to exercise their rights and rehabilitation and vocational potential).

Civil Rights Act of 1964, Title VII

The most important (or at least most pervasive) federal statute addressing employment discrimination and civil rights is Title VII of the Civil Rights Act of 1964.[44] This law was critically important for the full integration of racial and other minorities into the American workforce, yet its passage was stalled for years in the U.S. Senate by repeated filibusters.

President John Kennedy, Attorney General Robert Kennedy, and congressional Democratic leaders grounded the statute in the plenary power of Congress to regulate interstate commerce[45] rather than in constitutional due process or equal protection under law, believing that this was the only way that the law could survive a legal challenge by noncompliant private sector businesses. The legal premise justifying enactment of the Civil Rights Act of 1964 was that discrimination of minorities—especially of blacks—by business had an immeasurably adverse impact on interstate commerce and that Congress was empowered to remedy this by means of a federal nondiscrimination mandate to all public and private business entities.

Title VII specifically prohibits discrimination against job applicants and employees based on race/ethnicity, gender (as of 1972), religion, and national origin at all stages along the continuum of employment processes. The groups enumerated in Title VII are referred to in case and administrative law as "protected classes." Specifically, Title VII states in pertinent part that:

It shall be an unlawful employment practice for an employer:

1. To fail or refuse to hire or to discharge any individual, or otherwise to discriminate against any individual with respect to his compensation, terms, conditions, or privileges of employment, because of such individual's race, color, religion, sex, or national origin, or

2. To limit, segregate, or classify his employees or applicants for employment in any way which would deprive any individual of employment opportunities or otherwise adversely affect his status as an employee, because of such individual's race, color, religion, sex, or national origin.[46]

Title VII applies to all private sector businesses with 15 or more employees; labor unions; and federal, state, and local governmental entities. Title VII is administered and enforced by the EEOC. States are free to provide additional constitutional, statutory, judicial, and administrative protections to their citizens over and above that provided by federal law.

Employers are required by EEOC regulations to create, submit for review, and maintain records that evidence compliance with Title VII. For reporting purposes, race/ethnicity is divided into five classifications: white (non-Hispanic), black, Hispanic, Asian/Pacific Islander, and American Indian/Alaskan native.[47]

Title VII expressly permits employment discrimination against protected classes of persons based on bona fide occupational qualifications, or BFOQs.[48] A BFOQ must be based on business necessity, that is, reasonably necessary for the normal operation of a particular business. BFOQs are allowed for gender, religion, and national origin (and age under the ADEA) classifications, provided that employers can establish business necessity. (BFOQs based on race violate public policy and are generally disallowed.) An example of a legitimate gender-based BFOQ is the requirement, based on social mores, that dressing room attendants be of the same gender as patrons. An example of a legitimate religion-based BFOQ is the requirement that a parish priest for a Catholic church be Catholic.

Title VII prohibits intentional and unintentional employment discrimination. Intentional wrongful employment discrimination is referred to as "disparate treatment," whereas other employment practices, though they appear to be protected class–neutral on their face, have a particular adverse "disparate impact" on the employment rights of protected class members.

Civil Rights Act of 1991

The Civil Rights Act of 1991[49] was enacted to clarify congressional intent regarding employment discrimination, after the U.S. Supreme Court reportedly "weakened the scope and effectiveness of federal civil rights protections"[50] in its 1989 decision in *Wards Cove Packing Co.* v. *Atonio.*[51] The provisions of this federal statute affect the Civil Rights Act of 1964 and the Rehabilitation Act of 1973.

The Civil Rights Act of 1991 invalidates the Supreme Court's holding in *Wards Cove,* in part, by reshifting part of the burden of proof in disparate impact employment discrimination cases from plaintiffs to employers, to prove business necessity for any business practice that is proved (by a plaintiff) to have a disparate impact on a Title VII–protected class.

This statute amended several other statutes enforced by EEOC, substantively and procedurally. Previously, jury trials were possible only in cases brought under the Environmental Protection Act or the ADEA. The Civil Rights Act of 1991 permitted jury trials and recovery of compensatory and punitive damages under Title VII and the ADA for lawsuits involving intentional discrimination. The new law imposed statutory caps on the amount of damages that could be awarded for future monetary losses, pain and suffering, and punitive damages, based on employer size. The maximum award of compensatory and punitive damages combined was set at $300,000 for the largest employers (more than 500 employees).

In addition, the Civil Rights Act of 1991 added a new subsection to Title VII, codifying the disparate impact theory of discrimination, essentially putting the law back as it had been before *Wards Cove.* The act also provided that where the plaintiff shows that discrimination was a motivating factor for an employment decision, the employer may be held liable for injunctive relief, attorneys' fees, and costs (but not individual monetary or affirmative relief), even if the employer proves it would have made the same decision in the absence of a discriminatory motive. The act also provided employment discrimination protection to employees of Congress and some high-level political appointees. Title VII and ADA coverage was also extended to include American and American-controlled employers operating abroad.[52]

Drug-Free Workplace Act of 1988

The Drug-Free Workplace Act of 1988[53] requires that companies and individuals who enter into contracts with the federal government valued at $25,000 or more (and all federal grant recipients) certify that their facilities are drug-free workplaces. Federal contractors are required, at least, to do the following:

- Have in place an effective workplace drug education program
- Post and give to each employee a copy of the prohibition against the "unlawful manufacture, distribution, [use], or [possession] of controlled substances ... in the workplace,"[54] specifying potential disciplinary actions for violation of the prohibition
- Notify the federal contracting agency, within 10 days, of any drug-related criminal convictions of its employees

The Drug-Free Workplace Act of 1988 does not specifically mandate that employers carry out workplace drug testing; however, neither are they prohibited by the statute from doing so. Workplace drug testing is of relatively recent vintage. Workplace drug testing first began in the military during the 1970s and gradually extended to private sector businesses as drug abuse spread. In 2007, 73 percent of drug users were employed, consisting of some 8.1 million workers. These impaired workers have higher than average absenteeism, accident rates, and workers' compensation claims.[55]

Employee drug testing includes the following test types[56]:

- **Preemployment drug screening**, the most commonly used employee drug test type. Preemployment drug testing is recognized as a common law management right to promote an employer's legitimate business interests.
- **Reasonable suspicion drug testing**, done when a supervisor of an employee reasonably believes that the employee may be under the influence of mind-altering drugs. Legal bases for reasonable suspicion drug testing include the fact that employers are vicariously liable for the conduct of employees acting within the scope of employment and the statutory requirement under the Occupational Safety and Health Act of 1970 for employers to maintain a workplace free of serious safety hazards.
- **Periodic drug testing** of employees, such as during a periodic physical examination, or as part of a promotion into a position that requires the employee to handle classified documents or carry a firearm.
- **Postaccident drug testing**, after serious accidents (especially those involving injury), with or without suspicion of employee misconduct.
- **Random drug testing**, the least often used and most effective and controversial form of employee drug testing.
- **Exculpatory drug testing**,[57] designed to exculpate an employee who erroneously tests positive for illicit drug use, by comparing the blood types of the suspect and blood group substances found in the positive urine sample. Approximately 80 percent of the population are "secretors" of such substances, for whom exculpatory testing, based on ABO blood groups, is feasible.

Case law to date addressing the constitutionality and propriety of employee drug testing has generally upheld the practice, with one proviso. Except for military service members and prisoners, direct observation of a subject rendering a urine sample is universally considered to be repugnant and an unconscionably impermissible violation of personal human dignity and privacy. In business settings, therefore, only indirect observation of subjects rendering urine samples is permitted, such as the posting of a guard outside of a lavatory so that extraneous paraphernalia is not carried in by testees.

Effective January 1, 1996, all transit employers regulated by the U.S. Department of Transportation were required to have, in addition to drug awareness programs, alcohol abuse prevention programs that comply with the specific regulations of the department. These federal regulations preempt any conflicting state laws concerning alcohol misuse. Safety-sensitive employees, including truck and bus drivers, are prohibited from imbibing alcohol 4 hours before driving and are subject to testing to confirm that they are alcohol-free and (other) drug-free on the job.[58]

Employee Polygraph Protection Act of 1988

The Employee Polygraph Protection Act of 1988 (EPPA)[59] severely curtailed the use of polygraph examinations in the workplace. This federal statute, based on respect for individual privacy, prohibits the use of "lie detector" examinations of any kind by private sector employers, except for the following:

- Job applicants in the security industry
- Job applicants in companies that manufacture or market controlled drugs
- Current employees, as part of an investigation concerning a specific economic loss, such as theft from, or sabotage of, a firm

The polygraph is an instrument that measures the physiological responses of heart rate, respiration, and perspiration through a galvanic skin response. Physiological responses to "control" or background lies are compared with those of "relevant" lies to determine whether a polygrapher believes that a subject is truthful or deceptive. If no determination as to truthfulness can be made, the test is reported as inconclusive.

The congressional Office of Technological Assessment has concluded that a polygraph only has validity when the control question technique is used in the area of specific criminal investigations.[60] The EPPA correctly reflects the widely held belief that the use of polygraphs for other purposes constitutes an unwarranted invasion of individual privacy.

Results of private sector employment-related polygraph examinations may not be released to anyone except the employee tested and appropriate governmental agencies (such as the police), and then only with a court order. Employers are required to post conspicuously a notice of employee rights under the EPPA. The law is administered by the Employment Standards Division of the U.S. Department of Labor.

Employee Retirement Income Security Act of 1974

The Employee Retirement Income Security Act of 1974 (ERISA)[61] was enacted by Congress to regulate private pension and benefit plans. A key original intent behind the legislation was the desire to ensure that pensioners receive what is due them at the end of a working career. ERISA preempts all conflicting state laws (except for state insurance laws) concerning employee benefits and pensions.

Regarding employee health benefit plans, employer-sponsored health benefit plans fall outside of state jurisdiction because they are not legally considered to be insurance. This means that state laws such as health care malpractice case and statutory laws do not apply to such plans, which include two thirds of current employee health benefit plans. ERISA itself fails to address such issues, creating what has been called "the ERISA vacuum."[62]

Under ERISA, employer contributions to pension plans fully vest after 5 years of employment. The portability option is a voluntary option under ERISA under which employees can roll over vested pension benefits when they leave their current place of employment. Pensions are of two types: the traditional (and more costly) defined benefit plan and the defined contribution plan, including the popular 401(k) plan.

Companies and their pension insurers and trustees are legal fiduciaries to pension beneficiaries, meaning that they stand in a legal position of trust toward beneficiaries and must act prudently to safeguard the assets of the pension fund. Companies also have substantial disclosure (to beneficiaries) and reporting (to the federal government) requirements concerning employee pension plans. ERISA is coadministered by the Department of Labor and the Internal Revenue Service.

Equal Employment Opportunity Commission

The EEOC is a federal administrative agency created by Congress in the Civil Rights Act of 1964 to administer and enforce Title VII of that statute. The EEOC also administers and enforces the ADA, ADEA, and the Equal Pay Act of 1963[63] and provides oversight and coordination of all federal regulations, policies, and practices affecting equal employment opportunity.

The EEOC consists of five commissioners and a general counsel, all appointed by the president and confirmed by the Senate. The president designates the chairman, who acts as chief executive officer of the commission. All commissioners serve for 5-year, staggered terms. The commissioners make EEOC policy, whereas the general counsel supervises equal employment opportunity litigation brought on behalf of complainants.

EEOC staff process and investigate complaints of employment discrimination against private and public entities. In most instances, charges must be filed with the EEOC within 180 days of the alleged employment discrimination (extended to 300 days if the state has an antidiscrimination agency). If the EEOC investigation of a charge concludes that there is reasonable cause that actionable employment discrimination occurred, it will initiate conciliation procedures to try to resolve the charge to the reasonable satisfaction of the complainant at this lowest level of adjudication. That failing, the EEOC may sue the respondent in federal court on the alleged victim's behalf. (Only the Department of Justice may bring suit against a state or local governmental entity, however.) If the EEOC does not file a lawsuit, an aggrieved private party may file a private lawsuit against an offender within 90 days of dismissal of the case by the EEOC.[64]

Family and Medical Leave Act of 1993

The Family and Medical Leave Act of 1993 (FMLA)[65] was signed into law by President Clinton just after his inauguration and became effective on February 5, 1993. The FMLA requires covered employers to provide up to 12 weeks of unpaid, job- and benefit-protected leave per year to eligible employees for childbirth, adoption, and personal and family medical illnesses.

Employees eligible for FMLA protection are those who have worked for at least 1250 hours during the previous 12 months at a location in which their employer has 50 or more employees located within a 75-mile radius. Under Department of Labor administrative rules, which became effective in April 1995, covered illnesses under the FMLA include those conditions that incapacitate an employee or family member (spouse, child, or parent) for at least 3 days, require consultation with a health care professional, and are treated with prescription medications.

Under the administrative rules implementing the FMLA, an employee on FMLA leave of absence for personal illness is not required to accept an employer's offer of "light duty" or other reasonable accommodation. This rule is seemingly inconsistent with the ADA and probably results in significant confusion on the part of human resource managers who must coadminister the FMLA, ADA, and workers' compensation laws for their companies.

Although eligible employees must provide 30-day advance notices of covered leave except for emergency absences, employers continue to fear abuses of the system by employees and an adverse effect on productivity.[66] Employers may require the production of a medical certificate of illness and even a second opinion regarding a claimed covered illness (at the employer's expense). Employers may also compel employees invoking the FMLA to use accrued paid leave (vacation and sick days) for some or all of the FLMA period. Employer retaliation against an employee invoking the protection of the FMLA is prohibited. The law is enforced by the U.S. Department of Labor.

Ragsdale[67] was the first FLMA case decided by the U.S. Supreme Court. In that case, Ms. Ragsdale was granted 30 weeks of undesignated medical leave for cancer treatment. When she sought additional time off, it was denied, and she sued under the FMLA. In denying her petition for relief, the court invalidated a regulatory provision of the FLMA that required employers to notify employees taking medical leave that the absences would count against their annual 12-week FLMA entitlement.

Occupational Safety and Health Act of 1970; Occupational Safety and Health Administration

The Occupational Safety and Health Act of 1970[68] was enacted to establish and enforce workplace safety and health standards. The Occupational Safety and Health Administration is the federal administrative agency that promulgates rules and enforces the act. The rules of the administration, covering workplace issues from universal precautions to standards for the minimization of cumulative trauma disorders in industry, apply to almost all private sector employers, except family farmers and self-employed persons.

The Occupational Safety and Health Act is enforced by the U.S. Department of Labor, and compliance is monitored through mandatory reporting and scheduled and surprise (pursuant to a warrant) administrative inspections. Employers with more than 10 employees must make and maintain detailed occupational injury and illness records for their employees.

Pregnancy Discrimination Act of 1978

The Pregnancy Discrimination Act of 1978[69] is a codicil statute amending Title VII of the Civil Rights Act of 1964. Under the Pregnancy Discrimination Act the definition of unlawful gender-based employment discrimination is expanded to include discrimination based on pregnancy, childbirth, and related medical conditions (including complications of pregnancy and therapeutic abortions). The law does not mandate that employers covered by Title VII provide pregnancy-related medical benefits (or any benefits); however, if medical benefits are provided to employees, pregnancy must be treated in the same manner as any other covered disability. Pregnancy-related benefits may not be limited to married employees only.[70] If reasonable job accommodation is provided by an employer for other disabilities, it must also be provided for (temporary) disability related to pregnancy. Under the Pregnancy Discrimination Act, employers are also prohibited from mandating a specific numbers of days after which pregnant employees must return to work after childbirth.

Workers' Compensation Statutes

State workers' compensation statutes were first introduced on a voluntary basis in five states in 1911[71] to provide some degree of protection to industrial workers injured while on the job. Before that time, workers who were injured on the job, who almost universally had neither health nor disability insurance, were normally summarily discharged from their employment because they could no longer work. As a result, many industrial worker injury cases became the subject of lawsuits, most of which were won by employers, on theories ranging from the "fellow servant rule" (another worker, not the employer, was at fault) and "contributory negligence" on the part of the injured worker. This social injustice led to the enactment of mandatory workers' compensation statutes in all 50 states by 1948.[72]

Workers' compensation statutes provide for income continuation and payment of related medical and rehabilitation expenses for covered workers injured on the job. The issues adjudicated by state workers' compensation administrative agencies include (1) whether the employee was injured while functioning within the scope of employment and (2) the degree of resultant disability. Workers' compensation laws generally do not consider who was at fault for a covered incident resulting in employee injury. In that sense, workers' compensation laws are no-fault laws.

Because of a sense that workers' compensation laws are subject to abuse (despite the fact that few, if any, injured employees reap a financial windfall from workers' compensation benefits), many state legislatures have enacted workers' compensation reform measures.[73] Some of the reform measures include reducing the roles of personal injury attorneys in the administrative process, risk-shifting for minor job-related injuries, and case management of individual workers and their rehabilitation.

ETHICAL AND LEGAL ISSUES IN WORKPLACE SEXUAL HARASSMENT

Though sexual harassment has long been a widespread problem affecting productivity, morale, and every other aspect of interpersonal relations in the workplace, only recently have allegations of sexual harassment lodged against prominent public officials brought this problem out of the closet and into every boardroom, work setting, and living room in the United States and elsewhere.

The EEOC defines and describes[74] sexual harassment as follows:

> Sexual harassment is a form of sex discrimination that violates Title VII of the [Civil Rights Act] of 1964. Unwelcome sexual advances, requests for sexual favors, and other verbal or physical conduct of a sexual nature constitutes sexual harassment when submission to or rejection of this conduct explicitly or implicitly affects an individual's employment, unreasonably interferes with an individual's work performance or creates an intimidating, hostile or offensive work environment. Sexual harassment can occur in a variety of circumstances, including but not limited to the following:
> The victim as well as the harasser may be a woman or a man.
> The victim does not have to be of the opposite sex.
> The harasser can be the victim's supervisor, an agent of the employer, a supervisor in another area, a co-worker, or a non-employee.
> The victim does not have to be the person harassed but could be anyone affected by the offensive conduct.
> Unlawful sexual harassment may occur without economic injury to or discharge of the victim.
> The harasser's conduct must be unwelcome.

The EEOC definition of sexual harassment has a dual focus on (1) the types of inappropriate conduct that constitutes sexual harassment and (2) the possible adverse employment consequences for victims of sexual harassment and for others in the workplace. Conduct that constitutes sexual harassment could include the following:

- Unwelcome comments of a sexual nature about a victim's person or body parts
- Solicitation of others for sexual relations
- Inappropriate touching of another person on a private area of his or her body with the intent to arouse or gratify sexual desires (i.e., commission of sexual battery)

Employment consequences fall into two categories: adverse employment decisions resulting from *quid pro quo* situations and hostile work environments. *Quid pro quo* describes a situation in which a victim's response to sexual harassment is the basis for employment-related decisions involving the victim or other workers. A *quid pro quo* complaint typically is lodged by an employee who has been denied opportunities because he or she refused a perpetrator's sexual advances or by an employee who has been denied opportunities because another employee obtained those opportunities by submitting to a perpetrator's sexual advances. An example of a *quid pro quo* sexual harassment situation would be the case in which an employer's decision to fund a staff occupational therapist's attendance at a professional conference depended on whether the occupational therapist submitted to the employer's sexual advances.

Complaints related to hostile work environments can be made by any person in the workplace who is reasonably offended by a perpetrator's sexual harassment (of the complainant or of another person in the work setting) and whose work is impeded by that harassment.

In a hostile work environment scenario, sexual harassment unreasonably interferes with the victim's or another person's work performance. Complaints related to hostile work environments can be made by any person in the workplace who is reasonably offended by a perpetrator's sexual harassment (of the complainant or of another person in the work setting) and whose work is impeded by that harassment. An example of a hostile work environment sexual harassment situation would be the case in which a certified rehabilitation aide is unable to concentrate on patient care activities because of the misconduct of a licensed rehabilitation supervisory professional who is making sexual advances toward a patient.

The EEOC and the courts adjudicating sexual harassment cases traditionally have used the "ordinary reasonable person" standard to assess whether an individual's conduct constitutes sexual harassment. This is the same standard commonly used to determine whether a defendant in a civil tort (e.g., health care malpractice) case violated a duty owed to a plaintiff. Under this standard, as applied in a sexual harassment case, a trier of fact (judge or jury) places himself or herself into the shoes of an ethereal ordinary person and determines how such a person would be likely to perceive the conduct in issue and decides the case accordingly.

The problem with the traditional "ordinary reasonable person" standard is that it frequently is translated into a "reasonable man" standard, with the result that the trier of fact assesses interpersonal conduct exclusively from a male point of view. To ensure that a gender-neutral standard is applied in administrative and legal sexual harassment cases, some federal courts have established a modified standard that eventually may supplant the traditional standard of review. Under this modified standard, the trier of fact still places himself or herself into the shoes of an "ordinary reasonable person" when determining whether specific conduct constitutes sexual harassment, but the "ordinary reasonable person" must be of the same gender as the alleged victim of sexual harassment or misconduct.

Expert testimony has been presented in sexual harassment cases to support the notion that men and women view sexually oriented conduct—in the workplace and elsewhere—differently. Testifying in *Robinson* v. *Jacksonville Shipyards,*[75] Alison Wetherfield of the Legal Defense and Education Fund of the National Organization for Women cited a study in which 75 percent of men polled said that they were flattered by sexual advances by women in the workplace; only 15 percent claimed that they would be offended by such conduct. Of women surveyed, however, 75 percent stated that they would be offended by sexually oriented conduct in the workplace.[76] In *Robinson,* the court used an "ordinary reasonable woman" standard to hold an employer responsible for the sexually harassing conduct of male employees toward a female co-worker.

Supporting Alison Wetherfield's assertion that men and women view sexually oriented conduct differently is a recently reported study done by the spousal research team of Struckman-Johnson and Struckman-Johnson, reported in the journal *Sex Roles.*[77] In a study of 277 college men, subjects were asked to imagine that they were the target of unsolicited sexual advances from casual female acquaintances. Conduct to be imagined ranged from a gentle touch on the genitals, to a push, to coercion with and without a deadly weapon. Nearly 25 percent of the men stated that they would willingly continue sexual activity with an "attractive" female aggressor, even if coerced by the assailant with a deadly weapon.

In another legal case, *Ellison* v. *Brady*,[78] a federal appeals court evaluated what were described as "bizarre," repetitive, unwelcome love letters written by a male co-worker to a woman in a federal government office. The lower court found that the man's conduct did not constitute sexual harassment. In reversing that decision, the appellate court used an "ordinary reasonable woman" standard to assess whether the letters constituted sexual harassment.

An excellent model for assessing interpersonal conduct is the one developed by the U.S. Navy[79] after the Tailhook convention in which a number of male officers were accused of sexually harassing female colleagues at an aviator's convention at the Las Vegas Hilton Hotel. This model categorizes conduct as follows:

- "Green light," that is, interpersonal conduct that is clearly acceptable behavior in the eyes of an "ordinary reasonable person" of either gender
- "Yellow light," that is, conduct that may be unacceptable in the eyes of some "reasonable" persons of the same gender as the target of the conduct
- "Red light," that is, conduct that is always unacceptable in the eyes of an "ordinary reasonable person" of the same gender as the target of the conduct

Green light conduct might include things such as complimenting a colleague about his or her dress in an inoffensive and nondiscriminatory manner. Yellow light behavior might include soliciting a date with a co-worker for the first time. Red light behavior includes conduct such as repeated solicitations for a date after rejection, indecent exposure, and sexual assault or battery. Media depictions of workplace sexual assault and battery, such as presented in the film *Disclosure*,[80] promote the trivialization of serious sexual misconduct in the public's eye by labeling it merely as "sexual harassment." Such serious, felonious sexual misconduct involves conduct more egregious than simple "sexual harassment."

The following sexual harassment cases decided by the U.S. Supreme Court illustrate the evolution of victim protection under federal law. In *Oncale* v. *Sundowner Offshore Services*,[81] the court ruled for the first time that same-gender sexual harassment is legally actionable. In other words, it is the offensive nature of the conduct that makes it sexual harassment, irrespective of the gender or sexual orientation of the victim (or perpetrator). In *Burlington Industries* v. *Ellerth*[82] and *Faragher* v. *Boca Raton*,[83] the court held that employers face vicarious liability for supervisors' sexual harassment of workers if victims suffer tangible (significant) adverse job actions such as firing, nonpromotion, or loss of benefits. An employer may escape this vicarious liability if it can prove two things: (1) that the employer acted reasonably to prevent and promptly correct the sexual harassment at issue and (2) that the employee-victim unreasonably failed to use employer-sponsored initiatives to prevent and correct sexual harassment.

In the workplace then, managers bear the formidable responsibility of ferreting out, eliminating, and preventing sexual harassment. The buck *does* stop at the manager's desk. Managers may even be held liable for sexual harassment of which they are unaware, especially if the organization or work unit does not have in place a reporting or grievance mechanism for receiving and investigating complaints of sexual harassment. Specific management responsibilities regarding sexual harassment include the following:

- Sensitizing and educating employees about what constitutes sexual harassment; how men and women may differ in their attitudes toward sexual conduct; and the types of conduct that reasonable persons might find offensive. This process not only should be a part of new employee orientations but also should be regularly reinforced as continuing for all employees. Managers might wish to consult with human resource management specialists to lead sessions at which employees are given information about current administrative and legal sexual harassment cases and are asked to participate in group cooperative learning processes, such as brainstorming about what interpersonal conduct constitutes permissible and impermissible behavior in the workplace.[84]
- Expressing strong disapproval of sexual harassment and developing and enforcing appropriate sanctions to stop sexual harassment whenever it is found to exist. Managers are responsible for taking immediate action to stop known sexual harassment, regardless of who the perpetrator[85] or the victim might be. Reporting, investigation, and grievance procedures for internal resolution of sexual harassment complaints should be in place. Managers must be prompt, fair, and impartial in their investigations of such complaints, respecting the rights of all parties involved, to the maximum extent possible.[86] If employees and others view management's commitment as strong, the investigatory process as equitable, and the awarding of sanctions as appropriate, then minor complaints stand a better chance of being resolved at the organizational level instead of through the EEOC or the courts.
- Apprising employees, as required by federal law, of their right to initiate formal charges with the EEOC. Although victims of sexual harassment should be encouraged to resolve grievances at the lowest appropriate level, under the EEOC sex-discrimination guidelines, managers are responsible for making their employees aware of their right to pursue unresolved complaints at higher administrative or legal levels. Making employees aware of their rights could be done as part of the sensitization and ongoing educational processes. In addition, managers should ensure that a statement of employees' rights and the organizational policy statement on sexual harassment, with a clear description of the internal grievance process, is posted in a prominent place.

Special Issues in Health Care Professional Education Settings

Sexual harassment and misconduct issues in health care professional educational settings primarily involve student-professor, student–clinical instructor, student-student, and student-patient scenarios. Health care professional codes of ethics range from clarity to ambiguity in their treatment of these issues.

EXERCISE

Review the code of ethics of your discipline and any ethical guidance on implementation. How does your discipline address sexual behavior between and among licensed professionals, students, and patients? Compare how state licensing statutes and regulations (if applicable) address these parties' sexual behaviors.

Gutheil and Gabbard[87] described boundary theory as the bright line between appropriate and inappropriate interpersonal behavior. Boundary violations by health care professionals in professional relations with their patients may be positive (giving a patient a friendly pat on the back) or negative and wrongful (taking sexual advantage of a patient). An overly rigid application of boundary theory may harm patients, too, by compelling providers to be too formal with patients, discouraging them from sharing important personal health information with their providers.

Health care professional students are protected from sexual harassment and misconduct in educational settings not only by the Civil Rights Act of 1964 but also by Title IX of the Education Amendments of 1972.[88] Health care professional academic and clinical educators should maintain the same formality in relationships with professional students as they maintain with patients to avoid misunderstandings and the appearance of impropriety.

Students must also be cognizant of their ethical duties to maintain appropriate relationships with faculty and patients. Consider the reported federal health care malpractice legal case *Oslund* v. *United States*.[89] In this case a patient sued the United States for the alleged sexual misconduct of an occupational therapy intern at a Veterans Administration hospital. The alleged misconduct involved a meretricious relationship between the student intern and the psychiatric patient, during which time one transferred genital herpes to the other. The federal district court ruled, in part, that the intern's otherwise confidential medical records were to be opened for the patient's attorney to determine when she developed and first sought treatment for herpes.

Clinical managers and instructors must be sure to include health care professional students in the scope of coverage of their policy manuals prohibiting sexual contact between staff and patients and should orient students as to their responsibilities immediately upon arrival at the clinical sites. Also prudent is to have in place work rules prohibiting dating between staff and patients, as well as between students and supervising staff in the clinic.

Studies by McComas et al.[90] and deMayo[91] indicate that a majority of clinical health care professionals and students experience inappropriate patient-initiated sexual behaviors (PISBs). McComas et al.[90] studied 205 physical therapy students and clinical affiliates at the University of Ottawa. Of the 78% that responded, he reported that 66.2% of students and 92.9% of clinicians experienced some form of PISB incident to practice. He also found that 22.1% of students and 45.2% of clinicians reported experiencing severe PISBs, ranging from indecent exposure to sexual assault and battery. A statistically significant gender difference was noted, in that 83.1% of women, but only 56.3% of men, reported being victims of PISB. deMayo[91] distributed 733 random surveys to American Physical Therapy Association members, with 358 (48.6%) responding. In this study, 86% of respondents (81.5% of whom were females) reported being victims of PISB.

Farber et al.[92] surveyed 1000 internal medicine physicians about PISB, with 330 (33%) responding. Minor boundary violations by patients (including patients calling physicians by their first names) were reported by 75% of respondents. Use of sexually explicit language by patients was reported by 11% of respondents, and physical abuse by patients by less than 5% of respondents. White[93] surveyed 310 Australian medical students, with a high response rate of 293 completed surveys (94.5%). In this study, 47.9% of females and 24.6% of males reported being victims of inappropriate sexual behaviors, mostly by fellow students. However, with medical student–perpetrators removed from the data set, 73.3% of reports of unwanted physical contact were between male patients and female medical students. Comparing the findings of Farber et al. and White reveals that patients may be more prone to initiate sexual behavior against novice professional students than against seasoned health care professionals.

Hint: Although managers have the primary responsibility for preventing and eliminating sexual harassment, responsibility is ultimately shared by everyone in an organization.

HUMAN RESOURCE MANAGEMENT ISSUES

Recruitment and Selection

The same equal employment opportunity legal considerations that govern employment discrimination generally apply specifically to employee recruitment and selection procedures in the private and public sectors. Job applicants, like current employees, are protected from employment discrimination by federal statutes previously discussed, including the Civil Rights Acts of 1964 and 1991, the Equal Pay Act of 1963, ADEA, and ADA. Federal constitutional law, case law, and administrative law protections augment federal statutory protections. State anti–employment discrimination statutes and case and administrative law provide additional protection to job applicants.

Administrative guidelines promulgated by the EEOC offer employers specific guidance concerning prohibited and precautionary preemployment inquiries.[94] Prohibited inquiries generally include questions concerning the following:

- Race, ethnicity, national origin (Note that every employer has the right and legal duty to inquire about an applicant's legal right to work in the United States. This must be done for every job applicant.)
- Marital status, number of children, child care arrangements, existence of an opposite- or same-gender "domestic partner"
- Religious beliefs and practices
- Disabilities, whether obvious or perceived
- Age

Precautionary inquiries—that is, ones that must pass the threshold test of being specifically job-related in order to be legitimate—generally include questions concerning the following:

- Height, weight
- Educational level
- Criminal convictions
- Military discharge classification (if less than honorable)
- Financial status

Most or all of these precautionary inquiries have been found, in administrative and judicial cases, to have a disparate impact on federally protected classes of persons.

Employers may legally inquire about the existence of an applicant's criminal convictions but should include a disclaimer in the job application that an affirmative response will not necessarily preclude selection of the applicant but that the conviction will be considered in light of the totality of circumstances, including the nature of the offense, the applicant's age at the time the offense occurred, and indices of postconviction rehabilitation. Most of the prohibited and precautionary preemployment inquiries become legitimate areas of inquiry, for example, for activation of benefits,[95] EEOC demographic reporting requirements, and other legitimate business and legal requirements once an applicant is selected for employment.

Under what is known as the "four-fifths rule," the EEOC attributes as possible evidence of disparate discriminatory impact employee selection rates for protected classes that are less than 80 percent of the rate of the group with the highest selection rate. Consider the following example:

> *Thirty applicants are hired as home health aides for a managed care organization. Forty white males applied for employment with the managed care organization, as did 40 females (10 of whom are black). Twenty successful applicants are white males and 10 are females, three of whom are black. Is the EEOC's four-fifths rule violated? Yes. The selection rate for the group with the highest selection (white males) is 50 percent. To avoid closer scrutiny by the EEOC, the selection rates for females generally and blacks specifically must be at least 40 percent (80 percent of 50 percent). Here, only 25 percent of females (30 percent of black females) were selected.*

Employers, especially in occupations where employees are in close contact with clients (e.g., the health care professions), need to be concerned about liability exposure for negligent hiring, a claim that may arise when a client or other person is injured by an employee. **Negligent hiring** means that the employer may be liable for injury to others when the employer fails to take reasonable steps to ascertain that a job applicant poses a danger to others and, once employed, that an employee causes harm to the person or property of another in the course of employment.

Employers should take appropriate steps to screen for dangerousness through preemployment inquiries about criminal convictions and gaps in employment or education and by conducting appropriate background investigations, pursuant to signed releases by applicants[96] (including mandatory inquiries to the National Practitioner Data Bank for licensed primary health care professionals). In addition, employers should check as many employment references as is feasible and document the process and reference responses.

Employees Versus Independent Contractors

The distinction between employees and contract workers has enormous consequences for employers and workers. By definition, an independent contractor is a person who works independently of detailed control of an employer. The employer is not normally vicariously liable for the contractor's work-related conduct. Employers, however, may be vicariously liable for the conduct of contractors under ostensible agency, when contractors are indistinguishable from employees in the eyes of the public.

Employers are primarily liable for the negligent selection and retention of contractors, areas over which employers do have control. Health care employers are additionally subject to primary liability for the negligent failure to monitor the quality of health care delivery throughout their organizations, irrespective of whether the care is delivered by employees, contractors, or others.

Employers, employees, and independent contractors also incur tax liabilities for labeling workers as employees or contractors. Employers are required by law to withhold federal income tax and Social Security contributions from employees, but not from contract workers, who are responsible for their own withholding. The complex and admittedly (by the Internal Revenue Service) ambiguous set of criteria for distinguishing employees and contractors, based on common law, for example, classifies workers based on the nature, duration, and location of their work and on the degree of permissible supervision of their work product by employers.[97]

Employee Discipline and Termination

Two basic approaches to employee discipline are a punitive approach and a constructive, rehabilitative approach.[98] The constructive approach is always preferred when an employer wants to retain his or her employees because it promotes personal responsibility and self-correction by employees and a positive attitude and work ethic, which leads to enhanced productivity. Under either approach, employees are entitled to administrative due process or fundamental fairness consisting of the following:

• Procedural due process, that is, notice of an infraction and an opportunity to be heard on the matter before disciplinary action is taken.
• Substantive due process, that is, fair treatment. Under this prong of due process, the sanction(s) awarded for an offense must be reasonable in light of the totality of the circumstances. By analogy to criminal law, the punishment must fit the "crime."

In addition to being constructive and in compliance with due process standards, employee discipline should be progressive. This means that discipline takes place along a continuum of possible actions, ranging from no action at one extreme to discharge from employment at the other extreme. In between are progressive disciplinary steps, including a verbal warning, a written reprimand, a disciplinary transfer, and suspension from employment. For some offenses, the appropriate first step (after investigation) is discharge. Such offenses might include violent workplace behavior causing injury to others and sex offenses committed on the job.

Scenarios that may lead to disciplinary action against employees have recently been augmented by newly publicized ones, including resume fraud[99] and office romances.[100] Although employers are urged to have written policies making resume fraud grounds for dismissal from employment, the actual dismissal of an employee for resume fraud must be assessed case by case, taking into account the employee's whole record and the employer's financial and time investments in that employee. A survey conducted by the Society for Human Resource Management of its members revealed that 90 percent of human resource professionals believe that, unless a superior-subordinate relationship exists, dating among employees should not be prohibited.[101]

Discharge from employment has significant potential legal and financial consequences for employers and employees. The following procedural steps are recommended before executing disciplinary terminations of employees:

- Do not discharge an employee "on the spot" for any offense.
- Conduct a prompt and complete investigation of an alleged offense, affording all relevant parties (including the subject of the investigation) the opportunity to be heard.
- Consult with human resource management specialists and legal counsel for advice *ab initio* (Latin for "from the beginning") and throughout the process.
- If disciplinary termination is found to be warranted, ground it on a specific reason or reasons, and notify the employee in person, if feasible.
- Carefully and thoroughly document the investigatory process and retain it for at least the period of the legal statute of limitations for wrongful discharge,[102] along with all supporting documentation.

Health Care Professional Student Preemployment Contracts

The successful negotiation of preemployment contracts permits many health care professional students to contribute meaningfully toward self-funding their education, without being saddled with excessive loans upon entering the workforce. Employers also benefit from preemployment contracting with health care professional students in that their staffing processes are made more predictable, with relatively firm work commitments on the part of prospective scarce health care professionals.

Preemployment contracting also has several important potential disadvantages. The process of seeking out and negotiating preemployment contracts may foster excessive competition among students in selected job markets and practice settings. Employment contracts are formal legal instruments—just like any other business contract—with obligations incumbent on both parties, including penalties for breach of respective promises. Such contracts are often complex, containing elements such as conditions precedent to the receipt of employment bonuses and liquidated (preestablished) monetary damages provisions for nonperformance. Students who receive monetary bonuses from employers also incur tax liabilities. Health care professional program directors and student advisors should counsel students to have all preemployment agreements reviewed by legal counsel before signing them.

Students also should be counseled concerning potential ethical dilemmas associated with preemployment contracting. Potential issues include the hypothetical student who "shops" for other employment after having signed a contractual agreement with another entity from whom the student has received money. Students under contract to an employer may also be subject to preferential treatment in clinical affiliations and internship experiences vis-à-vis those not under contract by clinical faculty having undisclosed conflicts of interest.

Letters of Recommendation: To Write or Not to Write?

Employers, professors, clinical educators and managers, and other professionals are frequently asked to write letters of recommendation for employees, students, volunteers, and others. Prospective writers of recommendations may be torn ethically between the conflicting duties of helping someone whom they may like personally and conveying accurate information about the person. Cherrington[103] believes that letters of recommendation are biased and of little value and that "employers usually disregard such letters unless they contain negative information."

Writers of letters of recommendation often are constrained from making candid comments about candidates because of a fear of liability exposure. The legal morass surrounding letters of recommendation is indeed complex. Potential litigation over recommendations may include the following:

- **Defamation of character**, that is, the communication of false information injurious to a person's good reputation in the community. Slander is defamation communicated orally, and libel encompasses all other forms of defamation, including that conveyed in letters of recommendation.
- Invasion of privacy, that is, the public disclosure of private facts about a person, such as arrests, drug use, and sexual orientation. Courts have found liable and imposed punitive damages against employers who unlawfully release confidential employee information, such as a credit history, drug test results, and human immunodeficiency virus status.
- Intentional infliction of emotional distress, that is, unreasonable conduct (including the communication of information about a person) that results in severe physical and psychological injury.

At the opposite end of the legal spectrum, individuals may also face liability exposure for failing to provide a reference when they have agreed to do so, as may be spelled out in an employment contract or employee handbook. Litigation might also result if one candidate learns that an employer, or other official, has written a favorable reference for one candidate but has declined to do so for the litigant.

The growing concern over potential litigation over letters of recommendation has prompted many employers and individuals to change their policies on references. Many employers limit the information they convey to basic employment and salary data, even though, in some states, recommenders enjoy qualified immunity from liability as long as they act in good faith. Even with such protection, the burden of litigation over whether the writer is protected by qualified immunity is enough to prevent many individuals and companies from giving out information about others.

The following risk management suggestions are recommended for writers of letters of recommendation:

- Require a written request for information from a prospective employer or other requestor and a written release from the candidate (especially when the recommendation will be anything less than sterling) before releasing any information.
- Respond to requests for information about employees, students, or others only in writing, so that your words will not be misconstrued. Maintain file copies of correspondence for at least the length of time of the state statute of limitations on legal actions. (Check with your legal advisor regarding the length of the tort statute of limitations for your state.)
- If possible, centralize formal responses to reference requests. Have your human resource manager and/or legal advisor review and send out any responses to requests for information about current or former employees, students, volunteers, or others.

Restrictive Covenants in Employment Contracts

Restrictive covenants in employment contracts limit the ability of parties to act without restraint in specified ways. In health care contracts the principal types of restrictive covenants affecting employees are the nonsolicitation provision and the covenant not to compete. A nonsolicitation clause in an employment contract prevents a former professional employee from marketing his or her professional services to the employer's existing clients after termination of the employment relationship. A covenant not to compete is a contractual general promise made by an employee not to compete directly with a former employer.

A covenant not to compete is, in essence, a restraint on trade, which is generally considered to be against public policy. For that reason, a few states prohibit it altogether in employer-employee contracts. Even those states, however, permit such contractual provisions in cases involving the sale of an ongoing business to another professional in order to protect against exploitation of the "goodwill" value of the business being sold and during dissolution of a partnership. Most states allow covenants not to compete in employment contracts as a means to protect an employers' legitimate business interests.[104]

A covenant not to compete in an employment contract must meet four criteria in order to be valid and enforceable:

- It must be supported by consideration, that is, the covenant not to compete must have been made as part of a bargained-for exchange, and value must have been given by the employer in exchange for the employee's promise not to compete.
- A covenant not to compete must be reasonable in three areas in terms of the following:
  - The geographic area of practice restriction
  - Specific practice restrictions
  - Length of time

SUMMARY

Employment law is governed primarily by common and statutory law. The common law principle of employment at will governs most employment relationships and permits an employee or employer to terminate the business relationship at will without penalty. Exceptions to employment at will include employment under contract for a specific term and employment treated as contractual because of considerations such as language contained in employee handbooks and public policy considerations. The principle federal statute governing employment discrimination is Title VII of the Civil Rights Act of 1964, which prohibits employment discrimination against protected classes of workers based on race/ethnicity, gender, religion, and national origin. Supplementing Title VII, among other federal and state statutes, are the ADA and ADEA, which protect disabled and older workers from discrimination in employment.

Sexual misconduct is inclusive of all forms of sexual harassment, but not the other way around. Both forms of misconduct evidence disrespect for victims, and both are disparaging, not only of perpetrators in the health care environment but of the perpetrators' disciplines and health care in general. Sexual exploitation of patients, colleagues, students, and others is proscribed by law, customary practice, and professional ethical standards promulgated by professional associations of respective health care disciplines.

Three types of sexual misconduct involve health care providers and patients: nonconsensual sex, putative consensual sex, and PISBs that are not reciprocated by health care professionals. Because patients display transference emotions toward their caregivers, the concept of consent to sexual relations has no real meaning. All sexual conduct with patients is therefore nonconsensual. Clinicians and clinic managers must be ready to deal effectively with PISBs.

The two types of workplace sexual harassment are *quid pro quo,* or favorable employment considerations in exchange for sex, involving superiors and subordinates; and sexual harassment by a perpetrator of any person in the workplace, creating a hostile work environment and reasonably adversely affecting the work of a victim. The EEOC and federal courts have established legal standards regarding sexual harassment, which complement professional ethical standards promulgated by health care professional associations across many disciplines.

Anyone can be a victim of sexual harassment, and everyone can be a perpetrator. Therefore, every health care professional must be vigilant, but open, in professional relations with patients, colleagues, students, and others in the course of official duty.

The current complex work environment—especially under managed care—requires careful professional management of human resources. Human resource managers and legal counsel are key consultants to employers and employees.

Business ethics differ from health care professional ethics in that the former are largely driven by revenue, whereas the latter are focused on patient welfare. Under business ethics, business owners are not fiduciaries to their clients, whereas under health care professional ethics, clinicians clearly are.

CASES AND QUESTIONS

1. Develop five legitimate bona fide occupational qualifications that justify employment discrimination.
2. How can you reconcile the *Martin* and *Williams* Americans with Disabilities Acts case holdings?
3. Name five risk management measures specific to your practice setting that can be implemented to minimize the occurrence of sexual harassment of co-workers by employees.
4. P is a 36-year-old female physical therapist–MBA who is employed as a regional facilities manager for XYZ Company, a national rehabilitation services corporation. Q, an important business client of XYZ Company, makes an inappropriate pass at P during a business luncheon and subsequently fondles her breasts in the parking lot after lunch. What action(s) should P take?
5. X, a male medical student affiliated with ABC Hospital, solicits a date from Y, a female occupational therapy intern working at the facility. Is X's conduct, per se, improper? Is it appropriate for X and Y to date?

SUGGESTED ANSWERS TO CASES AND QUESTIONS

1. The following are examples of legitimate bona fide occupational qualifications that justify employment discrimination:
   a. Requirement that a religious minister be credentialed by the same denomination as the congregation.
   b. Requirement that a wet nurse be female.
   c. Requirement for male-only applicants for the position of attendant for a men's dressing room at a public swimming pool.
   d. Requirement for female-only applicants to play the role of Selena in the upcoming movie based on her life.
   e. Federal Aviation Administration regulations requiring airline pilots to retire at age 60.

2. *Martin* was a Title III case that specifically addressed the narrow issue of the use of a golf cart by a disabled professional during golf tournaments. *Williams* was a Title I case that addressed ambiguous disabilities in general.

3. The following are examples of risk management measures that can be implemented to minimize the occurrence of sexual harassment of co-workers by employees:
   a. Have in place and disseminate the clinic's policy recognizing sexual harassment as a prohibited behavior.
   b. Express a strong managerial commitment to preventing, investigating, and (where sexual harassment is established) punishing sexual harassment.
   c. Implement effective complaint and investigatory processes that are fair to all parties.
   d. In consultation with human resource management and legal consultants, establish orientation and ongoing training of the workforce concerning sexual harassment.
   e. Carry out systematic and *ad hoc* consultation and coordination with legal and human resource management specialists on sexual harassment issues.

4. P should immediately report Q's misconduct to her supervisors. Management then has the legal obligation to investigate and deal effectively with P's complaint. Although this case scenario does not exactly match the facts in the U.S. Supreme Court case *Ellerth* v. *Faragher* (1998), management has the ethical and legal duty to investigate P's complaint and take appropriate action, or face possible liability exposure. For an interesting analysis of a similar case and commentary from five business experts, see Magretta's "Will She Fit In?" (*Harvard Business Review* 75[2]:18, 1997.)

5. Based on these facts alone, X's solicitation of a date with Y and the process of dating between X and Y are not improper. ABC Hospital and the students' respective schools may not be legally empowered to impose and enforce a dating ban between students (although they would be so empowered to disallow students from dating patients and from dating supervising staff).

SUGGESTED READINGS

Armbruster KR, Ellard WM, Holtzclaw SR: ERISA preemption: state-law claims by health-care providers, *Health Lawyer* 8(2):12-14, 1995.

Assey JL, Hebert JM: Who is the seductive patient? *Am J Nurs* 83:530-532, 1983.

Berger E: Why does sexual activity climb in US? *San Antonio Express News* p 14A, March 9, 2005.

Cornell University Law School, Legal Information Institute: *Welcome to the LLI*. Retrieved March 18, 2007, from http://supct.law.cornell.edu/; an excellent ongoing free source of U.S. Supreme Court case decisions.

Davidson MJ: The Civil Rights Act of 1991, *Army Lawyer* pp 3-11, March 1992.

Employers face a difficult burden of proof when attempting to enforce a disability-based distinction in employee benefits, *Health Lawyer* 7(1):2, 1993.

Ensman RG: Don't ask! Twenty questions to avoid during employment interviews, *Advance for Health Information Professionals* p 15, Dec 13, 1993.

Fields G: Ten digit truth: fingerprinting of job seekers proliferates in private sector, *Wall Street Journal* p B1, June 7, 2005.

Fitzgerald LF: A new framework for sexual harassment cases, *Trial* pp 36-44, March 2003.

Fox MW: The changing face of discrimination law, *Texas Bar Journal* pp 564-569, June 2006.

Frye PR, Rose KC: Responsible representation of your first transgendered client, *Texas Bar Journal* pp 558-564, July 2003.

Furey MK, Ohnegian SA: Employee handbooks may be implied contracts, *National Law Journal* p B12, Oct 24, 1994.

Gostin LO, Widiss AI: What's wrong with the ERISA vacuum? Employers' freedom to limit health care coverage provided by risk retention plans, *JAMA* 269:2527-2532, 1993.

GPO Access: *Electronic Federal Code of Regulations*. Retrieved March 19, 2007, from http://www.ecfr.gpoaccess.gov.

Jackson S, Loftin A: Proactive practices avoid negligent hiring claims, *HR News* p 9, Sep 1995.

Korotkin MI: Damages in wrongful termination cases, *American Bar Association Journal* pp 84-87, May 1989.

Kruger P: See no evil, *Working Woman* pp 32-35, June 1995.

Legal report: cardinal rules for disciplinary terminations, Alexandria, Va, 1995, Society for Human Resource Management.

Lewis K: Physical therapy contracts, *Clinical Management* 12(6):14-18, 1992.

Lopez JA: Control the damage of a false accusation of sexual harassment, *Wall Street Journal* p B1, Jan 12, 1994.

Miller G: At-will employment doctrine: are patient care employers vulnerable? *Hosp Health Serv Adm* 36(2):257-270, 1991.

Niven D: The case of hidden harassment, *Harvard Business Review* pp 12-27, March/April 1992. The scenario presented in this case study involves a female office worker who is sexually harassed by her supervisor's superior. The victim's supervisor learns of the sexual harassment by chance, and when questioned about it, the victim does not want it to be reported. The case analysis offers the opinions of several human resource management and legal experts on how the victim's immediate supervisor should proceed.

O'Neal LL, Loftin AT: Consider context before firing for resume fraud, *HR News* p 13, Feb 1996.

Perry PM: Don't get sued for age discrimination, *Law Practice Management* pp 36-39, May/June 1995.

Perry R, Crist P: Strategies for negotiating preemployment agreements, *Am J Occup Ther* 48:824-831, 1994.

Phelan G: Reasonable accommodation: linchpin of ADA liability, *Trial* pp 40-44, Feb 1996.

Plevan BB, Borg JA: Expanded employer liability for supervisors' conduct in hostile work environments, *National Law Journal* pp B5-B10, Aug 8, 1994.

Rybski D: A quality implementation of Title I of the Americans with Disabilities Act of 1990, *Am J Occup Ther* 46:409-418, 1992.

Scott RW: Defending the apparently indefensible urinalysis client in nonjudicial proceedings, *Army Lawyer* pp 55-60, Nov 1986.

Scott RW: The ADA and you, *Clinical Management* 12(1):16-17, 1992.

A short history of the American labor movement, Washington, DC, 1981, American Federation of Labor–Congress of Industrial Organizations.

Shortell SM, Kaluzny AD: *Health care management: organization design and behavior,* ed 3, Albany, NY, 1994, Delmar.

US Department of Labor, Office of the Assistant Secretary for Administration and Management: *Title VII, Civil Rights Act of 1964, as amended.* Retrieved March 19, 2007, from www.dol.gov.

US Equal Employment Opportunity Commission: *Title VII, Civil Rights Act of 1964.* Retrieved March 25, 2007, from www.eeoc.gov.

Young RS: Managing medical leaves of absence, *HR Magazine* pp 23-30, Aug 1995.

Youngberg BJ: The Americans with Disabilities Act: meeting the challenge in the health care arena, *Quality & Risk Management in Health Care* 1(6):1-8, 1991.

REFERENCES

1. Knight D: Giving back, *Indianapolis Star* p D1, April 30, 2006.
2. Furey MK, Ohnegian SA: Employee handbooks may be implied contracts, *National Law Journal* p B12, Oct 24, 1994.
3. The Railway Labor Act of 1926, 45 United States Code Sections 151 et. seq.
4. The National Labor Relations Act of 1935 (Wagner Act), 29 United States Code Sections 151-187.
5. The Labor-Management Relations Act of 1947 (Taft-Hartley Act), 29 United States Code Sections 141 et. seq.
6. See Executive Order No. 10988, 1962.
7. 29 United States Code Sections 158, 183.
8. *American Hospital Association* v. *National Labor Relations Board,* 499 U.S. 606 (1991).
9. "33.2 percent of the total work force in the United States was unionized in 1955; 15.5 percent in 1994." *World Almanac and Book of Facts 1996,* Mahwah, NJ, 1995, World Almanac Books.
10. US Department of Labor, Bureau of Labor Statistics: *Union members summary.* Retrieved Jan 27, 2007, from www.bls.gov.
11. The Age Discrimination in Employment Act of 1967, 29 United States Code Sections 621-634.
12. The Older Workers Benefit Protection Act of 1990, 29 United States Code Section 623.
13. US Equal Employment Opportunity Commission: Discrimination by Type: Age. Retrieved Feb 21, 2007 from www.eeoc.gov.
14. The Americans with Disabilities Act of 1990, 42 United States Code Section 12101-12213.
15. Preamble, The Americans with Disabilities Act of 1990, Public Law 101-336, 104 Stat. 327, July 26, 1990.
16. The Rehabilitation Act of 1973, 29 United States Code Section 794a.
17. 42 United States Code Section 12187.
18. 42 United States Code Section 12111.
19. 42 United States Code Section 12102.
20. *The Americans with Disabilities Act: your responsibilities as an employer,* Pub No EEOC-BK-17, Washington, DC, 1991, Equal Employment Opportunity Commission (p 2).
21. 42 United States Code Section 12111.
22. US Equal Employment Opportunity Commission: *Discrimination by Type: Disability.* Retrieved Sept 7, 2007, from www.eeoc.gov.

23. *The Americans with Disabilities Act: your responsibilities as an employer,* Pub No EEOC-BK-17, Washington, DC, 1991, Equal Employment Opportunity Commission (p 6).

24. 42 United States Code Sections 12114, 12211.

25. *The Americans with Disabilities Act: your responsibilities as an employer,* Pub No EEOC-BK-17, Washington, DC, 1991, Equal Employment Opportunity Commission (p 15).

26. Enforcement Statistics and Litigation: ADA Cases. Retrieved Mar 8, 2007, from www.eeoc.gov.

27. *Borkowski* v. *Valley Central District,* 63 F.2d 131 (2d Cir. 1995).

28. *EEOC* v. *AIC Security Investigations, Ltd.,* 820 F. Supp. 1060 (N.D. III. 1993).

29. *Tuck* v. *HCA Health Services of Tennessee, Inc.,* 7 F.3d 465 (6th Cir. 1993).

30. *Langan* v. *Department of Health and Human Services,* 959 F.2d 1053 (D.C. Cir. 1992).

31. *Vande Zande* v. *Wisconsin Department of Administration,* 44 F.3d 538 (7th Cir. 1995).

32. *Harmer* v. *Virginia Electric & Power Company,* 831 F. Supp. 1300 (E.D. Va. 1993).

33. Phelan G: Reasonable accommodation: linchpin of ADA liability, *Trial* pp 40-44, Feb 1996. In this excellent overview article the author describes many additional reasonable ADA accommodation cases.

34. *U.S. Airways* v. *Barnett,* 535 U.S. 391 (2002).

35. *Chevron* v. *Echazabel,* 536 U.S. 73 (2002).

36. *Garrett* v. *University of Alabama,* 531 U.S. 356 (2001).

37. *Barnes* v. *Gorman,* 536 U.S. 181 (2002).

38. *Karracker* v. *Rent-A-Center,* 411 F.3d 831 (7th Cir. 2005).

39. *Albertsons Inc.* v. *Kirkenburg,* 527 U.S. 555 (1999). Based on this and related court cases, the Equal Employment Opportunity Commission amended its handbook *The Americans With Disabilities Act: Your Responsibilities as an Employer* to include the following material: "Since *The Americans with Disabilities Act: Your Responsibilities as an Employer* was published, the Supreme Court has ruled that the determination of whether a person has an ADA 'disability' must take into consideration whether the person is substantially limited in performing a major life activity when using a mitigating measure. This means that if a person has little or no difficulty performing any major life activity because s/he uses a mitigating measure, then that person will not meet the ADA's first definition of 'disability.' The Supreme Court's rulings were in *Sutton* v. *United Airlines, Inc.,* 527 U.S. 471 (1999), and *Murphy* v. *United Parcel Service, Inc.,* 527 U.S. 516 (1999)" (official page numbers of cases added by author).

As a result of the Supreme Court's ruling, the guidance from this handbook on mitigating measures, found in the section "Additional Questions and Answers on the Americans with Disabilities Act," is superseded. Following the Supreme Court's ruling, whether a person has an Americans with Disabilities Act "disability" is determined by taking into account the positive and negative effects of mitigating measures used by the individual. The Supreme Court's ruling does not change anything else in this document.

For more information on the Supreme Court rulings and their impact on determining whether specific individuals meet the definition of "disability," consult the *Instructions for Field Offices: Analyzing ADA Charges After Supreme Court Decisions Addressing "Disability" and "Qualified,"* which can be found on commission's website at www.eeoc.gov/policy/docs/field-ada.html.

40. *PGA Tour Inc.* v. *Martin,* 532 U.S. 661 (2001).

41. *Toyota Motor Manufacturing* v. *Williams,* 534 U.S. 184 (2002).

42. Wehman P, Revell W, Kregel J et al: Supported employment: an alternative model for vocational rehabilitation of persons with severe neurological, psychiatric, or physical disability, *Arch Phys Med Rehabil* 72(2):101-105, 1991.

43. Wilson JB: *ADA reform bill,* June 17, 2005. Retrieved March 12, 2007, from www.pointoflaw.com.

44. Civil Rights Act of 1964, Title VII, 42 United States Code Section 2000e-2000e-17.
45. U.S. Constitution, Article I, Section 8.
46. Civil Rights Act of 1964, Title VII, Section 703(a).
47. 29 Code of Federal Regulations Sections 1602.20(b), 1607.4(B), 1993.
48. Civil Rights Act of 1964, Title VII, Section 703(e).
49. The Civil Rights Act of 1991, Public Law 102-166, 105 Stat. 071, 42 United States Code Sections 1981a and 2000e.
50. 42 United States Code 1981 note.
51. *Wards Cove Packing Co.* v. *Atonio,* 490 U.S. 642 (1989).
52. Equal Employment Opportunity Commission: *The Civil Rights Act of 1991.* Retrieved March 19, 2007, from www.eeoc.gov/abouteeoc/35th/1990s/civilrights.html.
53. The Drug-Free Workplace Act of 1988, 41 United States Code Section 701-707.
54. Ibid., Section 701(a)(1)(A).
55. US Department of Labor: D*rug-free workplace advisor.* Retrieved March 20, 2007, from www.dol.gov/elaws/drugfree.htm.
56. Aalberts RJ, Rubin HW: A risk management analysis of employee drug abuse and testing, *Chartered Property and Casualty Underwriters Journal* 41(2):105-111, 1988.
57. Scott RW: Defending the apparently indefensible urinalysis client in nonjudicial proceedings, *Army Lawyer* pp 55-60, Nov 1986.
58. Allen TY: DOT drug-testing rules require detailed plans, *HR News* p 3, March 1996.
59. The Employee Polygraph Protection Act of 1988, 29 United States Code Section 2001-2009.
60. Scott RW: Defending the apparently indefensible urinalysis client in nonjudicial proceedings, *Army Lawyer* pp 55-60, Nov 1986 (at p 56, note 8).
61. The Employee Retirement Income Security Act of 1974, 29 United States Code Section 1001 et. seq.
62. Gostin LO, Widiss AI: What's wrong with the ERISA vacuum? Employers' freedom to limit health care coverage provided by risk retention plans, *JAMA* 269:2527-2532, 1993.
63. The Equal Pay Act of 1963, 29 United States Code Section 206, an amendment to the Fair Labor Standards Act, provides in pertinent part that "No employer shall discriminate between employees on the basis of sex by paying wages to employees less than the rate at which he pays wages to employees of the opposite sex for equal work on jobs which require equal skill, effort, and responsibility, and similar working conditions" (29 U.S.C. Section 206d[1]).
64. US Equal Employment Opportunity Commission: *EEOC's Charge Processing Procedures.* Retrieved Sep 7, 2007, from www.eeoc.gov.
65. The Family and Medical Leave Act of 1993, 29 United States Code Section 2601-2654.
66. Young RS: Managing medical leaves of absence, *HR Magazine* pp 23-30, August 1995. citing "Survey of 123 Fortune 500 companies by Labor Policy Association, Washington, DC."
67. *Ragsdale* v. *Wolverine Worldwide Inc.,* 535 U.S. 81 (2002).
68. The Occupational Safety and Health Act of 1970, 29 United States Code Section 651-678.
69. The Pregnancy Discrimination Act of 1978, 42 United States Code Section 2000e(k).
70. Equal Employment Opportunity Commission: *Facts about pregnancy discrimination,* Jan. 15, 2004. Retrieved March 22, 2007, from www.eeoc.gov/facts/fs-preg.html.
71. White B: Workers' compensation rates drop as reform legislation takes hold, *Houston Business Journal* p 30, Nov 29, 1993.
72. Cherrington DJ: *The management of human resources,* ed 4, Englewood Cliffs, NJ, 1995, Prentice Hall (p 509).

73. Besides being covered under state-sponsored workers' compensation insurance plans, employers in many states may self-insure against worker injuries. In three states—Texas, New Jersey, and South Carolina—employers may opt out of participation in state workers' compensation systems altogether but must otherwise insure against claims and lawsuits from injured employees. CCH/Wolters Kluwer Financial Services: *Nonsubscriber Workers' Compensation Plan*. Retrieved Mar 23, 2007, from www.insource.nlis.com.

74. Equal Employment Opportunity Commission: *Sex discrimination guidelines*, EEOC 29 Code of Federal Regulations 1604.11, Federal Register, 45:74677, 1980.

75. *Robinson* v. *Jacksonville Shipyards*, 760 F. Supp. 1486 (Middle District of Florida, 1991).

76. Hays AS: Courts concede that the sexes think in unlike ways, *Wall Street Journal* p B1, May 28, 1991.

77. Struckman-Johnson CS, Struckman-Johnson D: Men's reactions to hypothetical female sexual advances, *Sex Roles* 1:387, 1994. See also Wade N: Pas de deux of sexuality is written in the genes, *New York Times* p D1, April 10, 2007.

78. *Ellison* v. *Brady*, 924 F.2d 871 (9th Circuit 1991).

79. *Naval Personnel Bulletin 15620: Resolving conflict: following the light of personal behavior*, Washington, DC, 1993, US Government Printing Office.

80. *Disclosure*, 1995, Warner Bros.

81. *Oncale* v. *Sundowner Offshore Services*, 523 U.S. 75 (1998).

82. *Burlington Industries* v. *Ellerth*, 524 U.S. 742 (1998).

83. *Faragher* v. *Boca Raton*, 524 U.S. 775 (1998).

84. Graf LA, Hemmasi M: Risque humor: how it really affects the workplace, *HR Magazine* pp 64-69, Nov 1995.

85. Hays AS: Courts concede that the sexes think in unlike ways, *Wall Street Journal* p B1, May 28, 1991.

86. Hicks M: Love amid the cubicles, *San Francisco Examiner* p D1, Feb 12, 1995.

87. Gutheil TG, Gabbard GO: Misuses and misunderstandings of boundary theory in clinical and regulatory settings, *Am J Psychiatry* 155(3):409-414, 1998.

88. Title IX of the Education Amendments of 1972, 20 United States Code Sections 1681-1683. The case of *Jackson* v. *Birmingham School Board*, 544 U.S. 167 (2005) held that Title IX's private right of action includes retaliation claims by individuals who complain about sexual harassment.

89. *Oslund* v. *United States*, Civ. No. 4-88-323 (US District Court, District of Minnesota, Oct 23, 1989).

90. McComas J, Hebert C, Glacomin C et al: Experiences of student and practicing physical therapists with inappropriate patient sexual behavior, *Phys Ther* 73:762-769, 1993.

91. deMayo RA: Patient sexual behaviors and sexual harassment: a national survey of physical therapists, *Phys Ther* 77:739-744, 1997.

92. Farber N, Novack D, Silverstein J et al: Physicians' experiences with patients who transgress boundaries, *J Gen Intern Med* 15(11):770-775, 2000.

93. White G: Sexual harassment during medical training: the perceptions of medical students at a university medical school in Australia, *Med Educ* 34:980-986, 2000.

94. *Preemployment inquiries*, Washington, DC, 1991, Equal Employment Opportunity Commission.

95. Swoboda F: Extending the benefits umbrella to a wider world, *Washington Post* p H5, June 4, 1995.

96. Jackson S, Loftin A: Proactive practices avoid negligent hiring claims, *HR News* p 9, Sep 1995.

97. Internal Revenue Service: *Small business and self-employed one-stop resource*. Retrieved April 18, 2007, from www.irs.gov/businesses/small.

98. Cherrington DJ: *The management of human resources,* ed 4, Englewood Cliffs, NJ, 1995, Prentice Hall (p 594).

99. Strauss R: When the resume is not to be believed, *New York Times* p E2, Sep 12, 2006.

100. Fandray D: Office romances: to control love in the cubicles, put a policy in place, *Continental Vision* pp 25-26, June 2003.

101. *Legal report: cardinal rules for disciplinary terminations,* Alexandria, Va, 1995, Society for Human Resource Management.

102. Korotkin MI: Damages in wrongful termination cases, *American Bar Association Journal* pp 84-87, May 1989.

103. Cherrington DJ: *The management of human resources,* ed 4, Englewood Cliffs, NJ, 1995, Prentice Hall (p 228).

104. Koeppel D: Lose the employee. Keep the business, *New York Times* p C5, May 5, 2005.

NOTES

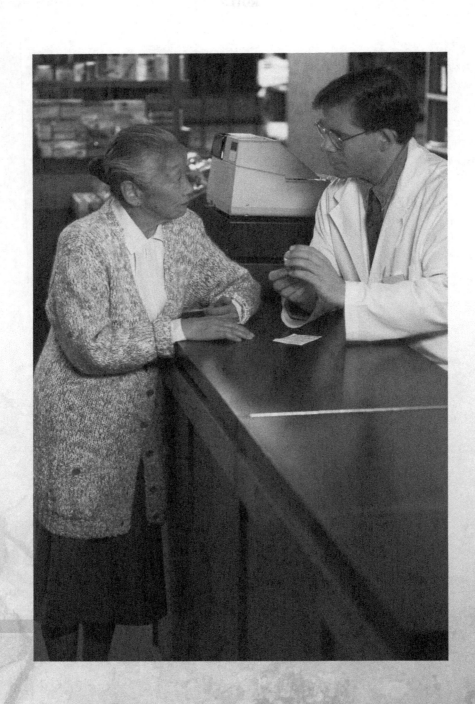

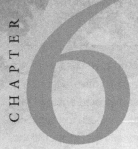
Business Law and Ethics

KEY TERMS

Acceptance

Administrative law

Advance directives

Agreement

Antitrust law

Bilateral contract

Borrowed servant rule

Business disparagement

Business torts

By operation of law

Capacity

Caveat emptor

Chattels

Claims-made

Clean hands doctrine

Clinical affiliation agreements

Conditions concurrent

Condition precedent

Conditions subsequent

Consequential damages

Consideration

Copyright

Corporation

Counteroffer

Damages at law

Depositions

Disaffirm

Durable power of attorney
for health care decisions

Enjoin

Equitable remedies

Executed

Expectancy damages

Express contract

Four-corners doctrine

General partnership

Good Samaritan

Guarantor

Implied contract

Implied-in-fact

Implied-in-law

Impossibility of performance

Incidental damages

Integration clause

Intellectual property

Interrogatories

Joint venture

Laissez faire

Legal benefit

Legality

Limited liability company

Liquidated damages

Living will

Material breach

Mutuality of assent

Offeree

Offeror

One-year rule

Parol evidence rule

Patent

Performance

Prima facie

Pro bono publico

Professional corporations

Promisee

Promisor

Quasi-contract

Ratification

Rejection

Reliance damages

Restitution damages

Risk pooling

Risk transfer

Service mark

Sole proprietorship

Status quo ante

Statutes of frauds

Subpoena duces tecum

Trademark

Treble

Unilateral contract

Void

Voidable

Wrongful interference with a
contractual relationship

INTRODUCTION

This chapter introduces basic business law concepts, beginning with a discussion of administrative law and the important roles of federal and state administrative agencies in overseeing health care business operations. Other concepts discussed include antitrust law, attorney-client relations (including deposition preparation and practice), business tort litigation, contracts, forms of business organizations (sole proprietorships, partnerships, corporations, and hybrid forms), good Samaritan laws, the Health Insurance Portability and Accountability Act, insurance, the Patient Self-Determination Act, professional advertising, the Safe Medical Devices Act, and the Sarbanes-Oxley Act.

ADMINISTRATIVE LAW

Administrative law encompasses all of the legal principles governing the activities and procedures of federal, state, and local governmental agencies, boards, commissions, and other similar entities. The influence of the hundreds of administrative agencies over business and professional affairs in the United States has become so pervasive over the past half century that administrative agencies have come to be referred to as the "fourth branch" of government. The late Professor Kenneth Culp Davis (1908-2003), administrative law scholar, noted that business professionals have greater interface with state and federal administrative agencies than with any other branch of government at all levels of interaction.[1] Health care professionals have continuous interaction with administrative agencies on issues such as licensure, reimbursement, taxation, and workplace safety.

Administrative agencies have grown in number and risen in prominence since World War II for several reasons. First and foremost, the complexity of modern-day society and the business environment has led generally to a perceived need for greater governmental assistance, oversight, and intervention in business and professional affairs. From environmental regulation and health care administration to labor relations and professional licensure, governmental administrative agencies at all levels have become ever more involved in rule making and regulation of business activities. In addition to becoming more complex, society also has become less averse to governmental regulation of business in the twenty-first century (although there currently is an equivocal counterswing of the pendulum of public opinion in this regard). The doctrine of *laissez faire* was replaced by an attitude of trust in the ability and integrity of government to protect the public from unethical and incompetent businesspersons.

Administrative agencies, especially at the federal level, possess attributes of all three traditional branches of government. Under a valid constitutional delegation of legislative authority (often under vague guidelines), administrative agencies make rules (a legislative function); investigate matters under their jurisdiction pursuant to broad discretionary powers (an executive function); and enforce their rules through adjudication and the award of sanctions against violators (a judicial function).

To survive legal scrutiny, the activities of administrative agencies must fall within the constitutionally permissible delegation of federal or state legislative authority. In addition to carrying out activities pursuant to a valid delegation of legislative authority, administrative agency activities also must afford procedural due process (notice; opportunity to be heard) to those under their jurisdiction.

When the meanings of statutes are not altogether clear, the rules and decisions of administrative agencies must be found by the courts to be reasonable interpretations of such statutes. Administrative rules and decisions must be reasonable and reasoned, not arbitrary or capricious. Courts typically defer to the proper exercise of administrative agency authority.[2]

Three important federal statutes warrant mentioning in this section. The Administrative Procedure Act of 1946[3] provides a statutory framework for most decision making by federal administrative agencies. The Freedom of Information Act of 1966[4] requires federal governmental agencies to make public documents available expeditiously to requesters, absent statutory exemptions to their release. There were 480,300 Freedom of Information Act requests processed in 2005, down from 520,300 in 1998.[5] The Privacy Act of 1974[6] requires federal agencies to inform individuals about the purposes and uses of information collected about them. Like the Freedom of Information Act, the Privacy Act contains a number of exceptions authorizing release of personal information about individuals to federal agencies and to entities outside the federal government without their consent. State governments commonly have similar statutory schemes for administrative procedure, release of public records, and protection of privacy.

ANTITRUST LAW

Antitrust law, consisting of statutes, case law, and administrative regulations and rulings, has as its primary purpose the promotion of competition among private sector businesses that benefits the general public. The three federal statutes that provide the framework for federal antitrust regulation are the Sherman Act of 1890,[7] the Clayton Act of 1914,[8] and the Federal Trade Commission Act of 1914.[9] States also enact antitrust laws, but the federal courts have exclusive jurisdiction over federal antitrust law.

The Sherman Act has two sections. Section One prohibits business agreements or arrangements that unreasonably interfere with interstate commerce (restraint of trade). Certain types of business practices are so blatantly anticompetitive that they are always considered to be illegal, such as agreements to fix prices and group boycotts of competitors (*per se* violations). The **legality** of other types of agreements are analyzed on case by case under the "rule of reason." Section Two prohibits the willful acquisition or maintenance of monopoly power in a given market or the attempt to achieve such control. Willful monopolization of a market or industry is done with the intent to affect competition adversely.

The Clayton Act prohibits specific anticompetitive business practices, including unjustified price discrimination by sellers and unreasonable mergers and acquisitions, among other practices. The Federal Trade Commission Act created the

Federal Trade Commission, an administrative agency that, along with the Department of Justice, administers federal antitrust law. The Department of Justice can bring criminal or civil legal actions against alleged violators of the Sherman Act. Private parties personally injured by such violations can sue civilly, and if successful, recover triple (**treble**) damages and the cost of their attorneys' fees.

Certain entities enjoy statutory or judicial exemptions from the enforcement of federal antitrust laws. Those of particular interest to health care professionals include the following:

- State governments and their political subdivisions, as well as private parties who are acting (with active state supervision) under clear statutory authority ("state action doctrine")[10]
- Activities of industries highly regulated by federal agencies, including transportation, communications, and banking
- The insurance industry
- Labor unions
- Cooperative research activities involving small businesses
- Concerted political action by private businesspersons (including professional associations) to affect or create law (the Noerr-Pennington doctrine)[11]

Health care is not exempt from compliance with antitrust laws, although health care was largely ignored for purposes of antitrust enforcement by government agencies and the courts until recently.[12] That changed in 1975 when the U.S. Supreme Court, in *Goldfarb* v. *Virginia State Bar*,[13] disallowed a "learned professions" exemption for health care and other professional services.

Since 1975, there have been a number of prominent applications of federal antitrust laws to health care service delivery. In 1988 in *Patrick* v. *Burget*,[14] the U.S. Supreme Court held that private medical staff privileging actions that are not actively supervised by state governmental agencies do not enjoy "state action" immunity from antitrust scrutiny. In 1990 the U.S. Supreme Court, in *Wilk* v. *American Medical Association*,[15] denied review of the decision of the Seventh Circuit Court of Appeals that the American Medical Association had carried out an illegal boycott of the chiropractic profession in violation of Section One of the Sherman Act. The Department of Health and Human Services has issued guidelines for health care professionals and entities, designed to create safe zones within which they can avoid potential civil and criminal liability involving hospital and physician joint ventures.[16] Stark I and II, addressing permissible and impermissible physician self-referral for ancillary services, was previously discussed in Chapter 4.

EXERCISE

Consider managed care. What antitrust (restraint of trade) considerations might apply to managed care practices?

ADVERTISING PROFESSIONAL SERVICES

When it comes to advertising professional health care services, the traditional adage of *caveat emptor* ("let the buyer beware") is tempered by legal and ethical considerations favoring patient rights. Until the late 1970s, health care professional ethics codes and that of the legal profession proscribed professional advertising.

Advertising in any form by health care and legal professionals was formerly considered inappropriate for a number of reasons. It was argued that advertising of health care and legal services had an adverse effect on professionalism, was misleading, and engendered undesirable economic consequences, including increased overhead cost passed on to consumers and creation of a substantial entry barrier to more junior professional colleagues attempting to enter or penetrate a market. In 1977, these arguments were systematically addressed and refuted by the U.S. Supreme Court in *Bates and Van O'Steen v. State Bar of Arizona,*[17] the landmark legal case involving professional advertising.

In *Bates,* the U.S. Supreme Court held that the advertising of professional services fell within the rubric of First Amendment free speech rights. Specifically, the court declared that truthful advertising about the availability and cost of professional service delivery serves an important societal interest—to ensure that consumers make informed decisions about professional services based on readily available, complete, and reliable information.

Because professional advertising is a form of "commercial speech," it does not enjoy the broadest constitutional protection otherwise afforded to political or literary speech under the First Amendment. Government entities are free to regulate professional advertising to prevent the dissemination of misleading, deceptive, or false advertising, and advertisements for illegal activities (such as regulated health services rendered by unauthorized providers). As with other forms of protected speech, states may impose reasonable restrictions on the time, place, and manner of professional advertising.

Forms of health care professional advertising that might be prohibited as misleading, deceptive, or false could include advertisements that compare the relative quality of services offered among competitors ("comparative competitor claims"). In addition to being subject to constitutionally permissible state regulation, such advertisements might expose the advertising professional to common law business tort liability (discussed subsequently).

Subsequent to *Bates,* primary health care disciplines revised their ethics codes to reflect the change in legal status of professional advertising. The advertising of professional services requires a balance between legal and ethical considerations and the right of professionals to free speech. Such a balance is not always easy to maintain.

EXERCISE

Examine the ethics code and guidelines of your discipline. What are the permissible parameters for professional advertising? Compare the provisions of your discipline to that of another health care professional discipline.

ATTORNEY–HEALTH CARE PROFESSIONAL CLIENT RELATIONS

How, When, and Where to Seek Legal Advice

In the potentially litigious business environment in which they work, health care professionals need to have available legal counsel for confidential advice. Providers need to consult with their attorneys, not only when a potentially compensable event such as patient injury arises but also for everyday business and personal affairs.

Every health care professional—whether self-employed or employed by another person or entity—should individually form a professional relationship with an attorney of choice. In no other professional relationship is a client able to discuss business and personal matters openly and know that, with few exceptions, the information conveyed to the advisor will be held in strict confidence. Such is the nature of the attorney-client relationship.

How does one locate an attorney? The best ways to find an attorney are through word-of-mouth recommendations of professional colleagues[19] and through communication with bar association lawyer referral services. Bar associations usually offer lawyer referral services at no fee or at a low fee for the initial consultation and refer only to highly reputable attorneys who are specialists in areas of client interest. One of the least effective ways to choose an attorney is randomly to select one from listings in a telephone directory.

An attorney representing a health care professional optimally should be intimately familiar with the legal issues pertinent to the client's discipline. To the extent that an attorney is not familiar with a health care professional client's discipline, it is the responsibility of the client to educate the attorney about the discipline and pertinent issues affecting the client. At all times, the client should be in control of the attorney-client relationship.[20]

Attorneys have frequently been the subject of humor and ridicule in recent times.[21] To a certain degree, the levity is harmless and the public's angst understandable.

RULE 1.6 OF THE *MODEL RULES OF PROFESSIONAL CONDUCT*

Confidentiality of Information

(A) A lawyer shall not reveal information relating to representation of a client unless the client consents after consultation, except for disclosures that are implicitly authorized in order to carry out the representation, and except as stated in paragraph (B).

(B) A lawyer may reveal such information to the extent the lawyer reasonably believes necessary:

(1) to prevent the client from committing a criminal act that the lawyer believes is likely to result in imminent death or substantial bodily harm; or

(2) to establish a claim or defense on behalf of the lawyer in a controversy between the lawyer and the client, to establish a defense to a criminal charge or civil claim against the lawyer based upon conduct in which the client was involved, or to respond to allegations in any proceeding concerning the lawyer's representation of the client.[18]

However, in their defense, attorneys have probably the most extensive history of *pro bono publico* (free of charge or reduced-fee) service to socioeconomically disadvantaged clients of any professionals.[22] In the best light, attorneys are champions for their clients and defenders of justice and order. In the least favorable light, attorneys are seen as personifications of societal problems.

> Every health care professional should form a professional relationship with an attorney of personal choice.

Pretrial Depositions: The Make or Break Point in Malpractice Litigation

Depositions are pretrial procedures in which parties and (fact and expert) witnesses are questioned by attorneys and give answers under oath concerning issues that are or may be pertinent to pending litigation. Everything said in a deposition is recorded and transcribed by a court reporter, and the transcript is reduced to written form for introduction at trial.

Health care professionals undergoing deposition must take them seriously. The adage, "A witness in deposition today may be a defendant tomorrow" is one that health care professional deponents should always remember.

No witness should undergo deposition without being prepared for the process by his or her attorney. Deposition preparation of a deponent by an attorney has been called "the most important trip to the woodshed."[23] The following are some important tips for prospective nonexpert deponents:

- Always remember that a deposition is serious business. Dress in business attire for your deposition. Do not make jokes with your attorney, the opposing attorney, or anyone else in the process.
- Keep in mind that a major purpose for a deposition is to find out or "discover" important information favorable to a party in litigation. The deposition process is sometimes referred to as a "fishing expedition."
- Do not bring any items with you to a deposition that are not demanded of you by opposing counsel in a *subpoena duces tecum*.
- Irrespective of how nice or friendly the opposing attorney appears, he or she is not a friend of the deponent. Treat opposing counsel with caution and respect.
- Wait for a question to be completely stated before answering. Consider pausing to think before answering. (Pauses before answering should not be reflected in a deposition transcript, unless they are also indicated in the record for the attorneys and others who speak during the deposition.)
- Do not argue with opposing counsel.
- Do not use statements such as "Do I have to answer that?" and "Can we go off the record?"
- If you do not understand a question, ask for it to be repeated. If you do not know an answer, state that you do not know the answer. Do not guess!
- Do not volunteer information. As a deponent, carefully limit your answers to respond only to the precise questions asked, and do so in as few words as possible.

- If your attorney objects on the record to a question, stop speaking immediately and do not resume until the objection is resolved by the attorneys.
- Do not let opposing counsel put words in your mouth by summarizing what you have testified. Carefully correct improper characterizations of your testimony.
- Freely admit, if asked, that you have been prepared for your deposition by your attorney.
- If, at any time, you need to take a break to use the restroom or get a drink of water, state that you need a break. Do not let opposing counsel question you for hours on end without taking a reasonable number of breaks. (A tired deponent becomes careless and shows anger with opposing counsel more easily than one who is refreshed. A jury may consider an agitated and argumentative deponent to be an untruthful person.)
- Exercise your rights to review and correct your deposition after it is transcribed. Carefully review, correct, and sign it with assistance of counsel.

Consider the following hypothetical deposition scenario:

T is an occupational therapist being sued by P, a patient, for professional negligence for injury incident to a functional capacity assessment. T's deposition is being taken by P's attorney in the attorney's law office. T, who is 8 ½ months pregnant, is represented at the deposition by her attorney. The deposition begins at 8:30 AM. After one morning restroom break, a 30-minute lunch break, and one afternoon restroom break, T is visibly physically and emotionally exhausted. She begins to argue with, and make sarcastic remarks to, P's attorney during questioning. What should T's attorney do? T's attorney should, considering the fact that T is 8 ½ months pregnant, demand that the session be suspended until the next day and state the reason for the demand on the record, and further inquire of the opposing counsel on the record about the projected length of the residual portion of T's deposition. (P's attorney may be deliberately trying to wear T down physiologically and emotionally so that T's testimony will favor P's case. Unless the deposition is videotaped, a jury will not know that T was pregnant while being deposed.)

Health care administrators and facility clinic and risk managers should consider implementing ongoing in-service education programs on legal issues targeted to specific disciplines or interdisciplinary groups of professionals. Discussions about, and even simulations of, depositions (under attorney guidance) should be included in such programs. Education about legal issues may enhance professionals' sense of confidence in their practices and reduce stress and costly defensive health care practice.

Health care professionals undergoing deposition must take the process seriously because "a witness in deposition today may be named as a defendant in the case tomorrow."

BUSINESS TORTS

Business torts are wrongs committed against the legitimate proprietary business interests of individuals, partnerships, or corporations. Actionable business torts vary from state to state. Three that have the potential to arise frequently in health care settings are discussed in this section. These torts are tortious interference with a contractual relationship, interference with a prospective business relationship, and business disparagement.

Tortious or **wrongful interference with a contractual relationship** involves wrongful conduct on the part of a person or business entity intentionally to induce another person or business to breach an existing contract. An example of wrongful interference with an existing contract would be the situation in which one managed health care organization wrongfully caused a physical therapist–employee, who is under contract with a competitor, to breach the contract and come to work for the tortfeasor. Keep in mind that, absent the existence of a valid, enforceable contract (normally including contracts terminable at the will of the parties), the tort of wrongful interference with a contractual relationship is not normally actionable. Absent predatory, malicious conduct by a party, competition by rivals for employees or other business interests constitutes legitimate business practice.

Wrongful interference with a prospective business relationship occurs when one party intentionally and wrongfully acts to interfere with a pending business relationship. Such a situation would include wrongfully inducing a party in contract negotiations with another party to break off negotiations.

Business disparagement involves the wrongful communication of false information about a businessperson or entity that causes injury to the victim's business reputation or interests. The tort of disparagement is also commonly known, in its various forms, as injurious falsehood, slander of quality or of title, and trade libel.

CONTRACTS

Contract law forms the foundation for all commercial transactions, including purchases of goods and services (including patient care services) and employment relationships. A majority of civil legal cases involve, not health care malpractice, but commercial, contractual disputes. A binding contract does not necessarily have to be in writing in order to be enforceable.

As much as with any area of law, issues involving commercial contracts have business, legal, and ethical considerations. For example, beyond the legalities of, say, a health care professional student accepting multiple interview opportunities in exotic locations (even though the student has already accepted a position locally and has no intention of accepting one of those positions), there are also ethical concerns to address. Is this sort of practice right or fair, and does it reflect disfavorably on the student's profession? In addition, a business consideration associated with the practice of accepting multiple job interviews for positions that a candidate has no intention of pursuing is that this practice may have adverse employment consequences in that the candidate's professional reputation may be tarnished by the practice. Also, the sojourner may find himself or herself without important future networking opportunities with professional colleagues.

The right of individuals and corporations (also legally considered to be "persons") to contract is fundamental in American law. This right is one of only a few private rights that are enumerated in the body of the U.S. Constitution. Article I, Section 10 of the Constitution states:

No state shall ... pass any ... Law impairing the Obligation of Contracts.[24]

The freedom of individuals to create contracts gives private citizens and corporations immense power over private business affairs. In essence, parties to business contracts are virtually free to create their own "private law," which the civil courts will enforce with few exceptions. Those exceptions to enforcement of private, contractual law generally involve agreements that involve illegal subject matter or contain provisions that violate public policy considerations.

Every professional interaction between a health care professional and a patient involves at least an **implied contract**. Even when there are no written or otherwise formally stated contractual terms to the patient care agreement, that is, an **express contract**, the law imposes certain obligations upon the health care provider and the patient.

When does a health care provider begin to owe a duty of special care to a patient? The special, implied contractual duty of special care arises when the health care provider agrees to accept the patient for evaluation and possible treatment. In simplified contractual terms, the patient presents himself or herself for care and makes an offer to become a patient. The health care professional, then, is normally free to accept or reject the patient's offer. **Acceptance** of the patient by the health care provider for care completes the **bilateral contract**, in which both parties incur legally enforceable obligations.

The health care professional has (at least) the following contractual obligations: to exercise sound professional judgment in order to reach a correct diagnosis and use his or her best professional skills to try to effect an optimal therapeutic result for the patient; to maintain a professional demeanor throughout the relationship; to refer the patient to other professionals, when warranted; and to safeguard confidential patient information, unless required by law to reveal such information.

The patient, too, has legally binding contractual obligations associated with the health care professional–patient relationship. These obligations normally include the obligation to pay for services rendered (personally or through a third-party intermediary) and to cooperate with the health care professional in charge of the patient's care, as well as the support staff carrying out the clinician's directives.

Definition of a "Contract"

A contractual promise, in its simplest terms, is one that a person (or corporation) makes that is legally enforceable. The American Law Institute formally defines a contract as "a promise or set of promises for the breach of which the law gives a remedy, [and] the performance of which the law in some way recognizes as a duty."[25] By a "promise," the legal system defines a contractual obligation as one that binds a party to a contract to perform some action, or refrain from action, presently or at some future time.

Contract: A promise enforceable as a legally binding obligation.

Bilateral Versus Unilateral Contracts

Most business contracts are bilateral contracts, meaning that there are two or more parties to an agreement who are legally bound to perform (or refrain from acting) in some way. In a bilateral contract, both parties exchange mutual contractual promises that by virtue of consideration (discussed subsequently) create legally binding obligations upon the parties. Contracts between health care professionals and patients for health care service delivery are examples of bilateral contracts.

A **unilateral contract** (relatively uncommon in business settings) is one in which one party can consummate a binding contract only by completing some action (or omission) requested by another party. In a unilateral contract, then, there is no formal exchange of contractual promises, only a contractual offer made by one person to another, that demands specific action on the part of the latter party. Consider the following hypothetical situation:

> *It is a Wednesday. A, a contract physical therapist working in a home health setting, is obligated to come to the home of B, a bedridden patient, for a treatment session on Saturday. A, however, is suddenly called away for an emergency out-of-town professional association meeting and knows that she cannot return by Saturday. A wants to ensure that she provides physical therapy coverage for her home patients, including B. A telephones C, a physical therapist colleague to whom she has made frequent referrals in the recent past. When A calls C at C's office, A is already at the airport, ready to board a flight for her meeting. C is not in, so A leaves the following message on C's answering machine: "If you make the home visit to B for me on Saturday for treatment, I will pay you $50.00." C returns to her office at the end of the day and hears the message. Once C completes performance of the patient visit to B, the unilateral contract is consummated, and A becomes legally bound to fulfill her promise to pay C for C's services.*

Under a unilateral contract, then, only the party making a contractual promise (A, in the hypothetical example) is contractually bound to act in a certain way (in this case, to pay money to C for C's services). The person to whom the offer and promise to perform are made (C) has no legal obligation to do anything. Only if the party to whom the offer and promise are made completes the requested performance does a contract exist. At that point, the promisor's duty is to perform as promised (e.g., by paying for what was requested or by performing a service in return).

Basic Elements of a Binding Contract

Four basic required elements are common to all contracts. These elements are (1) contractual agreement between or among the parties, (2) mutual consideration in support of parties' contractual promises, (3) recognized legal capacity on the part of the parties to enter into a binding contract, and (4) legality of the subject matter of the agreement.[26]

Parties to a Contract

Several legal terms are commonly used to describe the parties to a contract. These terms initially may appear confusing, but once learned, they aid in simplifying the discussion of contract issues with readers' business advisors and legal counsel. In a bilateral or unilateral contract, the party making an offer to be contractually bound to some performance is called the **offeror**, or **promisor**. The party to whom an offer is directed is called the **offeree**, or **promisee**.

Agreement

Agreement of the parties in a bilateral contract to be legally bound to perform their mutual promises is a fundamental element in the contractual process. The mutual agreement of parties to a bilateral contract to be bound to performance is often referred to as **mutuality of assent**.[27]

An offeror virtually controls the scope of duty that he or she incurs to an offeree by the way in which the offeror phrases the contractual offer. An offeror can restrict acceptance of the offer to specifically named persons. Restrictions can also be placed on acceptable time frames for accepting a contractual offer. Restrictions can even be placed on the permissible modes and forms of acceptance of an offer.

Special conditions can be attached to an offer as the offeror sees fit (within the bounds of law and public policy), and the occurrence (or nonoccurrence) of such conditions may discharge one or both parties' duty to perform under the contract. For example, an offeror can expressly condition his or her performance under a contract to the happening of some precondition, such as receipt of favorable financing for a business loan. Such a condition is called a **condition precedent**.

In the health care setting, it is generally illegal and unethical to condition patient care on the patient's signing of a waiver or limitation of liability. These exculpatory releases are generally unenforceable as conditions precedent because they violate public policy.[28] Bargained-for agreements that require providers and patients to resolve grievances through mediation and/or arbitration, rather than through litigation, however, are generally valid and enforceable.

Parties to a bilateral contract may also require simultaneous performance of their contractual obligations, such as might be the case in a contract between a health care continuing education course sponsor and presenter. Simultaneous performance conditions are called **conditions concurrent**.

Finally, the parties may condition their continuing performance under a contract to some future event, such as is exemplified by a "military relocation" discontinuance clause in a military health care provider's off-duty employment contract with a civilian health care agency. Such conditions are referred to as **conditions subsequent**.

Once an offer, the terms of which are reasonably certain, is properly accepted by an offeree, there is mutuality of assent, and a binding contract is formed. Remember that the making of a **counteroffer** by an offeree to an offer is normally considered as a **rejection** of the initial offer, not a conditional acceptance. The counteroffer then becomes a new offer, which the original offeror may be able to accept and thus form a bilateral contract.

Generally, certain basic elements must be present in every oral and written business contract. These elements are the following:

- Identification of the parties to the contract
- Identification of the subject matter of the contract
- The consideration, or value, given by each party to the other
- Time frames for performance of the parties and payment, when indicated

Consideration

Consideration can be thought of as the inducement that causes a party to a contract to allow himself or herself to become legally bound to perform under the agreement. Consideration does not always equate to money. Many health care and other business contracts (especially under the so-called barter system) call for mutual performance of professional services rather than the payment of any money.

Another common explanation for consideration in support of a party's contractual promise is that it can be construed as some legal detriment to the promisee or some **legal benefit** to the promisor.[29] That is, the party promising performance must be legally benefited in some way by the other party for having made a contractual promise, or the party to whom performance is promised must incur some legal detriment (such as forgoing another business opportunity).

> **Consideration:** Value given in exchange for another person's contractual promise.

In short, consideration is value given in exchange for another person's contractual promise. Courts do not normally critique whether what is exchanged is equivalent but rather normally leave contractual parties free to bargain as they see fit.

Capacity

Contractual **capacity** refers to the legal ability of prospective parties to enter into contracts that are enforceable. Most prospective parties to business contracts display obvious capacity to contract. Those who do not include minors, persons incapacitated by alcohol or psychotropic drugs, and persons who have been legally adjudicated as incompetent. The consequences of contracting with a person with no legal capacity, or with limited capacity, to contract include (1) the purported contract may be null and **void**, (2) the contract may be unilaterally **voidable** at the option of the party lacking capacity, or (3) the contract may be valid, if an exception to lack of contractual capacity applies.

As a general rule, minors in most states have the limited legal capacity to contract for any goods or services for which adults may contract. However, also in most cases, minors are permitted by law to **disaffirm**, or disavow, their contractual obligations any time before they reach the legal age of majority (18 to 21) and even for a limited time thereafter. To validate a contract made by a minor, the minor normally must continue to perform under a contract after the minor achieves the age of majority. This is called contract **ratification**.

When a minor properly disaffirms a contract, the minor normally only has to give back to the other party to the contract that property (including money) that the minor presently has in his or her possession. A minor may even disaffirm most contracts when the minor has misrepresented his or her age.

A minor, however, may be obligated by law to repay the reasonable value of necessary goods and services received under contract. Necessities, which require repayment for value, include food, health care services, and shelter.

Intoxicated or otherwise impaired persons have limited protection under law from contractual obligations, similar to those granted to minors. In most cases, an impaired person may elect to void a contract made while impaired; however, unlike minors, the impaired person must repay, in restitution, the reasonable value of any goods or services received.

Only those persons who are legally adjudicated as incompetent fully lack capacity to contract. For such persons, such as institutionalized patients with mental illnesses, contracts must be entered into with the incompetent persons' surrogate decision makers, that is, court-appointed conservators or guardians. A purported contract with a legally adjudicated incompetent person is void; that is, no contract exists.

Legality

In addition to all of the other requirements of a valid, enforceable contract, the subject matter of a contract must be legal and must not violate public policy. For example, a written contract among several health care professionals to provide health care services to patients that includes an unwritten understanding that the parties will defraud the Medicare and Medicaid programs is illegal and therefore null and void.

The law does not countenance an illegal contractual agreement. This is so because, under its equity (or fairness) powers, a court will only come to the aid of a contractual party who comes to court "with clean hands." This concept is known as the equitable **clean hands doctrine**.

> The law does not countenance an illegal contractual agreement, nor one that violates public policy.

Examples of contracts that are void because they violate public policy considerations include agreements grounded in immoral (but legal) or unconscionable behavior or unprofessional conduct. For example, a managed care contract that requires of participating health care providers that all outpatient physical and occupational therapy care be limited to a single visit, irrespective of patient diagnosis, might well be declared unconscionable by a court and thereby void as violative of public policy (Box 6-1).

Quasi-Contract

It was previously stated in the chapter that every health care professional–patient interaction involves at least an implied contract for service delivery. Such an implied contract is referred to in law as an **implied-in-fact** contract. The contract and its

> **BOX 6-1** ■ **Four Basic Elements of a Binding (Bilateral) Contract**
>
> - Agreement of the parties (mutuality of assent)
> - Consideration (mutuality of obligation)
> - Capacity (recognized legal status to contract)
> - Legality of subject matter

terms are implied from the conduct of the health care professional and of the patient. Certain other types of interaction are referred to legally as contracts **implied-in-law**. In such an arrangement, one party believes—reasonably or otherwise—that a contract exists with another party. However, there is no agreement or assent to be bound by the other party. Such a scenario is also called **quasi-contract** (Latin for "analogous to a contract").

Because there is no assent to be contractually bound by one side in a quasi-contractual situation, a court cannot award contractual damages for nonperformance by a party. However, using its equitable powers, a court can prevent unjust enrichment on the part of a party by compelling the party who receives goods or services from another to pay the fair value of the goods or services. Consider the following hypothetical example:

> *A, a trauma surgeon, is driving along a country road when she comes upon a one-automobile crash victim, B, on the side of the road. A renders emergency medical treatment to B, who is unconscious. Under quasi-contract principles, A is entitled to recover the reasonable value of her medical services to B.*

Oral and Written Agreements

Only specific types of contracts must be in writing in order to be legally enforceable. State laws requiring that certain contracts be in writing to be enforceable are called **statutes of frauds**. In this case, the word *fraud* does not refer to deceptive misrepresentation.

Although statutes of frauds differ from jurisdiction to jurisdiction, there are common types of contracts that usually require a writing. These contracts include the following:

- A contractual promise to serve as a surety (or **guarantor**) for another person's debts, that is, a cosigner
- Contracts for the transfer of long-term interests in real property
- Promises in consideration of marriage, for example, prenuptial agreements
- Contracts for the sale of goods (under the Uniform Commercial Code) for purchases for more than $500[30]
- Contracts that cannot be performed (**executed**) within 1 year from the making of the agreement

The provision requiring contracts that cannot objectively be performed within 1 year to be in writing is called the **one-year rule**. Consider the following hypothetical examples:

1. It is June 1. Q, a student nurse who will graduate on June 15, receives an offer of employment from R, a human resources manager at XYZ Hospital, for a period of 1 year commencing on June 16. Q accepts the offer without condition.
2. It is June 1. O, an occupational therapist, receives an employment offer from R for a period of 1 year commencing immediately. O accepts the offer without condition.

In which example, if either, is the statute of frauds applicable?

The one-year rule of the statute of frauds requires that the employment offer in example 1 be in writing in order to be enforceable. In example 2, no writing is required to enforce the agreement because the 1-year period does not begin to run until the next calendar day (June 2) and the employment contract in this example will be fully executed within 1 year.

Interpretation of Contracts

Although contracts that are not required to be in writing by the statute of frauds or other laws may be written or oral, the existence and interpretation of an agreement is certainly easier to ascertain and make if the contract is in writing. One admonition that readers should take from this chapter is that all business agreements should be reduced to writing.

As a general rule, courts asked to interpret written contracts will only interpret the understandings memorialized by the parties to the agreement in writing. This is often referred to as the **four-corners doctrine**. Like the adage concerning patient care documentation that "if it isn't written, it wasn't done," with contracts one can say, "if it isn't written, it wasn't part of the agreement," with limited exceptions.

A corollary rule to the four-corners rule is the parol ("spoken") evidence rule. Under this rule of interpretation of a written contract, a court will not normally permit the introduction into evidence of any purported prior or contemporaneous "understandings" by the contractual parties that were not incorporated into the written agreement. The **parol evidence rule** exists, in part, to protect the integrity of written contractual agreements and, in part, to give legal effect to the clear meaning of the parties as stated in their written agreement.

Many written agreements contain (usually at the end of the contract) an **integration clause**, which restates that there are no contractual understandings or obligations that are not included in the written agreement. Check out the bill of sale for your next new car for an excellent example of an integration clause.

Defenses to Performance of Contractual Obligations

Contracts may be executed, or fully performed, in one of several ways. Most often, parties to contracts complete their contractual obligations by legal **performance**. For example, a nurse practitioner contracts with a home health agency to render home services to specified patients for a 3-month period. The contractual duties of the parties are fully discharged when (1) the advanced practice nurse fully performs the duties under the contract for 3 months and (2) the agency pays for professional services rendered.

Occasionally, full or even substantial performance of contractual obligations by parties is made impossible by circumstances such as the death or bankruptcy of one of the parties or unforeseeable destruction of equipment necessary to complete the contract. Such circumstances are referred to as **impossibility of performance** and discharge contractual obligations **by operation of law**.

Finally, a contract may be terminated by agreement (Get it in writing!) of the parties or by the **material breach**, or failure of even substantial performance, of one of the contractual parties. A material breach of contract equates to a lack of legal consideration and normally excuses the nonbreaching party from further performance under the contract.

Breach of Contract and Contractual Remedies

In addition to a material breach of contract, a contractual party may commit a minor breach of contract. In the case of a minor breach of contract, the party in compliance may often have the right to suspend his or her continued performance until the minor breach has been corrected. Consider the following hypothetical example:

> *D, an occupational therapist and bioethicist, lectures extensively on biomedical ethics to occupational therapy professional students across the country. As part of one contract to lecture, D agrees with E, the full-time instructor in a management course in an occupational therapy program, to lecture to E's students for a 4-hour period. D finishes with the lecture after 2 hours and releases the students on a break. Is D's breach of contract a minor or a material breach? The answer probably depends on whether D can cure the breach by calling the students together and substantially completing the 4-hour period of instruction.*

Remedies for Breach of Contract

In addition to suspending performance under an existing contract, an aggrieved party in a breach of contract situation can sue for monetary damages and other legal and equitable remedies. Consider the case of *Sullivan* v. *O'Connor*,[31] a medical malpractice contract-based lawsuit concerning a surgeon's alleged breach of promise to improve the plaintiff-patient's facial appearance with a rhinoplasty. The court in this case distinguished three possible ways to calculate monetary damages in contractual lawsuits. These three types of contract damages are **restitution damages**, **reliance damages**, and **expectancy damages**.

An award of restitution damages provides sufficient monetary recovery only to restore the aggrieved party to the *status quo ante*, or the position he or she occupied before beginning performance under the contract. Restitution damages, then, compensate a plaintiff only for labor and materials expended in support of the plaintiff's performance under the contract.

Reliance damages operate not only to restore a contract plaintiff to the *status quo ante* but also to give the aggrieved party reasonable monetary damages to compensate for the breach. The court in *Sullivan* endorsed reliance damages as the most appropriate measure of contractual monetary damages in health care cases.

Expectancy (or compensatory) damages give a contract plaintiff the full "benefit of the contractual bargain," as contemplated by the parties when they formed the contract. That is, expectancy damages serve to place the plaintiff in exactly the same position in which he or she would have been had the defendant not breached the contract. Elements of damages included in expectancy recoveries include (1) incidental (direct) damages and (2) consequential (indirect) damages. **Incidental damages** include things such as travel and other out-of-pocket expenses. **Consequential damages** include lost profits (provable to a reasonable certainty) and pain and suffering. Subtracted from an expectancy award is the sum that the plaintiff saved by not having to perform further under the contract after the defendant's breach of contract.

In addition to monetary damages, or **damages at law**, contract plaintiffs may seek **equitable remedies** in litigation. The most common types of equitable contract remedies are (1) injunctions and (2) orders for specific performance of contractual obligations.

An injunction is an order issued by a court to a defendant to cease some offensive activity. By way of example, a health care professional–presenter of continuing education courses, who is under an exclusive contract with an educational group to make presentations, may be **enjoined** by a court from comparing his independent, but competitive courses, to those sponsored by the plaintiff.

Specific performance involves an equitable order by a court directed to a party, ordering that party to perform as required under a contract. Courts will not order specific performance of personal services contracts (including health care services delivery contracts) on the ground that such an order violates the Thirteenth Amendment to the Constitution, which reads as follows:

Section 1. Neither slavery nor involuntary servitude *[emphasis added], except as a punishment for crime whereof the party shall have been duly convicted, shall exist within the United States, or any place subject to their jurisdiction.*

Section 2. Congress shall have the power to enforce this article by appropriate legislation.[32]

Two final points about contractual damages warrant mention. First, punitive (or punishment) damages are seldom, if ever, awarded or appropriate in contract litigation cases. The concept of punitive damages is a tort concept, reflecting public policy considerations other than respect for the lawful private law made by parties to contracts. In contract litigation, punitive damages are normally only awarded when there is egregious misconduct by a defendant that constitutes a mixed tort-contract action. Second, **liquidated damages**, preagreed default damages specified in a contract, may be enforced by a court, provided that they are adjudged as reasonable and bargained for.

Breach of Warranty

Breach of warranty involves contractual liability for the failure of a product to meet reasonable or expressly agreed-on performance standards. In most states an injured party has the right to sue any distributor (including health care professionals) along the chain of commercial distribution. Courts disfavor imposing breach of warranty liability on health care professionals because courts view health care principally as a professional service. Normally, only when health care professionals regularly market products in clinical practice, such as optometrists, orthotists, and prosthetists (and others who sell equipment in their clinical practices) will courts allow breach of warranty cases to proceed.

Types of warranties include express and implied warranties. Express warranties involve statements of purported fact about the performance or potential of a product, which become part of the consideration, or benefit of the bargain. There is no legal requirement that express warranties be made, and they may be expressly disclaimed in contracts.

Implied warranties are of two types: implied warranties of merchantability and implied warranties of fitness for particular purposes. Merchantability means that products are generally suitable for expected uses. Fitness for particular purposes implies that products are especially appropriate for buyers' stated needs. The laws of many states prohibit the disclaimer of implied warranties of merchantability.

Clinical Affiliation Agreements

Relevant clinical experiences are integral component parts of professional health care education programs. Contracts between academic institutions and clinical sites for student placement are known as **clinical affiliation agreements**. Such agreements normally spell out in varying detail the major rights and responsibilities of the respective parties. One principal duty incumbent upon academic institutions is to certify that professional students participating in clinical experiences have had appropriate academic preparation for their particular assignments before arriving at clinical sites. A principal duty of clinical sites is to provide relevant learning experiences for affiliates, under appropriate guidance and supervision, consistent with individual student competency and agreed-on learning objectives.

Clinical affiliation agreements may or may not delineate who bears vicarious legal responsibility for student malpractice or ordinary negligence over and above that covered by student liability insurance. For many reasons, clinical sites may refuse to accept financial responsibility for professional student affiliates. Similarly, many public academic institutions are immune from liability under state sovereign immunity. It is incumbent upon all parties to clinical affiliation contracts to have them thoroughly reviewed before signing them.

In the absence of express provisions fixing financial responsibility for student conduct in clinical affiliation agreements, courts may use a legal concept called the **borrowed servant rule** to affix vicarious liability for student conduct. Under this ancient rule of law, liability attaches to the party whose interests are most being served by the student at the time of legally actionable conduct. For health care professional students, vicarious liability under the borrowed servant rule might logically attach to the academic institution early in a student's education (when the student is primarily serving the objectives of the academic institution) and to the clinical site late in a student's education (when the student is primarily serving the needs of the clinic).

Continuing Education Courses: A Special Case of Contractual Duties

In health care professional continuing education settings,[33] breach of contract liability issues can arise in at least three ways:

1. Involving continuing education course presenters and sponsors, based on compensation or presentation performance disputes. This type of contract legal action typically involves straightforward interpretation of express contractual language.
2. Involving continuing education course presenters or sponsors and course participants, based on the content or perceived value of particular presentations or courses. This type of contract legal action is often complex and may require that a court examine the language in course brochures, announcements, and other correspondence. To prevent these kinds of disputes from arising, continuing education course sponsors and presenters are urged to review the language in their marketing materials carefully—particularly course objectives—to ensure that what is promised to participants is substantially delivered.
3. Involving continuing education course presenters and demonstration subjects (patients), based on the scope and duration of professional (treatment) intervention. This type of contract legal action may involve the issue of patient abandonment by the presenter; that is, did the termination of professional care comport with the parties' understandings? Another question may be whether treatment by a presenter meets licensure and practice standards.

Continuing education presenters who treat patients at courses are strongly advised always to consider the following recommendations:

- Determine the legal requirements regarding practice and continuation of care in the state where the treatment takes place.
- Clearly define the scope and duration of treatment in a written agreement signed by presenter and patient(s) to prevent misunderstandings and patient dissatisfaction.

FORMS OF BUSINESS ORGANIZATIONS

When one or more persons create a business, they can form one of several legal forms of business organization. The forms of business organization, with various hybrids, include sole proprietorship, partnership, corporation, and limited liability company.

In a **sole proprietorship**—the simplest form for a business—an individual business owner personally makes all decisions and receives all of the profits generated by the business. In this scenario, the owner/entrepreneur is truly a one-person show. This form of business organization has maximal flexibility and minimal legal constraints on the formation and operation of the business. Business income and deductions are reported on the owner's individual tax returns.

The principal disadvantage of a sole proprietorship is that the owner personally bears the entire financial risk of loss, ranging from business losses to liability incident to claims and lawsuits. (Of course, the owner can and should transfer liability risks through the purchase of insurance.) Other relative disadvantages of the sole proprietorship include potential difficulty in attracting funds and discontinuity of operations in the event of serious illness or the death of the proprietor.

A **general partnership** is a contractual agreement between two or more persons or other legal entities to establish and operate a business for profit. The partnership contractual agreement may be express (oral or written) or implied. Like the sole proprietorship, partnership law is based in common rather than statutory law.

Absent other agreement, partners manage the business equally and share in and pay taxes individually on their proportional share of profits. (The partnership itself reports income but does not pay income tax.) Each partner is the agent for the other partner(s), and all partners are joint and severally liable for partnership business debts and tort liability.

The principle advantages of the general partnership are the sharing of business expenses and the availability of multiple sources of input for business decision making. The main disadvantage is the unlimited personal liability of each partner for partnership activities.

The limited partnership is a statutorily created form of business that consists of at least one general partner and one or more limited partners. The limited partnership is a business arrangement under which the limited partners do not manage the operational affairs of a business but share in its profits. The personal liability of limited partners is normally limited to the amount of their investment in the business.

A **joint venture** is much like a general partnership, with two important differences. A joint venture is formed for a specific, limited purpose, and the members of the venture have only limited agency authority to bind their fellow members.

A **corporation** is a form of business organization that is recognized as a legal person apart from its owners (shareholders) with most of the rights and duties of natural persons. Corporations are governed by statutory law, which varies from state to state. All states have relatively strict statutory requirements associated with the formation and administration of corporations that do not apply to proprietorships and partnerships.

The personal liability of corporate shareholders for the debts of the corporation is normally limited to the amount of their investment in the business, unless a court "pierces the corporate veil" to reach additional assets of shareholders when they have ignored corporate statutory formalities or have failed adequately to capitalize the business.[34] Piercing of the corporate veil is only rarely done by courts.

In addition to limited shareholder liability, another advantage of the corporate form of business is perpetual existence. A corporation, unlike a proprietorship or partnership, does not cease to exist upon the death of its owner(s). A major disadvantage to incorporating is double taxation on the net profits of a corporation and on its shareholders for disbursed dividends.[34]

Many states require licensed professionals to incorporate under special professional corporation statutes. Under the Texas Professional Corporation Act,[35] for example, certain health care professionals licensed by the state may incorporate under the statute and be shielded from personal liability (beyond their proportional share of the assets of the corporation) for the conduct of other corporate owners. Of course, being in a corporation does not shield a professional from liability for his or her own conduct.

Professional corporations may operate for profit or be nonprofit entities, in which case they do not issue stock. In some states, physicians form distinct professional associations,[36] which share characteristics with professional corporations.

The **limited liability company,**[36] a relatively recent hybrid form of business organization, is becoming increasingly popular. The limited liability company shares characteristics of professional corporations and partnerships. Like a corporation, its owners have the benefit of limited personal liability for contract and tort actions against the company. Like a partnership, company income is passed through to the owners for unitary taxation at the individual level.

The decision of which form of business organization to adopt is a complicated one. Health care professional entrepreneurs are urged to consult proactively with legal counsel for advice regarding such a decision.

GOOD SAMARITAN LAWS

The *American College Dictionary* defines **good Samaritan** as "a person who is compassionate and helpful to one in distress," citing a biblical passage, Luke 10:30-37, as authority. A more jurisprudential definition is found in *Black's Law Dictionary,* in which good Samaritan is defined as one who aids another person in imminent or serious peril. Under law, a good Samaritan rendering aid to another may be granted immunity from civil liability for negligence incident to such assistance.

Under the laws of the United States (unlike those of many other nations), unless there is some preexisting duty to come to another's aid, no one is obligated to help another person in peril.[37] One may have a moral duty to do so—especially where the rescuer faces no personal danger—but not a legal duty. Clinical health care professionals, of course, have a preexisting duty to patients under their care and must come to their aid in emergencies to the extent of their professional competence.

Good Samaritan Statutes

After World War II, state legislatures became concerned that physicians and other competent rescuers would refrain from assisting strangers in emergency situations out of fear of liability exposure. As a result, first California (in 1959) and then every other state and the District of Columbia enacted good Samaritan statutes to shield physicians and others from liability for emergency medical treatment, as long as specific statutory requirements were met.

Certain common guidelines pervade these good Samaritan statutes, including the following:

- The requirement that an emergency exist for statutory protections to apply
- Identification of who is protected from liability under the statute
- Delineation of the degree of culpability that causes a rescuer to lose statutory immunity from liability
- Determination of whether the statute applies to emergency aid rendered within a medical facility
- Determination of whether a statutorily protected rescuer must act without the expectation of compensation

Emergency and Good Faith

The two requirements most commonly observed in good Samaritan statutes are that a bona fide emergency exist and that the rescuer act in good faith in administering assistance. Few statutes, however, clearly define "emergency" or "good faith," and there is little case law addressing these points.

Most statutes also require that protected aid be rendered at or near the scene of an accident or emergency. Some allow for immunity even when aid is provided in a hospital or other health care facility setting, so long as the good Samaritan does not have a professional-patient relationship with the victim.

Culpability and Gratuitous Aid

Two other parameters of good Samaritan statutes concern (1) the effect of gross negligence or more culpable conduct on the part of a person rendering emergency aid and (2) the requirement that a rescuer offer assistance without expectation of compensation. The overwhelming majority of good Samaritan statutes deny immunity when a rescuer acts in a grossly negligent, reckless, or malicious way and causes injury to an accident victim. A majority of statutes require gratuitous assistance for protection; however, almost half of the statutes do not disallow reasonable compensation for services rendered. The legislative intent behind the statutes that disallow compensation for emergency services presumably is to foster altruistic behavior on the part of would-be rescuers. The legislative intent behind the statutes that are silent on the issue of compensation may be to prevent unjust enrichment by accident victims who receive valuable services.

Need for Reform and Professional Education

The lack of uniformity among the states regarding good Samaritan immunity from liability[38] creates significant confusion and may dissuade competent health care professionals and others from rendering emergency aid to victims, a consequence clearly contrary to the intent of these statutes. A legislative solution to this dilemma is to create a uniform good Samaritan statute that could be adopted nationwide, similar to uniform laws and guidance currently in effect governing commercial transactions and partnership and probate matters. Any uniform law should provide for immunity from liability for simple negligence for any rescuer who acts reasonably within the scope of his or her competency.

All health care professionals, support personnel, clinical managers, and facility administrators should become knowledgeable about their particular state laws providing

EXERCISE

Research the good Samaritan laws for your state. Is your discipline specifically addressed in these laws? Make a copy of the laws uncovered in your search, and share results with professional colleagues.

good Samaritan immunity before they find themselves in situations in which they are required to render emergency aid to patients or others. Periodic presentations by facility attorneys or legal consultants concerning good Samaritan laws makes an excellent addition to any health care facility in-service education program.

HEALTH INSURANCE PORTABILITY AND ACCOUNTABILITY ACT

The Health Insurance Portability and Accountability Act (HIPAA)[39] has two broad purposes: to facilitate the transferability of employee health insurance benefits between public sector and private sector jobs and to safeguard the sanctity and privacy of individual protected health information (PHI). Because Congress procrastinated and did not enact enabling privacy legislation by August 1999, the Department of Health and Human Services went on to create and implement privacy regulations pursuant to HIPAA. After the required comment period, these regulations became law on April 14, 2001, with an effective date of April 23, 2003.

The privacy rules do several important things for patients. These rules afford patients greater autonomy over their private health data. The rules also set strict limits on how individual health information is gathered, stored, and released by health care providers and organizations and hold covered providers and health care organizations legally accountable for impermissible breaches of patient privacy. Patient informed consent, although not required in writing, is a prerequisite to the use or dissemination of patient PHI for purposes of treatment, payment, or operations.

The privacy standards of HIPAA represent the first comprehensive federal guidelines for protection of PHI. Health care systems, plans, providers, and clearinghouses that conduct financial transactions electronically must comply with HIPAA in receiving, processing, storing, transmitting, and otherwise handling patient/client PHI. Protection extends to any individually identifiable health information maintained or transmitted in any medium and held by any covered entity or business associate of a covered entity. Supplemental guidance and protections are found in state and local case law, statutes, and administrative rules and regulations.

Covered entities must also obtain adequate contractual assurances from business associates that the latter will appropriately safeguard patient PHI that comes to them. Examples of activities that may be conducted by business associates include benefit management, billing, claims processing, data analysis, quality improvement management, practice management, and utilization review. If a business associate is found to have violated HIPAA, the covered entity must first attempt to "cure" (correct) the violation and, if unsuccessful, terminate the contract with the noncompliant business associate and report the matter to the secretary of the Department of Health and Human Services for follow-on administrative action.

Each employee, contractor, and consultant is a fiduciary, owing a personal duty to patients to take all reasonable steps pursuant to HIPAA to safeguard their PHI. All employees and other providers must receive HIPAA training during initial orientation and periodically thereafter to update their knowledge base about HIPAA. Providers and entities covered by HIPAA must exercise reasonable caution under all circumstances to disclose only the minimum necessary amount of PHI in order to comply with their legal duties owed to patients and others.

On the first visit to any covered provider, all patients must be made aware of the HIPAA privacy policy of the facility. Direct care providers must issue a patient notice of privacy practices to all patients at first contact and must make a good faith attempt to obtain patients' written acknowledgment of receipt of the document. In addition, providers must post their entire patient notice of privacy practices in their facility in a prominent location for patients to see. Normally, a covered entity (any provider filing reimbursement claims electronically) may use and disclose a patient's PHI for purposes of treatment, payment for services, and internal health care operations of the business, without the patient's authorization or consent. These disclosures are called "routine uses."

Regarding patient informed consent for routine uses of PHI, providers are required only to make a good faith effort to obtain patient/client informed consent for treatment, payment, and health care operations. Covered entities have wide discretion to design processes that mesh with their individual practices. Patients/clients have the right to request restrictions on the use or disclosure of their PHI, but covered entities are not required to agree to such restrictions.

Three general classifications of PHI disclosures exist under HIPAA. These classifications are permissive, mandatory (without patient authorization or consent), and authorized. Permissive disclosures include those necessary for treatment, payment, and operations. These disclosures include communication between and among treatment team members, determination of coverage for health services, and peer/utilization review activities.

Required disclosures are those made pursuant to legal mandates, such as a court order or state reporting statutes (for suspected abuse; communicable diseases (including sexually transmitted diseases), and gunshot wounds. Authorized disclosures encompass broad disclosure authority pursuant to valid written and signed patient authorization. Regarding minors' PHI, the Privacy Rule generally allows a parent to have access to the medical records about his or her child, as his or her minor child's personal representative when such access is not inconsistent with state or other laws. In three situations the parent would not be the minor's personal representative under the Privacy Rule. These exceptions are (1) when the minor is the one who consents to care and the consent of the parent is not required under state or other applicable law, for example, when the minor is emancipated; (2) when the minor obtains care at the direction of a court or a person appointed by the court; and (3) when, and to the extent that, the parent agrees that the minor and the health care provider may have a confidential relationship. However, even in these exceptional situations, the parent may have access to the health record of the minor related to this treatment when state or other applicable law requires or permits such parental access. HIPAA does not cover workers' compensation entities.

The following are suggested standard operating procedures for clinics that are covered entities under the HIPAA Privacy Rule. The following list is not intended to be comprehensive. In addition to appointing and adequately training a clinic privacy officer, the staffs of covered entities should brainstorm on lists of standard operating procedures to be implemented for their individual practices.

Providers covered by HIPAA may still use sign-in sheets for patients and call out their names in waiting rooms, so long as PHI is not disclosed in these processes. Seeing someone in a waiting room and hearing one's name called constitute "incidental" disclosures that do not violate HIPAA, according to the Department of Health and Human Services. A sign-in sheet may not, however, list patients' diagnoses.

STANDARD OPERATING PROCEDURES PURSUANT TO THE HIPAA PRIVACY RULE

1. Staff will not allow patient records to be placed or to remain in open (public) view.
2. Staff will not discuss patient PHI within the hearing/perceptive range of third parties not involved in the patient's care.
3. Patients and other nonemployees/contractors/consultants are not permitted access to the patient records room.
4. Except where authorized, permitted, or required by law, PHI disclosures require HIPAA-compliant written patient/client authorizations and written requests by requestors for information.
5. Patient records may not be removed from the facility, except for transit to and from secure storage, or otherwise as authorized, permitted, or required by law.
6. Written requests by patients for their health records will be expeditiously honored.
7. Patient/client records may be placed in chart holders for clinic providers, provided that the following reasonable and appropriate measures are taken to protect the patient's privacy: limiting access to patient care areas and escorting nonemployees in the area, ensuring that the areas are supervised, and placing patient/client charts in chart holders with the front cover facing the wall rather than having PHI about the patient visible to anyone who walks by.
8. Providers may leave telephone messages for patients on their answering machines. Limit the amount of information disclosed on the answering machine to clinic name and number, and any other information necessary to confirm an appointment, asking the individual to call back. It is permissible to leave a similar message with a family member or other person who answers the telephone when the patient is not home.
9. The clinic is required to give the notice of its privacy policy to every individual receiving treatment no later than the date of first service delivery and to make a good faith effort to obtain the individual's written acknowledgment of receipt of the notice.
10. The clinic also must post its entire privacy policy in the facility in a clear and prominent location where individuals are likely to see it and to make the notice available to those who ask for a copy. Copies of the clinic privacy notice are maintained in English and Spanish.

Providers may also transmit patient health records to other providers without patient authorization or consent, if the gaining providers are treating the patient for the same condition as the sending provider. This includes transfer of an entire patient health record (including documentation created by other providers), if reasonably necessary for treatment.

Providers are not normally required to document a "disclosure history" unless patient authorization is required for disclosure; however, it would be prudent risk management to create and maintain such a history. What is required is that covered providers and entities exercise reasonable caution under all circumstances to disclose only the minimum necessary amount of PHI in order to comply with their legal duties owed to patients and others.

HIPAA-related patient complaints should first be directed to the HIPAA privacy officer of an organization. A complaint may also be filed with the Office of Civil Rights, U.S. Department of Health and Human Services.

The Department of Health and Human Services requires the following in a written complaint:

1. Complainant's full name and residential and e-mail addresses, home and work telephone numbers
2. Name, address, and telephone number of entity violating complainant's PHI
3. Description of the PHI violation
4. Complainant's signature and date
5. Necessary reasonable accommodations, as applicable

An alleged PHI violator is prohibited from taking retaliatory action against a complainant. Potential sanctions for HIPAA Privacy Rule violations include civil and criminal penalties. Civil penalties of between $100 and $25,000 per violation are enforced by the Office of Civil Rights, Department of Health and Human Services. Criminal sanctions of 1 to 10 years' imprisonment and $50,000 to $250,000 fines are enforced by the Department of Justice.[40]

INSURANCE LAW

Nature of Insurance

Virtually every business undertaking—including the rendering of health care delivery services—carries with it a degree of risk of financial loss. Such is the nature of business. Financial losses may be incurred by business owners, investors, and professionals from fire damage and other natural disasters, spoilage of goods, theft of goods and services, and claims and litigation. The purchase of insurance is one of the most important ways that professionals can minimize their business-related financial losses, by transferring the legal responsibility to pay for covered outlays to third-party insurance professionals.

Several of the common types of insurance are familiar to health care professionals. As part of their employee benefits programs, most health care professionals enjoy employer-paid or subsidized health and life insurance. Many professional employees also have employer-paid or subsidized employment-related short- or long-term disability insurance coverage. Those who own homes and are encumbered with mortgages are required by their mortgagees (and by good business sense) to take out homeowner's insurance for the mutual protection of mortgagees and mortgagors (homeowners). Personal property insurance protects the insurable interests of persons and businesses in **chattels**, or movable items of personal property.

General liability and, for corporations, directors and officers liability insurance cover insured persons and businesses against losses from claims and litigation brought by parties against policyholders for monetary damages incident to personal injury or property damage for which the policyholders are legally responsible to pay. Automobile liability insurance is a special form of liability insurance with which most drivers are familiar.

All types of insurance have several key elements in common. All types of insurance have as their primary purpose the protection of persons or entities with insurable legal interests in specific property or persons. All types of insurance are characterized by the concepts of **risk pooling** and **risk transfer**. Risk pooling means that neither the innocent victims of misfortune nor those who negligently or otherwise wrongfully cause injury to other persons or their property bear the financial losses of their misfortunes personally. All of those who are jointly insured by an insurance company share in each payable loss through their payment of insurance premiums. The larger the pool of insured contributors, the greater the spread of risk of financial loss. Risk transfer means that the specific responsibility to pay for insured losses rests with insurance companies, rather than with individuals responsible for occasioning such losses.

Insurance law is largely a matter of state rather than federal law.[1] State legislatures enact applicable statutes governing insurance activities conducted within their states. State administrative agencies establish applicable insurance rules and regulations and enforce compliance. Litigation over insurance matters is generally under the jurisdiction of state courts (absent diversity of citizenship or a relevant federal question).

Insurer-Insured Relationship

The relationship between insured and insurer is a contractual one, with the policy representing the contractual legal instrument. The same rules that govern the formation, administration, and execution of business contracts in general also govern insurance policies.

The parties to the insurance contract are the insured and the insurer. The insured is legally considered to be the offerer of an application for insurance. The insurer, or insurance company, as offeree accepts the prospective insured's offer to purchase insurance and issues a policy. Intermediaries potentially involved in insurance contracts include brokers (representing insured persons) and underwriters and agents (representing insurance companies).

The mutual consideration in support of the validity of a health care professional liability insurance policy includes the insured party's promise to pay (in the form of a lump sum payment or periodic insurance premiums) and the insurer's promise to indemnify the insured against personal liability for covered losses. Indemnification means that the insurer "holds" the insured financially "harmless" by guaranteeing competent legal representation of the insured to defend the parties' mutual interests, up to the amount of insurance coverage, and by guaranteeing payment up to the maximum amount of insurance coverage in the event of settlement or an adverse judgment in court.

Health care professional liability insurance policies, reflecting state law requirements and public policy considerations, do not normally insure against liability for malicious intentional misconduct (such as malicious battery or sexual battery committed against patients). Nor do most such policies insure against liability for wanton reckless conduct, such as the conscious disregard of known contraindications to selected interventions in the course of treatment. These circumstances and other exclusions are stated in the exclusions section of an insurance policy.

Health care professional liability insurance policies, however, normally insure against liability arising from nonmalicious intentional treatment-related conduct generally, as long as such conduct does not involve a specific intent to cause harm to a patient. The inclusion of coverage for intentional conduct is critically important to health care professionals because their professional interventions necessarily involve the "laying on of hands."

Consider the following hypothetical example of a case in which coverage and indemnification for intentional treatment-related conduct by a health care professional should be allowable under a typical professional liability insurance policy:

A board-certified orthopedic physical therapist evaluates a patient with a diagnosis of cervical facet syndrome. The family practice physician who referred the patient for physical therapy requested only that the physical therapist "evaluate and treat" the patient. The accompanying full cervical radiographic series taken just 2 days before physical therapy evaluation is negative. In the course of the physical therapy evaluation, the physical therapist reaches a diagnosis of a mild, chronic right-sided C6-C7 facet subluxation. The therapist chooses to manipulate the patient's neck to resolve the patient's moderate local pain symptoms. As a result of manipulation, the patient's condition worsens. The patient's local pain begins to radiate to the right arm. Eventually, a C6-C7 diskectomy is required. The patient sues the physical therapist for professional negligence. The state physical therapy practice act is silent on whether physical therapists are privileged to carry out cervical orthopedic manipulation, as is the state medical practice act.

Does the defendant–physical therapist's individual professional liability insurance policy protect him against personal liability in the event of an adverse judgment? Yes. Spinal manipulation is clearly within the customary scope of practice of orthopedic physical therapy, unless expressly disallowed by a state practice act. The physical therapist did not violate the provisions of the referral order. The facts of the case, as stated, do not support the contention that the physical therapist acted maliciously or recklessly. The defendant–physical therapist's professional liability insurer should defend and indemnify the physical therapist against personal liability, to the maximum coverage limit of the policy. Remember, however, that once the insurer pays money to the plaintiff in settlement or judgment on an insured's behalf, the defendant–licensed health care professional's name must be reported for inclusion in the National Practitioner Data Bank.

State insurance law may also prohibit indemnification of a health care professional's liability for punitive damages, also on public policy grounds. Insurance entities normally, however, may insure for and indemnify against employers' vicarious liability for punitive damages levied against their employees who were acting within the scope of employment at the time of alleged wrongdoing because no public policy is normally violated in such circumstances.

Although an insurer's duty to indemnify an insured party against personal liability may be greatly affected by public policy considerations, its legal duty to defend its insured clients is governed largely by contract law (i.e., the private law of the parties). In most cases, an insurer has the contractual obligation to defend an insured client in a legal action against the client whenever there is a potential reasonable basis for indemnification of the insured by the insurer. (The customary practice is for an insurer to contract with outside legal counsel, who are civil trial experts, to represent its insured on behalf of the insurer.) In such cases, however, an insurer defends an insured party under an express reservation that indemnification is conditioned on a finding that permits indemnification under the insurance contract.

Both parties to an insurance contract are charged with the mutual implied duty of good faith. Consider the following hypothetical example:

An insured nurse practitioner is sued by a patient for alleged professional negligence incident to independent practice. In the course of managing the legal case, the defendant–nurse practitioner has the affirmative duty to cooperate with the insurer, including the following considerations:

- *Giving timely notice of the adverse patient event (i.e., P.C.E., or potentially compensable event)*
- *Cooperating with appointed legal counsel representing the insured and insurer's mutual interests, especially in formulating a legitimate case strategy most favorable to the defense*
- *Cooperating with legal counsel (for both sides) in pre-trial processes (including answering* **interrogatories** *and attending depositions)*
- *Appearing and testifying at trial, if the case proceeds to that point*

The insurer also has affirmative good faith contractual duties, including the following:

- *Using its best professional judgment and expending its best efforts to achieve a result most favorable for the insured*
- *Working closely with the insured (and the insured party's personal legal counsel, if one or more are involved in the case) and keeping the insured apprised of developments in the case*
- *Attempting to settle a claim or lawsuit within policy limits so as to avoid exposing the insured to personal liability for amounts in excess of insurance coverage*

State law may require that an insurer obtain an insured party's reasonable consent before settling a high-dollar claim. In one case an insured health care professional was allowed to bring a breach of contract legal case against his professional liability insurer (and the law firm that the insurer hired to defend the case) for settling a case against the insured without the insured's consent, as was required under the policy.[41]

Because an attorney retained by an insurer to defend a health care professional in a malpractice case represents the insured and the insurer, there is always the potential for a conflict of interest. The same potential for a conflict of interest exists when an employer's (vicarious) liability insurer corepresents the employer and a health care professional employee charged with negligence or wrongdoing incident to employment. Attorneys in such circumstances are required by law to inform the insured of the nature of the dual representation and to obtain the insured party's informed consent to the relationship.

If an actual conflict of interest between the parties represented arises, then the attorney is legally and ethically obligated to sever representation of the health care professional and advise the health care professional to retain substitute legal counsel. The attorney severing the attorney-client relationship with the health care professional is then precluded from revealing to anyone (except substitute counsel) prejudicial confidential communications made to him or her by the health care professional–client.

Because of the potential for a conflict of interest in health care malpractice litigation, health care professionals should consider retaining personal legal counsel to assist them in defense of their personal interests if they are claimed against or sued. The exercise of this option has several advantages and disadvantages.

Personal legal counsel exclusively represents the legal interests of the health care professional–client, not those of an employer or insurance company. Hence, there is no potential conflict of interest, and personal counsel may be in a better position to recommend a course of action most favorable to the health care professional. Health care professionals may feel more at ease with such corepresentation, especially if they have long-standing relationships with their personal legal counsel. The resultant diminution in the health care professional's stress level should work to everyone's advantage on the defense team because the defendant will probably be a more effective witness in deposition and at trial.

Two principal disadvantages arise to employing personal legal counsel to assist in health care malpractice defense cases in which insurance counsel is involved. First, the cost to retain personal counsel is potentially great. Second, the provider's personal and insurance counsel may not agree on case strategies and disposition. If such a disagreement is irreconcilable, then the provider's insurer may attempt to withdraw from representation, alleging failure on the part of the insured to cooperate with the insurer.

Occurrence Versus Claims-Made Professional Liability Insurance

During the 1970s, there was a substantial increase in the number and severity of health care malpractice claims and lawsuits. As a result, a health care professional liability insurance crisis ensued, leading first to decreased availability and later to decreased affordability of professional liability insurance. By the mid-1980s, health care professional liability insurers turned to writing claims-made, rather than occurrence coverage, professional liability insurance policies.[42]

Occurrence coverage means that a health care professional is indemnified for covered adverse incidents that occurred while the professional was insured by the insurer, irrespective of when a claim is filed. It does not matter, under occurrence coverage, whether the health care professional is still insured by the insurer at the time the claim is filed.

Before the advent of the insurance affordability crisis of the 1980s, occurrence coverage for health care professional liability insurance was the industry standard. However, as the numbers of health care malpractice claims and lawsuits rose precipitously during the 1970s and 1980s, the "tail" period for liability and indemnity exposure grew very long. Health care malpractice claims and legal judgments can take years to come to fruition, leading to significant uncertainty for health care professionals and their professional liability insurers.

As a result, most health care professional liability insurers began to write exclusively claims-made policies, reflecting their fear of uncertainty under the health care and global litigation crises. Under **claims-made** health care professional liability policies, claims brought against insurers for covered adverse incidents must be made while the health care professional is still insured by the insurer in order to be payable under the policy.

To minimize personal liability exposure incident to health care practice, health care professionals who are insured under claims-made policies must purchase an endorsement to their professional liability insurance policies called "tail coverage." The purchase of tail coverage, in essence, converts a claims-made professional liability insurance policy into an occurrence policy.

A sometimes costly alternative to tail coverage is "prior acts" coverage, also referred to as "nose coverage." Prior acts coverage consists of an endorsement to a new professional liability insurance policy offered by a new insurer for yet-to-be-claimed adverse incidents that may have occurred while the insured was covered under a previous policy. Prior acts coverage is not only more expensive than tail coverage but also is a less certain option for insured professionals and may be fraught with additional limitations and exclusions.[43]

The relative advantages of claims-made health care professional liability insurance policies are that (1) their cost is lower than for occurrence coverage policies and (2) liability limits can be modified from year to year. The relative advantage of an occurrence coverage policy is its longer-term (i.e., "tail") protection.[44]

Need for Professional Liability Insurance

Who needs professional liability insurance? Almost everyone does. Every health care professional involved in clinical practice, with the exception of those professionals who are federal employees (or state employees, under similar circumstances), need the protection of professional liability insurance coverage. Federal health care professionals enjoy worldwide protection from personal monetary liability for official acts incident to their federal duties under the Federal Employees Liability Reform and Tort Compensation Act of 1988.[45]

Experts disagree over whether health care professionals should carry individual professional liability insurance or should be content to rely on the coverage in liability policies carried by their employers.[46] In support of not purchasing individual professional liability insurance, it has been argued that knowledge on the part of a health care malpractice plaintiff of the existence of individual professional liability insurance makes it more likely that the patient will sue. However, the peace of mind associated with the security that individual professional liability insurance coverage provides more than offsets this consideration. In addition, an individual providers' insurance legal counsel can contribute significantly in defense of a health care malpractice legal case and may actually decrease the likelihood of a finding of liability (with all of its adverse consequences to the defendant-provider).

INTELLECTUAL PROPERTY

Intellectual property refers to writings, computer software, depictions, inventions, symbols, and other intangible creations of the mind. Federal law protects the legitimate rights of creators of such contributions. The federal courts have exclusive jurisdiction over patent, trademark, and copyright matters.

A **patent** is an exclusive grant to an original inventor (or inventors jointly) to make, sell, and use an invention for a period of years. Currently, the U.S. Patent and Trademark Office grants utility patents on new, nonobvious, useful processes, machines, and compositions of matter for a period of 20 years. An inventor must file a patent application with U.S. Patent and Trademark Office within 1 year after public use of an invention or be statutorily barred from obtaining a patent for the invention.[47] Absent a contractual agreement otherwise, an employee personally owns the patent rights to inventions made by the employee during the course of employment.

Like most areas of the law, patent law is ever evolving. In April 2007 the U.S. Supreme Court ruled definitively for the first time in *KSR* v. *Teleflex* that purported inventions that merely combine existing design features and technology from other products are not nonobvious innovations worthy of being patented.[48] Fundamental patent law may undergo even more radical change in the near future. Federal legislation introduced in 2007 would change the U.S. patent system from one that awards patents to actual inventors to one that rewards the first entity to file for patent protection.[49] This probusiness legal approach is the one used throughout most of the world.

A **trademark** is a distinctive symbol, word, or group of letters representing a particular product. A **service mark** is a distinctive symbol, word, or group of letters representing a professional service. The grant of an exclusive trademark or service mark to a businessperson serves to protect the proprietary and quality interests of the owner of these distinctive product and service representations. Trademarks and service marks should be registered with the U.S. Patent and Trademark Office in order to ensure universal protection; they are renewable indefinitely as long as they remain distinctive and are used by the owner.

A **copyright** protects an author's expression of a creative idea. That expression can be in the form of a writing, painting, computer program, or some other tangible means of expression. The owner of a copyright is legally entitled to exclusive rights in a work for the life of the author plus 50 years. A corporation that owns a copyright is granted exclusive rights in a work for 75 years.

Registration of a creative work with the U.S. Copyright Office is not a prerequisite to statutory copyright protection. Any original creative work in a tangible form is protected upon its creation. Nor are creators of copyrighted works required to affix the copyright symbol, ©, to their works in order to enjoy statutory protection. Registration of a copyright, however, provides *prima facie* evidence of the validity of the copyright and facilitates enforcement of the copyright holder's rights against unlawful infringement.

Unlike with patents, copyright ownership for a work created by an employee in the scope of employment resides in an employer, absent agreement otherwise. The copyright to a "work for hire," written by a contractor for another person, is owned by the party commissioning the creation of the work. The "fair use" doctrine entitles use or reproduction of copyrighted materials without the permission of copyright owners for limited purposes enumerated in the Copyright Act,[50] including criticism, comment, news reporting, teaching (including multiple copies for classroom use), scholarship, and research.[51]

Information in the public domain, including government documents, is not subject to copyright protection. Recitations of publicly known facts are also not protected; however, unique compilations or presentations of existing facts may enjoy copyright protection.

In 2006, 11,514 intellectual property dispute cases were decided by federal district courts. Of that number, 4944 were copyright cases, 3740 were trademark cases, and 2830 were patent cases.[52]

NURSING HOME ISSUES

Health care malpractice civil cases and criminal prosecutions involving providers in long-term care settings are increasing. Common allegations against long-term care providers and facilities include a pattern of substandard care and/or neglect of residents and intentional misconduct, including intentional infliction of emotional distress incident to verbal abuse, improper restraint, and battery.

The Centers for Medicare and Medicaid Services survey long-term care facilities for Medicare and Medicaid certification based on compliance with more than 100 requirements delineated in the Nursing Home Reform Act, part of the Omnibus Budget Reconciliation Act of 1987 (OBRA).[53] OBRA greatly expanded the rights of long-term care residents and included the right to be free from improper physical restraint.

OBRA prohibits the use of physical restraints on long-term care residents, except as adjuncts to treatment for specific medical conditions. Restraints include not only traditional arm and leg cuffs and lap belts but also bedding materials such as sheets, when they are used to limit a patient's free movement. Whenever physical restraints are to be used, providers must justify their use through clear documentation in a patient's treatment records, including clinical justification and a statement that less restrictive alternatives to physical restraint have been tried and found to be inadequate. A multistate post-OBRA implementation study of 2075 residents found that restraint reduction of 90 percent was accompanied by a 59 percent reduction in moderate to serious resident injuries.[54]

PATIENT SELF-DETERMINATION ACT

The Patient Self-Determination Act of 1990 (PSDA)[55] is a federal statute that codifies patients' right to control treatment-related decisions, routine and extraordinary. The PSDA obligates hospitals, health maintenance organizations, long-term care facilities, home health agencies, hospices, and other health care organizations receiving Medicare and Medicaid funds to its provisions.

A fundamental purpose of the PSDA is to educate patients about their rights to formulate **advance directives**. Advance directives are legal instruments that memorialize a patient's desires concerning life-sustaining measures to be undertaken in the event of the patient's incapacitation, which a patient executes while still legally competent. Common varieties of advance directives include living wills and durable powers of attorney for health care decisions.

A **living will** is a legal document, signed by a patient, which states the patient's wishes concerning life-sustaining measures to be undertaken in the event of the patient's subsequent incompetence. Statutory "natural death acts" are forms of living wills in effect in many states. Most states require that a patient be legally incompetent and terminally ill in order for a living will to become operative. Some states allow a living will to become operative when a patient is in a persistent vegetative state. A **durable power of attorney for health care decisions**, a special power of attorney, is a legal document signed by a patient, which delegates health care decision making to an agent of the patient's choice. The power becomes operative upon the patient's legal incompetence to make such decisions for himself or herself. The patient normally may designate anyone—a spouse, relative, friend, attorney, or other trusted person—as the surrogate health care decision maker.

The principle premise underlying the PSDA is respect for a patient's inherent right to self-determination and control over treatment decision making. According to this premise, a health care provider must disclose to a patient sufficient information about a proposed course of treatment—that is, the nature of the recommended intervention; its material risks, if any; reasonable alternatives to the proposed intervention; and expected benefits of treatment—to empower the patient to analyze the options and make an informed choice about whether to undergo or reject treatment.

The PSDA does not create any new substantive patient rights. Instead, the PSDA imposes affirmative procedural obligations on health care providers and facilities to which the law applies. Among other requirements, the PSDA requires providers and facilities to do the following:

- Provide written information to patients concerning their rights under state law to give informed consent to, or refusal of, treatment and to make advance directives
- Provide patients with copies of institutional policies concerning informed patient decision making and advance directives
- Document in patient records whether patients have executed advance directives concerning treatment[56]

Larsen and Eaton[57] did an exhaustive investigative analysis of the PSDA and reported that the law has enjoyed only limited success since its enactment. The reasons for its limited success include the facts that many patients are unaware of their right to make enforceable advance directives, many patients are unwilling to execute advance directives, and physicians do not know of or fail to comply with valid patient advance directives.

SAFE MEDICAL DEVICES ACT

The Safe Medical Devices Act of 1990,[58] administered by the Food and Drug Administration (FDA), requires health care facilities to report incidents involving serious patient injury, illness, or death resulting from defective medical equipment. Under the Safe Medical Devices Act, a designee of the facility (typically the facility risk manager) must submit a report directly to the FDA within 10 working days whenever a death occurs and to the product manufacturer (or directly to the FDA, if the name of the product manufacturer is not known) for cases involving injury or illness.

Such reports enjoy limited qualified immunity from use against the facility in civil litigation, unless the facility intentionally makes a false report.[59] In addition to generating an agency report under the Safe Medical Devices Act, the clinical manager for the area in which patient injury from equipment occurred should turn off and sequester the allegedly defective equipment; generate an internal incident report concerning the event; and ensure that documentation of the patient's postinjury evaluation and care are retained by medical records personnel as potential litigation documents.

SARBANES-OXLEY ACT

The Sarbanes-Oxley Act of 2002[60] is a federal statute enacted by Congress in the aftermath of the Enron and WorldCom corporate scandals that took down prominent corporations and their leaders and left thousands of employees without promised pensions. Sarbanes-Oxley, or "SOX" as it is commonly known, is designed to strengthen federal regulation of public companies. SOX increases corporate responsibility by making corporate executives and corporate legal counsel personally responsible for accurate public reporting of financial information about their businesses.

Section 404 of SOX is designed to assist investors and the general public by making transparent the internal controls of public companies for financial reporting. Corporate leaders are responsible under this section for annually reviewing, documenting, and having audited their internal controls and financial reports. These internal controls include information technology systems and procedures and authorizations that support accurate, dependable financial information reporting.

SOX requires personal certification by chief executive officer and chief financial officer of the public company of the accuracy of financial data submitted to the Securities and Exchange Commission.

SOX also added specific legal duties to in-house corporate legal counsel. The law mandates that corporate legal counsel report suspected material violations of the law to their corporate chief legal counsel or qualified legal compliance committee for further action. SOX clarifies that corporate legal counsel owe their duty of confidentiality to the corporation, not to officers, directors, and employees of the corporation. SOX also establishes for the first time federal rules of professional conduct for attorneys practicing before the Securities and Exchange Commission.[62] These rules augment existing state attorney regulations but, in case of conflict, should supersede them.

SOX has been challenged recently by business as excessively costly. One report stated that the cost of doing business for a publicly traded company with less than $1 billion in revenue increased 230 percent since SOX came into effect.[63] SOX has set the stage for expanded ethical and legal responsibilities in the future for nonprofit and other private business organizations.

SECTION 1350, SUBSECTION C OF TITLE 18 (THE FEDERAL CRIMINAL CODE)

(1) Whoever certifies any statement set forth in subsections (a) and (b) of this section knowing that the periodic report accompanying the statement does not comport with all of the requirements set forth in this section shall be fined not more than $1,000,000 or imprisoned not more than 10 years, or both, or

(2) willfully certifies any statement set forth in subsections (a) and (b) of this section knowing that the periodic report accompanying the statement does not comport with all of the requirements set forth in this section shall be fined not more than $5,000,000 or imprisoned not more than 20 years, or both[61]

SUMMARY

A key component of a proactive liability risk management program in business is regularly recurring education of professional, support, and administrative personnel of the basic principles of, and developments in, business law. Business law is extremely complex and in near-constant flux, requiring that continuing legal education in this area be given by attorneys, rather than nonattorneys.

The arm of government that health care business entrepreneurs interact with most often is the administrative branch, consisting of federal and state administrative agencies such as the Equal Employment Opportunity Commission, Health Care Financing Administration, Internal Revenue Service, and Occupational Safety and Health Administration. Complex federal statutory laws, such as HIPAA and SOX, make regular and proactive consultation with attorneys indispensable for business leaders. Similarly, every health care professional contemplating the formation of a business should consult proactively with an attorney of choice for early and ongoing advice.

CASES AND QUESTIONS

1. A physical therapist who has treated a patient for postoperative spinal rehabilitation exercises is being deposed as a fact witness in the patient's medical malpractice case against the patient's orthopedic surgeon. The patient's attorney asks the physical therapist to describe the lumbar intervertebral disk. The witness explains, at length, how the lumbar intervertebral disk is like a jelly doughnut. The patient's attorney impeaches (challenges the credibility of) the witness by saying, "You don't really mean to say that the lumbar intervertebral disk in human beings is similar to a jelly doughnut, do you?" After that exchange, the patient's attorney asks the witness to concede that a particular orthopedic physical therapy text is generally recognized as an authoritative work. The witness concedes that the text is authoritative. The patient's attorney then proceeds to impeach the witness using remote passages from the text that recite propositions with which the witness does not agree. How should the witness have approached these two trick questions?
2. A patient undergoing a physical examination in a physician assistant's office allegedly sustains a minor musculoskeletal arm injury from contact with a piece of medical equipment. What legal reporting responsibilities, if any, does the provider's medical service have?

SUGGESTED ANSWERS TO CASES AND QUESTIONS

1. First and foremost, this witness should have been thoroughly prepared for deposition by an attorney because a fact witness today may be named as a malpractice defendant tomorrow. The witness should not have attempted to describe in detail the anatomy and physiology of the lumbar intervertebral disk in the deposition unless the witness is an anatomist or physiologist. Instead, the witness should have declined to give a detailed description of the disk, based on the fact that such a description is beyond the scope of the witness's professional competence. Similarly, the question asking the witness to declare a text authoritative was designed to enable the patient's attorney to impeach the witness using remote textual passages. This witness should have stated that, although the text in question may be a legitimate reference text, without further review, the witness is

unwilling casually to declare it to be authoritative. (By "authoritative," the witness concedes that the work is accurate from cover to cover.)

2. The physician's assistant should report the incident to her or his supervising physician and generate an incident report. The report should include information about the postinjury evaluation, care of the patient, and detailed identification of the equipment involved. The incident report must be forwarded to the facility risk manager for review and retention. In this care there is no legal requirement to make a report to the equipment manufacturer or to the Food and Drug Administration under the Safe Medical Devices Act because neither serious injury/illness nor death occurred. (It might be prudent, however, to notify the equipment manufacturer of the incident but not to release a copy of the internal incident report.)

SUGGESTED READINGS

Helminski F: Ghosts from Samaria: good Samaritan laws in the hospital, *Mayo Clin Proc* 68:400-401, 1993.

Herzlinger RE: Why innovation in health care is so hard, *Harvard Business Review* pp 58-66, May 2006.

Jirank AL, Baker SD: Any willing provider laws: regulating the health care provider's contractual relationship with the insurance company, *Health Lawyer* 7(4):1, 1994.

Kang C: A primer on nonimmigrant and immigrant visa processing, *Texas Bar Journal* pp 870-882, Nov 2003.

Lisanter JE: Okay! I'm getting a lawyer, *Washington Post* p C4, July 20, 1999.

Markey ML, Markey M, Canton MI, Wisner C: Attorney-client privilege in the parent-subsidiary relationship, *Health Lawyers News* 6(5):5-10, 2002.

Nolo: www.nolo.com (legal information for consumers).

Osborne DE, Martinec JD, Johnson MW, Sauceda G: Asset protection planning after the bankruptcy act, *Texas Bar Journal* 68(11):1006-1011, 2005.

Public opinion survey reveals Texas' perception of justice system, *State Bar of Texas Update* p 1, Jan 1999.

Scott RW: Good Samaritan immunity, *Clinical Management* 11(4):11-12, 1991.

REFERENCES

1. Davis KC, Pierce RJ Jr: *Administrative law treatise,* ed 3, vol 1, Boston, 1994, Little, Brown.
2. *Chevron, USA, Inc.* v. *Natural Resources Defense Council,* 467 U.S. 837 (1984).
3. The Administrative Procedure Act of 1946, 5 United States Code Sections 551-559, 701-706.
4. The Freedom of Information Act, 5 United States Code Section 552.
5. Smith L: Freedom of information is a fundamental American right, *Herald-Zeitung* p 4A, March 22, 2007.
6. The Privacy Act, 5 United States Code Section 552a.
7. The Sherman Act of 1890, 15 United States Code Sections 1-3.
8. The Clayton Act of 1914, 15 United States Code Sections 15a, 19.
9. The Federal Trade Commission Act of 1914, 15 United States Code Section 41 et seq.

10. Marx D Jr, Laing MA: The state action doctrine: can it be applied to a private hospital's acquisition of a public hospital? *Health Lawyer* 8(3):1, 1995.

11. *Eastern Railroad Presidents Conference* v. *Noerr Motor Freight,* 365 U.S. 127. (1961); *United Mine Workers of America* v. *Penning,* 381 U.S. 657 (1965).

12. Furrow BR, Johnson SH, Jost TS, Schwartz RL: Health law: cases, materials and problems, ed 2, St Paul, Minn, 1991, West Publishing.

13. *Goldfarb* v. *Virginia State Bar,* 421 U.S. 773 (1975).

14. *Patrick* v. *Burget,* 486 U.S. 94 (1988).

15. *Wilk* v. *American Medical Association,* 895 F.2d 3-52, cert, denied, 498 U.S. 982 (1990).

16. Bernick DM: Medicine and the Law, *Permissible physician-hospital joint ventures.* Retrieved May 7, 2007, from, http://physiciansnews.com.

17. *Bates and Van O'Steen* v. *State Bar of Arizona,* 433 U.S. 350 (1977).

18. Rule 1.6. In *Annotated model rules of professional conduct,* ed 2, Chicago, Ill, 1992, American Bar Association.

19. Ginsburg WH: How to evaluate a lawyer, *Physicians Manage* pp 90-99, Dec 1991.

20. Overman S: How to work with your lawyer, *HR Magazine* pp 41-15, July 1992.

21. Frels K: Destroying the negative lawyer myth: act now on lawyer bashing, *Texas Bar Journal* pp 930, Dec 2004.

22. Standing Committee on Pro Bono & Public Service, American Bar Association: *Directory of pro bono programs.* Retrieved May 7, 2007, from www.abanet.org/legalservices/probono/directory.html.

23. McElaney JW: Preparing witnesses for depositions, *Journal of the American Bar Association* pp 84-86, June 1992.

24. U.S. Constitution, Article I, Section 10.

25. Restatement (Second) of Contracts, Section 1.

26. Calamari JD, Perillo JM: *Contracts,* ed 2, St Paul, Minn, 1977, West Publishing. (See Chapters 2, 4, 8, and 22).

27. Restatement (Second) of Contracts, Section 22.

28. See *Tunkl* v. *Regents of the University of California,* 60 Cal. 2d 92 (1963).

29. Calamari JD, Perillo JM: *Contracts* ed 2, St Paul, Minn, 1977, West Publishing.

30. Uniform Commercial Code, Section 2-201.

31. *Sullivan* v. *O'Connor,* 296 N.E. 2d 183 (Mass. 1973).

32. U.S. Constitution, Thirteenth Amendment.

33. Scott RW: Liability considerations in continuing education, *PT Magazine* pp 54-57, May 1994.

34. Huckstep A, Wilson JC, Carmody RP: *Corporate law for the healthcare provider: organization, operation, merger and bankruptcy,* Washington, DC, 1993, National Health Lawyers Association.

35. Texas Professional Corporation Act, Texas Rev. Civ. Stat. Ann. art. 1528e.

36. Internal Revenue Service: *Small business and self-employed one-stop resource.* Retrieved May 8, 2007, from www.irs.gov/businesses/small.

37. Minow M: Libraries, latchkey children and the law, *California Libraries* 10(6):1-2, 2000.

38. Mason R: Good Samaritan laws, legal disarray: an update, *Mercer Law Review* 38:1339-1375, 1987.

39. Health Insurance Portability and Accountability Act, 42 U.S.C. 1320d-2.

40. US Department of Health and Human Services: *Office for Civil Rights—HIPAA.* Retrieved May 8, 2007 from www.hhs.gov/ocr/hipaa/privacy.html.

41. Court rules physician may sue lawyer for malpractice settlement, *PT Bulletin* p 5, Sep 14, 1988.

42. Johnson KB, Hatlie MJ, Johnson ID: *The guide to medical professional liability insurance,* Chicago, Ill, 1991, American Medical Association.

43. Occurrence vs claims-made medical professional liability insurance policies: fundamental differences in the concept of coverage, *JAMA* 266:1570-1572, 1991.

44. Kelley K: In practice: occurrence vs claims-made policies, *PT Magazine* 2(7):17, 1994.

45. The Federal Employees Liability Reform and Tort Compensation Act of 1988, 28 United States Code Section 2679(b)(1).

46. Aiken TD: *Legal, ethical, and political issues in nursing,* Philadelphia, Pa, 1994, Davis.

47. 35 United States Code Section 102(b).

48. *KSR* v. *Teleflex,* U.S. Supreme Court, No. 04-1350, Apr. 30, 2007.

49. Copp T: Patent law legislation elicits calls for changes, *Austin American Statesman* p D1, April 27, 2007.

50. The Copyright Act, 17 United States Code Section 101 et seq.

51. Ibid., Section 107.

52. Bravin J: Patent holders' grip weakens, *Wall Street Journal* p A3, May 1, 2007.

53. Omnibus Budget Reconciliation Act of 1987, Public Law 100-203, 101 Stat. 1330, 42 United States Code Sections 1395i-3 and 1396. et seq.

54. Neufeld RR, Libow LS, Foley WJ et al: Restraint reduction reduces serious injury among nursing home residents, *J Am Geriatr Soc* 47(10):1202-1207, 1999.

55. The Patient Self-Determination Act of 1990, 42 United States Code Sections 1395cc and 1396a.

56. Patient Self-Determination Act, Section 1395cc(f).

57. Larsen EJ, Eaton TA: The limits of advance directives: a history and assessment of the Patient Self-Determination Act, *Wake Forest Law Review* 32(2):249, 1997.

58. The Safe Medical Devices Act of 1990, 21 United States Code Sections 301 note, 321, 360d, 360hh et seq.

59. The Safe Medical Devices Act: does it increase hospital liability? *Hosp Risk Manage* pp 55-58, May 1991.

60. The Sarbanes-Oxley Act of 2002, 15 United States Code Section 7201, et seq.

61. 18 United States Code Section 1350 (Failure of corporate officers to certify financial reports).

62. Godfrey CM: The revised role of lawyers after Sarbanes-Oxley, *Texas Bar Journal* 68(10):932-948, 2005.

63. Fowler T: Taking an account of reform, *Houston Chronicle* p D1, Jan 26, 2006.

NOTES

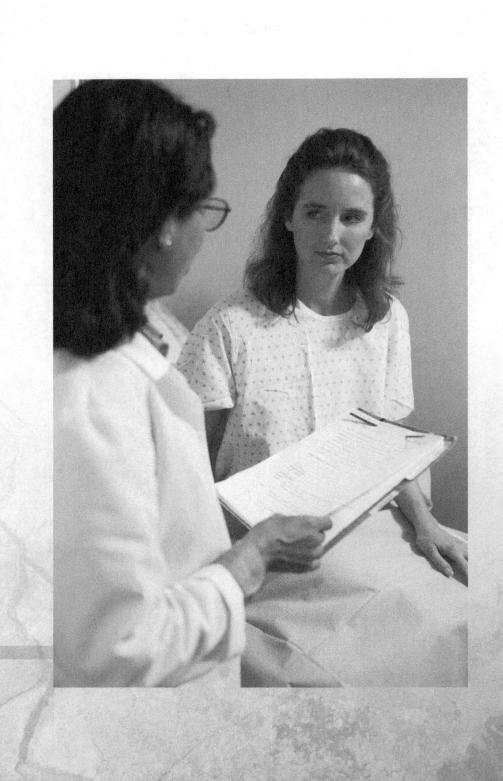

7

Legal and Ethical Issues in Education

KEY TERMS

Equal protection
Probable cause
Privacy
Reasonable suspicion

INTRODUCTION

This chapter introduces basic concepts related to legal and ethical aspects of education. Important federal statutory laws—including the Americans with Disabilities Act (Titles II and III), the Buckley Amendment, the Individuals with Disabilities Education Act, the No Child Left Behind Act, Title VI of the Civil Rights Act of 1964, and Title IX of the 1972 Educational Amendments—are discussed. Legal and ethical issues associated with academic discipline and dismissal are explored, as well as how such issues relate to academic program admissions. The chapter concludes with a discussion of legal responsibility for health care professional student conduct in the clinic.

Education, training, and development are related concepts that in health care education and delivery systems affect the conduct of academicians, professional students, clinical and administrative professionals, and support personnel. The process of "education" involves the acquisition of general or specific knowledge, with or without specific learning goals. "Training," however, encompasses the acquisition of focused, job-specific or job-related proficiency skills. "Development" embraces the furtherance of knowledge or skill under education or training.

A constitutional right to public education in the United States is a common belief. Although there may be such a right under selected state constitutions, there is no express right to public education in the federal Constitution. Under federal law, educational rights largely fall under limited federal statutes addressing educational issues within the restricted domain of federal jurisdiction (interests). Other federal educational rights derive from case law based on interpretation of federal constitutional provisions such as equal protection, privacy, and due process.

Education law is composed of federal and state laws. Education law may be grounded in federal and/or state constitutions, statutes, case law, and administrative rules and regulations.

SELECTED FEDERAL STATUTES AFFECTING EDUCATION

Congress has enacted a number of statutes designed to assist state and local government educational agencies to meet the many special needs of students at all levels in the education process: preschool, elementary, secondary, collegiate, graduate, and professional. For example, the original Elementary and Secondary Education Act of 1965[1] addressed bilingual and drug education, high school completion, and other issues within the purview of interests of the federal government.

The No Child Left Behind Act (NCLB) of 2002 amended the Elementary and Secondary Education Act. NCLB established new content and academic achievement standards for public schools. NCLB mandates periodic standardized assessment of progress for all students, especially including at-risk and disabled students. The law requires supplemental educational services, such as tutoring, for struggling low-income students. NCLB also requires public accountability for schools, allowing students to transfer from schools not achieving adequate yearly progress.[2] As of May 2007, Congress was working toward reauthorization of NCLB.[3]

Other federal statutes place specific mandates on the states based on federal constitutional authority, including equal protection, privacy, due process, and the plenary power of Congress to regulate interstate commerce. Title VI of the Civil Rights Act of 1964,[4] for example, prohibits discrimination against students by schools receiving federal financial assistance (i.e., almost all schools) based on race or national origin. The statute reads as follows:

No person in the United States shall, on the ground of race, color, or national origin, be excluded from participation in, be denied the benefits of, or be subjected to discrimination under any program or activity receiving Federal financial assistance.

Title IX of the Educational Amendments of 1972,[5] patterned after Title VI of the Civil Rights Act of 1964, prohibits gender discrimination in educational programs and activities that receive federal funds. This law, enacted in the same year that gender was added as a protected class to the Civil Rights Act of 1964, was intended to "round out" federal educational antidiscrimination policy by including as prohibited conduct gender discrimination in educational programs and activities receiving federal dollars. The statute reads in pertinent part as follows:

Section 1681 (a). No person in the United States shall, on the basis of sex, be excluded from participation in, be denied the benefits of, or be subjected to discrimination under any education program or activity receiving Federal financial assistance, except that:

(1) in regards to admissions to educational institutions, this section shall apply only to institutions of vocational education, professional education, and graduate higher education, and to public institutions of undergraduate higher education;

(2) in regards to admissions to educational institutions, this section shall not apply ... (B) for seven years from the date an educational institution begins the process of changing from being an institution which admits only students of one sex to being an institution which admits students of both sexes ...

(3) this section shall not apply to an educational institution which is controlled by a religious organization if the application of this subsection would not be consistent with the religious tenets of such organization;

(4) this section shall not apply to an educational institution whose primary purpose is the training of individuals for the military service of the United States, or the merchant marine; ...

(h) this section shall not apply to membership practices—(A) of a social fraternity or social sorority which is exempt from taxation under section 501(a) of Title 26, the active membership of which consists primarily of students in attendance at an institution of higher education, or (B) of the Young Men's Christian Association, Young Women's Christian Association, Girl Scouts, Boy Scouts, Camp Fire Girls, and voluntary youth service organizations which are so exempt, the membership of which has traditionally been limited to persons of one sex and principally to persons of less than nineteen years of age ...

Although there was initially some ambiguity over whether only specific programs receiving federal funds or entire educational institutions were bound not to discriminate based on gender, this issue was resolved in 1987 when Congress enacted the Civil Rights Restoration Act,[6] which applied Title IX to entire institutions, not just to specific programs or activities receiving federal funds. Subsequent federal case law applied Title IX protections not just to female students, but to female faculty and staff as well.[7]

The Family Educational Rights and Privacy Act of 1974,[8] popularly known as the Buckley Amendment, established uniform standards for educational institutions concerning the privacy of student records. This federal statute was enacted contemporaneously with the federal Privacy and the Freedom of Information Acts,[9] which regulate the confidentiality of and access to information about individuals that is in the possession of the federal government. The Buckley

Amendment gave students and their parents access to official school records and the right to challenge the accuracy of information contained in them. The amendment also required that student records be kept confidential and that they be released only with the written consent of students over age 18 or of parents of students under age 18.

This law also established a 5-year retention requirement for official student records. Clinical affiliation reports on health care professional students are official student records for purposes of the Buckley Amendment.

Under case law interpreting the Buckley Amendment, personal notes made by teachers about students are not considered to be official education records and are exempt from maintenance and disclosure requirements. Case law also established as permissible practice the posting of student grades for examinations, so long as students cannot be individually identified in such postings.

The Education for All Handicapped Children Act of 1975[10] was one of the first federal statutes to address the educational needs of disabled children. Signed into law by President Ford, the act mandated equal educational opportunity for disabled children between the ages of 3 and 21. This statute was subsequently amended and eventually incorporated into a successor federal statute titled the Individuals with Disabilities Education Act of 1990 (IDEA).[11]

IDEA built upon the Vocational Rehabilitation Act of 1973, Section 504,[12] and the Education for All Handicapped Children Act by specifically enumerating qualifying disabilities in children. IDEA clearly established the right of disabled children to free public education irrespective of parents' financial status.

IDEA established the concept of inclusion ("mainstreaming") of physically and mentally challenged students into regular classes and other educational experiences to the extent feasible in order optimally to normalize the education of disabled students. Under the law, individualized student educational program plans must be developed. School districts are also required to provide supportive "related services" to disabled students including transportation services; assistive technology devices; medical, psychological, physical, and occupational therapy; and audiology and speech-language evaluative services required to assist disabled students to benefit from special education.[13]

IDEA was reauthorized in 1997[14] and amended in 2004.[15] The 1997 version of the law built on the principle that all children ages 3 to 22 with disabilities are entitled to free and appropriate education within the least restrictive environment. The reauthorized act focused on improving special education curricula and preparing students for independent living and employment.

The 2004 amendment added a process called Response to Intervention, which shifts first-responder responsibility for addressing student academic and behavioral problems to general education classroom teachers before such students can be considered for special education intervention. This three-tiered process resulted because Congress thought that too many limited-English-proficiency and minority students were being labeled as "disabled."

The Equal Access Act of 1984,[16] enacted into law by Congress during President Ronald Reagan's first term, made public (secondary) schools into limited public fora by requiring that schools that receive federal funds allow use of their facilities for religious extracurricular clubs and activities if they allow them for nonreligious extra-curricular clubs and activities. The statute reads in pertinent part as follows:

> *It shall be unlawful for any public secondary school which receives Federal financial assistance and which has a limited open forum to deny equal access or a fair opportunity to, or [to] discriminate against, any students who wish to conduct a meeting within that limited open forum on the basis of* religious, political, philo-sophical, or other content of the speech *at such meetings. [emphasis added]*

The Americans with Disabilities Act of 1990 (ADA)[17] was a landmark federal civil rights statute that empowered disabled Americans. The Title I employment aspects were discussed in Chapter 5. The ADA mandates equality in opportunity for the disabled in employment (Title I) and access to public services (including education) and public transportation services (Title II), public accommodations and services operated by private entities (including private schools; Title III), and telecommunications services (Title IV).

The ADA expanded the scope of the Rehabilitation Act of 1973 to include under its jurisdiction all business entities, in the public and private sectors, having 15 or more employees. The Rehabilitation Act of 1973 was similarly amended to exclude these conditions from the definition of "handicap."[18]

A number of judicial ADA higher education cases have been reported.[19] Issues addressed include accommodation of testees in admissions tests, student disabilities unknown to school officials, requirements for sign language interpreters for deaf students, and the nature of "undue (financial) hardship" regarding modifications to school sites for disabled students. In general, if educational institutions take reason-able measures to accommodate known student disabilities so as to give qualified disabled students and applicants equal opportunity vis-à-vis nondisabled students and applicants, then they are complying with the letter and spirit of Titles II and III of the ADA, as applicable.

> Under the ADA, educational institutions are required to take reasonable measures to accommodate known student disabilities so as to give qualified disabled students and applicants equal opportunity in admissions, education, and services vis-a-vis nondisabled students and applicants.

FEDERAL EDUCATION LAW PREMISED ON FEDERAL CONSTITUTIONAL PROTECTIONS

Federal and applicable state constitutional protections apply to persons and actions in school settings with equal force as to any other place or circumstances. Due process of law, applicable to the states under the Fourteenth Amendment and to the federal government under the Fifth Amendment, requires that school officials treat students with substantive fairness in all aspects of educational processes and particularly that they procedurally give adequate notice to students and their parents or guardians of potential adverse administrative actions (such as suspension or expulsion) and afford students an opportunity to be heard on such issues before final decisions are made. The amount of "process" that is "due" turns on the severity of the disciplinary action in issue.

Equal protection under law, also applicable to the states under the Fourteenth Amendment and to the federal government under the Fifth Amendment, requires (at least) that school officials treat similarly situated students in a similar way. The Equal Protection Clause of the Fourteenth Amendment was a post–Civil War federal constitutional amendment designed to eliminate government-endorsed racial discrimination in the United States.

Although the "similarly situated" standard applies to treatment of students generally by school officials, school actions or policies that intentionally discriminate against, or even have a disparate adverse impact on protected minorities—including women and racial or ethnic minorities—are judged by courts under higher standards of review. Actions that adversely affect women, for example, such as the creation or maintenance of all-male schools or programs, must be proved to be substantially related to important governmental interests in order to survive judicial scrutiny. In recent times, all-male educational institutions of higher learning have become all but nonexistent because they cannot meet this intermediate-tier legal standard of scrutiny.

School actions or policies that discriminate against students based on race/ethnicity or religion are judged under the highest judicial standard of review. To be upheld, such actions or policies must directly advance compelling state interests, such as the preservation of life, health, or public safety. Because no school policy conceivably is justifiable under this highest-tier judicial standard of review, public school-based racial and religious discrimination, such as the maintenance of racially segregated schools,[20] is prohibited.

The constitutional right of (student) **privacy** applies with nearly equal force in the school setting as in other settings. The courts have ruled that the right of privacy under the Fourth Amendment applies in school settings. However, the courts have also held that, in order to conduct searches of students or their property, school officials need have only **reasonable** ("common sense") **suspicion** of wrongdoing, not **probable cause** (i.e., substantial, objective, credible evidence that a particular suspect committed a specific offense), which is the higher standard of justification required for searches by police.

The First Amendment to the Constitution simultaneously requires the official separation of church and state and governmental tolerance of the free exercise of individual and group religious beliefs. The balance struck between these two dichotomous mandates is that no religious instruction (of any faith) may be included in official public educational curricula, yet to the extent that secular extracurricular activities are supported by schools, religious activities must be supported as well.

ACADEMIC DISCIPLINARY ISSUES INVOLVING HEALTH CARE PROFESSIONAL STUDENTS

Official conduct on the part of public university faculty and administration is considered "state action," triggering the protections of individual liberty and property interests under the federal Constitution. Constitutional safeguards entitle public university students facing academic disciplinary action to substantive and procedural due process protection in adjudication of their cases. Under substantive due process, the key question is "Does the student facing discipline have a protected property or liberty interest in continued, unconditional enrollment in the institution of higher learning?" The procedural due process question is "Was the student given clear notice of specific academic or disciplinary noted deficiencies and a reasonable opportunity to respond to charges?" An additional procedural due process question for courts on reviews may be "Was the deficient student afforded a reasonable opportunity to improve his or her performance before execution of adverse administrative action?"

Disciplinary actions taken by private universities against students are subject to less judicial scrutiny than in public settings. Because there is no "state action" with private university actions, the questions to be answered on judicial review of private university disciplinary actions against students are "Did the private university have reasonable academic disciplinary rules in place and well-publicized?" and "Did the university follow its own procedures in deciding whether to discipline or dismiss a student for academic or disciplinary reasons?"

Several noted legal cases concern the propriety of academic dismissal by colleges and universities. In all of the following cases, courts displayed substantial deference to the professional judgments of school administrators and faculty.

In *Board of Curators of the University of Missouri* v. *Horowitz,*[21] the U.S. Supreme Court reviewed an academic dismissal decision involving a medical student from a state university. The student in question failed a major examination and reportedly had a poor overall academic record. In finding in favor of the university on procedural and substantive due process grounds, the court found that the student had adequate notice of poor academic performance and reasonable opportunities for improvement and that the decision of school administrators to dismiss the student was careful, deliberate, and fair. The opinion held the following:

> *Like the decision of an individual professor as to the proper grade for a student in his course, the determination whether to dismiss a student for academic reasons requires an expert evaluation of cumulative information as is not readily adapted to the procedural tools of judicial or administrative decision making. ... Courts are particularly ill-equipped to evaluate academic performance.*[22]

In a concurring opinion, Justice Powell added that "university faculty must have the widest range of discretion in making judgments as to the academic performance of students."[23]

In *Regents of the University of Michigan* v. *Ewing,*[24] the U.S. Supreme Court again deferred to academicians in affirming the academic dismissal of a medical student attending a state university Inteflex (combined undergraduate and medical education) program. In this case the student was dismissed after failing a National Board of Medical Examiners qualifying examination for clinical rotations after his fourth year of study. Because the dismissal was based on the student's overall academic record, it was deemed to be fair and not arbitrary and capricious, as the student had claimed.

In *Tobias* v. *University of Texas,*[25] the Texas Court of Appeals reviewed the case of a nursing student who was dismissed for academic deficiency after twice failing a required course titled "Nursing During the Childbearing Experience." The student appealed his failing grades through academic channels, invoking the grievance procedure of the university outlined in its catalog. When he was not permitted to take the course for a third time, the former student sued the university (and three professors individually, as state officials, under 42 U.S.C. Section 1983, for violation of his civil rights), claiming due process and equal protection violations under the federal and Texas constitutions and breach of contract. The appellate court affirmed the lower court decision of summary judgment in favor of the university, rejecting all of the former student's claims. In his opinion, Justice Lattimore held the following:

> *Substantive due process protection in the academic arena protects an individual from actions that are arbitrary and capricious. A judge may not override the faculty's professional judgment in academic affairs unless [their judgment] is such a substantial departure from accepted academic norms as to demonstrate that the person or committee responsible did not actually exercise professional judgment. Where a reviewing court has found* minimal *[emphasis added] evidence of professional judgment, such evidence has been considered sufficient to justify judgment against a student as a matter of law.*

Based on the case decisions cited, the following risk management measures are recommended for health care professional collegiate programs in order to protect student, faculty, and administration rights and to minimize litigation exposure incident to student disciplinary actions:

- Identify deficient academic performance by a student as early as possible, and promptly notify the affected student.
- Afford reasonable opportunity for the student to be heard on the matter. (These first two elements together constitute procedural due process.)
- Offer the deficient student specific recommendations for improvement. Explain the adverse consequences of continued unsatisfactory performance. Allow adequate time for remediation and improvement.
- Have in place in the institution clear, well-disseminated standards for minimally acceptable academic and clinical performance on the part of students. Have in place grievance and appeals processes for student use. Always follow these processes when adjudicating cases. Post procedures for filing grievances and appeals of adverse actions in institutional catalogs and/or student handbooks.
- Consider (after consulting with institutional legal counsel) including a disclaimer in catalogs and handbooks that no contractual agreement concerning student continuation in, or graduation from, the institution exists as a result of catalog or handbook information or language.
- Document student counseling sessions. Maintain documentation in a secure location.
- Involve institutional legal counsel in student disciplinary matters *ab initio*.

ACADEMIC ADMISSIONS ISSUES

The same considerations concerning student constitutional and common law rights that apply to academic disciplinary processes also apply to admissions decisions in public institutions, including substantive and procedural due process, equal protection, and antidiscrimination considerations. Because admissions to public colleges and universities constitute "state action," admissions committees, their staff, and institutional administration must ensure that processes are fundamentally fair to all applicants.

Under Title VI of the Civil Rights Act of 1964,[26] certain questions on applications and in interviews are prohibited, including questions about the following:

- Race or ethnicity
- Religious affiliation or beliefs
- Nationality
- Marital status
- Existence of dependent family members
- Perceived disabilities
- Military discharge classification
- Economic status

In addition to inquiries prohibited by law, certain questions and comments should not be asked or made because they can reasonably be misconstrued as discriminatory. For example, avoid the following:

- Offering compliments, criticism, or suggestions about personal appearance
- Questions concerning foreign language ability or region of the state or country in which an applicant grew up
- Inquiring about social organizations to which the applicant may belong, unless directly related to the applicant's abilities as a health care professional

During interviews of multiple applicants, remember to ask each applicant questions from the same basic shell of questions, allowing some latitude for specific inquiries to individual applicants. This promotes uniform treatment of applicants and should meet the equal protection requirement to treat similarly situated persons similarly.

LIABILITY FOR STUDENT CONDUCT IN CLINICAL SETTINGS

An important consideration for academic and clinical faculty who supervise health care professional students is who bears legal responsibility for liability-generating conduct on the part of students. Faculty and clinical supervisors may incur primary liability for their own liability-generating conduct that results in patient injury. One or more of them may also be vicariously, or indirectly, liable for student liability-generating conduct, even when faculty and supervisors themselves do not directly cause patient injury.

Any licensed or certified health care professional who has the legal duty to care for a patient may be primarily liable for physical and mental injury incurred by a patient as a result of (1) professional negligence (substandard care delivery), (2) intentional (mis)conduct, (3) breach of a contractual therapeutic promise made to a patient, and (4) patient injury that results from the use of a dangerously defective modality or product. A clinical faculty member who supervises the official activities of students, assistants, aids, and others may be vicariously, or indirectly, liable for patient injury resulting from the liability-generating conduct of these persons when it occurs within the scope of their employment or affiliation.

The party vicariously liable for health care professional student conduct usually is the party who has accepted such legal responsibility under a clinical affiliation agreement, or contract. The clinical affiliation contract should clearly delineate the scope of vicarious liability for the clinical site and the academic institution and should only be created in close consultation with both parties' legal counsel. As an additional protective measure for the clinical site and school, such a contract may also include express language that memorializes the mutual understanding of the parties that the academic institution will send to the clinical site only those students who are adequately prepared to participate in clinical experiences.

In the absence of clear contractual language spelling out who (or rather whose liability insurer) is responsible for student conduct, a court may invoke a common law doctrine called the "borrowed servant rule" to assign liability, based on whose interests (the school or clinical site) the student was primarily serving at the time of an adverse patient incident.

In addition to vicarious liability, clinical sites and academic institutions may incur primary liability for their own negligence in supervising and preparing students who injure patients, respectively. An academic institution, for example, may incur primary liability for the negligent instruction or academic preparation of a student and/or for the negligent or intentional misrepresentation of a student's competency or status.

A clinical instructor or site may incur primary liability for the negligent failure to review a referral order, a patient's treatment records, or a student's evaluation note before allowing the student to treat a patient. Clinical instructors and sites may also be primarily liable for the negligent failure to provide on-site and, when appropriate, direct supervision of a student during patient intake, evaluation, and treatment. State practice acts usually define the degree of supervision of students required of clinical instructors.

Failure to supervise primary liability is often couched in legal terms of art, such as patient or student abandonment. A clinical instructor who permits a health care professional student to evaluate and/or care for patients without the degree of supervision required by law may face, in addition to civil malpractice liability, a criminal legal action for the aiding and abetting unlawful professional practice by an unlicensed practitioner, as well as possible adverse administrative action affecting professional licensure and professional association action for ethics violations.

Malpractice exposure may also occur when a clinical instructor imparts negligent instruction or guidance to a student that results in patient injury, or when there is a negligent or intentional failure to include students in systematic quality oversight activities, such as peer review of patient care activities carried out in the clinic.

Center coordinators for clinical education (CCCEs) and clinic managers must ensure that clinical instructors thoroughly understand the rules of appropriate supervision of students. Clinical instructors must also exercise sound professional judgment when assigning patients to students, based on factors such as student competence and special considerations associated with particular patients.

It is essential that clinical instructors review all student evaluations and countersign their notes (as required) before allowing students to carry out initial treatment of patients. This precaution helps to protect all participants in the treatment process—the patient, the student, the clinical instructor, and the clinical site. Because health care professional students are not licensed providers, the "student note" is not valid without clinical instructor review and approval. The clinical instructor adopts, or is deemed legally to have adopted, all evaluation and treatment notes written by students under his or her supervision as his or her own notes. Whenever a health care malpractice case from an intervention involving a health care professional student results in the payment of a monetary settlement or judgment, it is normally the supervising clinical instructor's name—not the student's name—that is reported for permanent inclusion in the National Practitioner Data Bank.

Clinical instructors have not only the ethical responsibility but also a legal duty to evaluate and report honestly and accurately on a health care professional student's clinical performance to academic coordinators of clinical education. Any critical, candid comments about a student should be accurate, fair, objective, and well-supported by prior written counseling statements in which the student was given clear notice of deficient performance, an opportunity to respond to the allegation(s), and the opportunity to remedy any deficiencies. A clinical instructor who misrepresents a student's level of competence may be held legally accountable for directly related patient injury when that student enters professional practice.

Remember that federal and state statutory law and common law and customary practice require that clinical site personnel, as well as academicians, treat official information concerning health care professional students as confidential. Everyone who has official knowledge about students and their performance must understand the gravity of this responsibility and not disseminate confidential student information outside of the chain of those who have an official need to know, and the legal right to receive, the information.

SPECIAL INFORMED CONSENT CONSIDERATIONS WHEN STUDENTS ARE INVOLVED IN PATIENT CARE

The basic legal and ethical rule is that all health care professionals have the duty to make sufficient disclosure of treatment-related information to patients so as to enable them to make informed choices about care. Informed consent to treatment is premised on respect for the patient rights of autonomy and self-determination.

The disclosure elements for legally sufficient patient informed consent to evaluation and treatment when students are involved in patient care include the following:

- The type of treatment recommended or ordered
- Any material (decisional) risks of serious harm or complication associated with the proposed treatment
- The expected benefits of the proposed treatment, that is, patient goals
- Information about any reasonable alternatives to the proposed treatment, including their relative material risks and benefits
- The identification and role of a student or students in the patient's examination and treatment

In addition to the foregoing disclosure elements, the health care professional clinician must solicit and satisfactorily answer all patient questions about the treatment process. Clinical instructors should remember that it is their personal legal responsibility—not the student's—to obtain patient informed consent to treatment. (Similarly, this professional responsibility cannot legally be delegated to assistants, aides, or others.)

STUDENT RESPONSIBILITY

A student is always personally legally responsible for his or her own negligence or wrongdoing in the clinic. A student may be singularly responsible for patient injury when the student fails to comply with clear and reasonable instructions given by his or her clinical instructor. A student also may be held singularly liable when the student engages in reckless or malicious injurious conduct.

Just as with licensed health care professionals, students may be (and have been) charged with committing, against patients, intentional liability-generating misconduct. For example, a student may commit or be accused of battery (inappropriate or offensive touching of a patient), defamation (false assertions about a patient that harm the patient's good personal reputation), invasion of patient privacy, breach of patient confidentiality, or sexual harassment and misconduct.

LIABILITY RISK MANAGEMENT STRATEGIES FOR CLINICAL INSTRUCTORS AND AFFILIATION SITES

The following clinical risk management strategies represent a basic framework of ideas to which other strategies and practices may be added to form a comprehensive clinical risk management program.

Center coordinators of clinical education should consider implementing a policy that requires student affiliates to wear name badges that clearly identify them as health care professional students. Similarly, student-generated evaluation and treatment notation should bear, after the student's name, an identifier showing that the provider is a student.

Clinical site managers should also have a policy in place that assigns only seasoned clinicians as CCCEs and clinical instructors. Information about the selection process and copies of documentation concerning specific selection of CCCE and clinical instructor personnel should be generated and retained as legal documents.

Upon their arrival to the clinic, CCCEs and/or clinical instructors should thoroughly orient all students to the physical facility and its written policies, protocols, treatment guidelines, and other standardized operating procedures before students are asked to commence even supervised patient evaluation and treatment. Similarly, students should be thoroughly oriented to clinic equipment and supplies that they may use in their patient care duties during their affiliations. The student orientation process itself should be documented in a procedures manual, and CCCEs should consider having students sign off that they have read and understand all applicable clinic policies and procedures and are familiar with clinic equipment.

Taking these minimally burdensome steps is not practicing defensive health care clinical education. These measures are established for the protection of all participants in the health care professional student clinical education process—students, clinical site, CCCE, clinical instructor, and most importantly, patients.

SUMMARY

As with professional health care clinical practice, the academic and clinical components of health care professional student education are governed by legal and ethical rules of conduct with which academicians and clinical faculty and managers are bound to comply. This chapter summarizes important federal statutes, case law, and risk management strategies for minimizing liability exposure in academic and clinical education settings.

Governmental influence over public education (at all levels) resides primarily with state governments, but with strong federal influence. Significant federal educational statutes have been enacted in recent decades. The Civil Rights Act of 1964, Title VI, mandates nondiscrimination based on race or national origin in educational programs and activities that received federal funds. Title IX of the 1972 Educational Amendments added gender nondiscrimination to existing protections. The IDEA, 2004 amendment, is the most recent version of the Education for All Handicapped Children Act of 1975, which established as national policy that students with disabilities are entitled to free, mainstreamed (whenever possible) public education. The ADA further codified the rights of the disabled in educational and all other public and private settings.

The Family Educational Rights and Privacy Act of 1974,[8] popularly known as the Buckley Amendment, established uniform standards for educational institutions concerning the privacy and maintenance of official student records. The Equal Access Act of 1984 made public educational institutions into limited public fora for purposes of access to its facilities by religious, political, and other extracurricular special interest groups.

In addition to federal statutes, federal constitutional protections apply to governmental actions in educational settings. These rights include the right to due process of law (fairness, notice and opportunity to be heard), equal protection under the law, and the right to privacy.

Regarding academic discipline, educators and administrators must take reasonable steps to ensure that their reasonable disciplinary processes are disseminated to all those who potentially might be adversely affected by them and in particular must abide by their own rules and policies when disciplining students. Before adverse administrative action against a student may be taken in public educational institutions, the student is entitled to due notice of an infraction and the opportunity to state his or her side of the case.

Responsibility for health care professional student liability-generating conduct in clinical settings is normally preestablished in clinical affiliation agreements or contracts. Students are always personally legally responsible for their own conduct. In addition to vicarious, or indirect, liability, academic faculty and institutions may be primarily liable for failing adequately to prepare students for clinical experiences. Clinical instructors and sites may incur primary liability for failing to supervise or for negligently supervising students placed in their facilities.

CASES AND QUESTIONS

1. Z, a clinical instructor at XYZ Community Hospital, conducts a cursory review of an evaluation note for a patient with a diagnosis of herniated lumbar disk lesion, L4-L5, written by X, a student physical therapist. X's proposed treatment plan includes the administration of Williams' flexion exercises, not the prone-lying extension exercises that were ordered by the referring neurosurgeon. Z countersigns X's note. The treatment is carried out, resulting in acute exacerbation of the patient's right lower limb radicular signs and symptoms. As a result of the worsening of the patient's condition, the neurosurgeon performs a laminectomy-diskectomy the next day. What are the liability issues in this scenario?

2. B, a senior nursing student, is on a clinical affiliation at ABC Med Center, Anytown, USA. On the last week of her affiliation (which has been stellar), she comes to her clinical preceptor C and confesses that she has the "hots" for him. How does C handle this "thing about Mary"?

3. D, an occupational therapy student on an internship at X-O Hospital, is not progressing well in the viewpoint of his clinical instructor. The clinical instructor shares her concerns about D's affective conduct with the academic coordinator of clinical education and indicates that she plans to fail the student for the affiliation, based primarily on his spotty attendance and poor attitude. The clinical instructor ends up passing D, without making any adverse comments on his evaluation sheet. The clinical instructor does, however, inform C's future employer, with whom D is contractually bound to work after graduation, of her concerns about this student's affect. What are the liability issues in this scenario?

SUGGESTED ANSWERS TO CASES AND QUESTIONS

1. Although X is personally legally responsible for his or her own negligence, Z also faces probable liability in this scenario. Z is primarily responsible for negligent supervision of X's evaluation and negligent failure to check the referral order for specific instructions. Once Z countersigned X's evaluation note, it became Z's note for legal purposes.

2. Over the past two decades during which I have presented this case, I have been surprised by the range of "reasonable" options exercised by decision makers. Along a continuum of reasonableness, sanctions can range from no action to an oral warning to reporting the matter to the academic institution to dismissing the student from the affiliation. When resolving this problem, consider the fact that the student has performed in a stellar manner; that she has not acted on her emotions; and that she, like many patients, is probably displaying transference of emotions. For a legal perspective on psychological transference and countertransference, see *Simmons v. United States*, 804 F.2d 1363 (9th Cir. 1986).

3. D's clinical instructor had the legal and ethical duty to report D's performance accurately during D's affiliation. The clinical instructor violated this duty. The clinical instructor, however, had no right to discuss D's alleged poor performance with D's prospective employer. This breach of confidentiality violates the federal Buckley Amendment and constitutes a common law invasion of privacy (public disclosure of private facts).

SUGGESTED READINGS

Adverse academic, disciplinary and licensing decisions, *Journal of College and University Law* 20(2):198-201, 1993.

Fein B: A review of the legal issues surrounding academic dismissal, *Journal of Physical Therapy Education* 15(1):64-68, 2001.

Garcia G: Ball of confusion: Title IX advocates brace for a new round of threats to the gender-equality law, *San Antonio Current* p 6, Aug 25-31, 2005.

Gordon DJ: The duties of a clinical instructor, *Clinical Management,* 9(5):39-41, 1989.

Gostin LO, Beyer HA: *Implementing the Americans with Disabilities Act: rights and responsibilities of all Americans,* Baltimore, 1993, Brooks.

Scott RW: CIs and liability, *PT Magazine* 3(2):30-31, 1995.

Smith HG: Introduction to legal risks associated with clinical education, *Journal of Physical Therapy Education* 8(2):67-70, 1994.

REFERENCES

1. The Elementary and Secondary Education Act of 1965, 20 United States Code Section 2701 et. seq.
2. US Department of Education: *Reauthorization of No Child Left Behind.* Retrieved May 9, 2007, from www.ed.gov.
3. NCLB watch, *American Teacher* p 10, May/June 2007.
4. The Civil Rights Act of 1964, Title VI, 42 United States Code Section 2000d-1.
5. Title IX of the Educational Amendments of 1972, 20 United States Code Sections 1681-1683.
6. The Civil Rights Restoration Act of 1987, 20 United States Code Section 1687.
7. *Oslund* v. *United States,* Civ. No. 4-88-323 (US District Court, District of Minnesota, Oct 23, 1989).
8. The Family Educational Rights and Privacy Act of 1974, 20 United States Code Section 1232g.
9. Title 5, United States Code, Section 552.
10. The Education for All Handicapped Children Act of 1975, 20 United States Code Section 1401.
11. The Individuals with Disabilities Education Act of 1990, 20 United States Code Sections 1400-1485.
12. The Vocational Rehabilitation Act of 1973, 29 United States Code Section 706(8), Section 504, which prohibits discrimination against qualified "handicapped" persons by federal executive agencies and by the approximately 50 percent of American businesses that contract with the federal government, reads in pertinent part, "'Qualified handicapped person' means ... with respect to ... elementary and secondary ... education services, a handicapped person (i) of an age during which nonhandicapped persons are provided such services, (ii) of any age during which it is mandatory under state law to provide such services to handicapped persons, or (iii) to whom a state is required to provide a free appropriate public education under Section 612 of the Education of the Handicapped Act. 34 Code of Federal Regulations Section 104.3(k)(2), 1988."
13. The Individuals with Disabilities Education Act of 1990, 20 United States Code, Section 1401(17).
14. Patterson K: What classroom teachers need to know about IDEA '97, *Kappa Delta Pi Record* pp 62-67, Winter 2000.

15. Gallegos EM, Noland CD: School reform, *TEPSA Journal* pp 6-14, Winter 2007.

16. The Equal Access Act of 1984, 20 United States Code Section 4071.

17. The Americans with Disabilities Act of 1990, 42 United States Code, Sections 12101-12213.

18. For example, the new subsection 7(8)(C)(i) reads: "For purposes of programs and activities providing educational services, local educational agencies may take disciplinary action pertaining to the use or possession of illegal drugs or alcohol against any handicapped student who currently is engaging in the illegal use of drugs or in the use of alcohol to the same extent that such disciplinary action is taken against nonhandicapped students. Furthermore, the due process procedures at 34 C.F.R. 104.36 shall not apply to such disciplinary actions."

19. RIT: National Technical Institute for the Deaf: *Nondiscrimination in higher education*. Retrieved May 9, 2007, from www.netac.rit.edu/publication/tipsheet/ADA.html.

20. It was only just over 50 years ago, in *Brown v. Board of Education of Topeka, Kansas,* 347 U.S. 483 (1954), that the U.S. Supreme Court ruled that separate-but-equal public schools constituted unconstitutionally illegal, intentional racial discrimination.

21. *Board of Curators of the University of Missouri v. Horowitz,* 435 U.S. 78 (1978).

22. Ibid. at 89-90.

23. Ibid. at 96, note 6.

24. *Regents of the University of Michigan v. Ewing,* 474 U.S. 214(1985).

25. *Tobias v. University of Texas,* 824 S.W. 2d 201 (Tex. App. Ft. Worth 1991).

26. The Civil Rights Act of 1964, Title VI, 42 United States Code Section 2000d-1.

NOTES

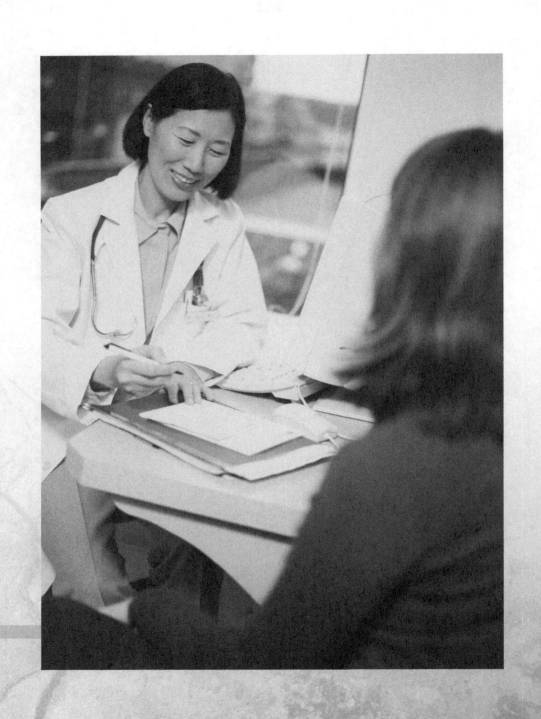

Ethics in Focus

INTRODUCTION

This chapter begins with an overview of patient informed consent to intervention. Life and death decision making is addressed next, followed by considerations of nondiscrimination against participants in health care delivery. The chapter next covers *pro bono* health care services, using attorney *pro bono* services as a model. Next, select professional practice issues are addressed, including financial responsibility, gifts, impaired providers, and professional relations. The chapter concludes with discussion of ethical issues in research.

PATIENT INFORMED CONSENT TO INTERVENTION

Patient informed consent to intervention is one of the most important mixed ethical and legal issues affecting health care professional clinical practice. Every health care clinician has the ethical duty and, in the overwhelming majority of cases, the legal duty to obtain patient or surrogate informed consent to health care interventions. This obligation is incumbent not only upon surgeons, anesthesiologists, and nurse anesthetists but also on all other primary health care professionals. Incidentally, the obligation to obtain patient informed consent applies irrespective of whether a non-physician health care professional evaluates and treats a patient with or without physician or other provider referral.

Ethical Duty to Obtain Patient Informed Consent

The ethical obligation universally to obtain patient or surrogate informed consent to health care evaluation and treatment is founded on the foundational ethical principle of autonomy.[1] Making relevant disclosure of information about evaluation and treatment and involving the patient in health care decision making evidences respect for patient autonomy and self-determination.

Every health care professional has an ethical and legal duty to obtain patient informed consent to evaluation and intervention.

All competent adult patients have the right to control the health care treatment decision-making process under the foundational ethical principle of autonomy.[2] Patients not considered legally competent to make such decisions—those who are legally adjudicated as incompetent, and minors, in some cases—have the right to have a surrogate decision maker or other legal representative receive the same disclosure information that would be imparted to a competent patient and to make decisions for them.

For many centuries the foundational ethical principle of respect for patient autonomy was not the preeminent guiding ethical principle governing health care delivery. Rather, physicians and other primary health care professionals conformed their conduct to another foundational ethical principle, beneficence, under which the health care professionals make and execute professional judgments that they believe to be in patients' best interests but do not routinely involve patients in decision making regarding interventions to be used.[3]

The history of the development of the law and ethics of patient informed consent demonstrates that, until recently, health care professionals practiced their professions largely without involving their patients in treatment-related decision making. Many explanations—some seemingly reasonable—have been proffered by medical and other health care professions to justify unilateral decision making regarding health care interventions. The ancient Greeks believed that to involve patients in medical decision making would impair patients' confidence in the ability of their health care providers to make professional judgments. By the Middle Ages, it was widely believed that the use of deception was necessary to ensure patient compliance with prescribed medical treatment that was deemed to be in the patient's best interests.[4] Modernly, there is legitimate concern among health care professionals that patients will not understand and will be confused by the myriad of complex pieces of information that must be imparted as part of informed consent disclosure. Finally, with streamlined managed heath care delivery, there is even a sense among some health care providers that routinely obtaining patient consent to treatment is just too time-consuming.

The customary health care professional practice of not including patients as partners in health care decision making began to change in the early and mid-1900s. Several phenomena accelerated the rise in importance of respect for patient autonomy in health care decision making. First, courts began to mandate that health care professionals respect patient autonomy and impart "legally sufficient" disclosure to permit patients to make knowing, intelligent, voluntary, and unequivocal elections of recommended treatment. The advent of this trend in judicial activism is exemplified by the 1914 New York case, *Schloendorf* v. *Society of New York Hospital*,[5] that expanded intentional tort liability in battery of health care providers who failed to respect the right of patients knowingly to consent to treatment. In 1965 in *Natanson* v. *Kline*,[6] the Kansas Supreme Court also ruled as follows:

> *The courts frequently state that the relationship between the physician and his patient is a fiduciary one, and therefore the physician has the obligation to make a full and frank disclosure to the patient of all pertinent facts related to his illness. We are here concerned with a case where the physician is charged with treating the patient without consent on the grounds that the patient was not fully informed of the nature of the treatment or its consequences, and therefore "consent" obtained was ineffective.*

In another leading informed consent case in 1972, *Canterbury* v. *Spence*,[7] Judge Spotswood Robinson III of the U.S. Court of Appeals for the District of Columbia further refined the nature of the ethical duty owed by health care professionals toward their patients. He stated,

> *The patient's reliance upon the physician is a trust of the kind which traditionally has exacted obligations beyond those associated with arms length transactions. [The patient's] dependence upon the physician for information affecting his well-being, in terms of contemplated treatment, is well-nigh abject.*

Other twentieth-century developments that furthered the recognition of patient autonomy over decision making and the need for patient informed consent in health care service delivery include the growth in postsecondary education after World War II and the concomitant rise of the consumerism movement in the United States and Canada and later in Western Europe. As consumers became more aware of their power over merchants in the retail industry, the age-old adage *caveat emptor* (Latin for "let the buyer beware") became whittled away as the public forcefully lobbied federal and state legislators for the enactment of consumer protection laws. As a result of consumer protection legislation, the doctrine of *caveat emptor* largely came to have little meaning in retail consumer business transactions. About the same time, it was realized that this doctrine was even less appropriately applied in the delivery of health care services to patients. Many health care professional association codes of ethics expressly recognize an ethical duty on the part of professional members to make sufficient disclosure of pertinent information to patients under their care to permit patients to make informed elections about treatment.

EXERCISE

Examine the ethics code of your discipline for express language requiring patient informed consent for health care service delivery. Compare the ethical standards of your discipline to the ethics codes of two other disciplines.

Legal Aspects of Patient Informed Consent to Treatment

Failure to Obtain Patient Informed Consent Is a Form of Health Care Malpractice

Failure on the part of health care professionals to make necessary disclosure of examination and treatment-related information so as to enable patients to make informed decisions about treatment options constitutes professional negligence—the most common variety of health care malpractice. Until recently, lack of informed consent tort cases in health care settings were treated as intentional tort actions and were processed through the civil legal system as battery cases.[8] The rationale for labeling lack of informed consent health care malpractice cases as battery cases was that physicians and other health care professionals charged with such malpractice actions were considered by law to have had harmful physical contact with their patients without such patients' consent. By 1965, when the *Natanson* v. *Kline* decision was announced, courts began to realize that there was a fundamental distinction between consent-related cases that involved intentional wrongs (i.e., based on a lack of authorization) and those that involved unintentional wrongs (i.e., based on a lack of understanding); the courts began correctly to classify lack of informed consent health care malpractice cases as professional negligence actions because patients treated without informed consent probably would have given at least nominal (albeit uninformed) consent to the treatment that led to injury.[9]

Certain consent-related actions still are properly brought as intentional battery cases. For example, when a surgeon operates on a patient and amputates the wrong limb or excises the wrong breast or testicle during a mastectomy or orchiectomy, respectively, or when a nurse administers the wrong medication to a patient, causing patient injury, the proper designation for the ensuing legal action is a "battery." This is so because the defendant–health care professional involved had absolutely no authorization from the injured patient to carry out inappropriate and harmful treatment.

The professional negligence designation for lack of informed consent health care malpractice cases takes into account the fact that patients injured in such cases probably gave nominal consent to treatment, but their health care providers failed to conform to acceptable practice standards by neglecting to respect patient autonomy by involving the patients in treatment-related decision making. Therefore, failure to obtain patient informed consent to treatment equates to substandard care—the essence of health care professional negligence.

Failure to obtain patient informed consent to treatment equates to substandard care.

Legal Recognition of the Obligation to Obtain Patient Informed Consent

The courts have ruled on at least two occasions that informed consent in the health care setting is a concept reserved exclusively for surgical and operative procedures—not for routine health care delivery.[10,11] In *Spence* v. *Todaro,*[10] the U.S. District Court for the Eastern District of Pennsylvania, interpreting Pennsylvania state law, specifically held that the doctrine of informed consent to treatment does not apply to postoperative physical therapy rehabilitation. This case concerned a postoperative orthopedic patient who was referred to physical therapy for rotator cuff rehabilitation. The patient claimed injury incident to physical therapy and sued the physical therapist for malpractice, citing a lack of informed consent as the basis for his lawsuit. The federal court held that, under Pennsylvania statutory law, the doctrine of patient informed consent to treatment applies only to surgical interventions—not to routine (nonsurgical) health care delivery. The court went on to reject the plaintiff-patient's contention that, because his physical therapy followed directly from his rotator cuff repair, it was legally part of the surgery, thereby making his lack of informed consent a valid issue for judicial review.

In all other health care legal cases, however, the doctrine of patient informed consent to treatment has been found applicable, expressly or by implication, to nonsurgical cases and to nonphysician primary health care providers. For example, in *Flores* v. *Center for Spinal Evaluation,*[12] a physical and occupational therapy malpractice case involving an allegation of professional negligence incident to postinjury rehabilitation, the court held in dismissing the case that, despite limited legal precedent on physical and occupational therapy malpractice, these health care professionals (and by analogy, other rehabilitation professionals) should be treated exactly like their physician colleagues when they are health care malpractice defendants.

Recent U.S. Supreme Court case decisions interpreting the Constitution have reflected the deference of the court to and respect for patient self-determination regarding important health care decision making. For example, U.S. Supreme Court case decisions (and those of state supreme and appellate courts) based on the fundamental right of privacy have favored patients in their decisions to compel removal of life support apparatus[13] and even the withdrawal of nutrition and hydration.[14,15]

In many states, legislatures have enacted statutes that mandate the specific informed consent disclosure required for surgical procedures and anesthesia administration as a matter of law. In these states, compliance with statutory disclosure, coupled with the signature of a patient on a statutory form, creates a rebuttable presumption that the patient gave informed consent to care. The burden of persuasion to dispute or rebut that presumption in litigation then shifts to the patient.

The Patient Self-Determination Act[16] (discussed in Chapter 6) codifies the rights of hospitalized inpatients and long-term care residents to participate in treatment decision making and to control the use of extraordinary treatment measures, such as artificial life support. The Patient Self-Determination Act, although not creating any new substantive legal requirements for health care organizations or rights for patients, binds all health care facilities that receive Medicare or Medicaid funding to inform patients about their existing substantive rights under state law and to respect legitimate patients' advance directives concerning treatment. Regarding informed consent, the law provides in pertinent part[17] the following:

> *[A] provider [must] maintain written policies and procedures with respect to all adult individuals receiving medical care ... to provide written information to each such individual concerning an individual's rights under state law (whether statutory or as recognized by the courts of the state) to make decisions concerning ... medical care, including the right to accept or refuse medical or surgical treatment.*

Another source of legal obligation to obtain patient informed consent is the patient bill of rights and responsibilities, a document customarily posted in patient treatment areas in health care facilities across the United States. The patient bill of rights and responsibilities for Brooke Army Medical Center, San Antonio, Texas,[18] states in pertinent part the following:

> *You have the right to freedom of expression, to make your own decisions, and to know that your human rights will be preserved and respected. We will make sure that you know which physician or care provider is primarily responsible for you care. We will explain the professional status and the role of persons who help in your care. We will keep you fully informed about your condition, the results of tests we perform, and the treatment you receive. We will clearly explain to you any treatments or procedures that we propose. We will request your written consent for procedures that carry more than minimal risk. We will make sure that you are part of the decision-making process in your care. When there are dilemmas or differences over care decisions, we will include you in resolving them. We will honor your right to refuse the care that we advise. We will honor your Advance Directive or Medical Power of Attorney, regarding limits to the care that you wish to receive.*

The Joint Commission, like other private accreditation entities, imposes similar requirements on its member health care organizations. Specifically, the Joint Commission standards require appropriate evidence in patient health records of informed consent to treatment, as well as institutional policy statements on patient informed consent.[19]

Finally, health care organizations and networks can create legally binding standards regarding patient informed consent in their organizational procedures manuals, protocols, and clinical practice guidelines, over and above those otherwise required by law. Administrators and clinical managers are urged to review these documents to ensure that what is written therein reflects desired practice standards for the organization.

When Is Lack of Patient Informed Consent Legally Actionable?

Even though every single unexcused and unjustified omission of patient informed consent is an example of professional negligence, only a limited number of instances are legally actionable. Professional negligence malpractice litigation premised on a lack of informed consent is legally actionable only in the following cases:

- An undisclosed risk materializes, resulting in patient injury; and
- The plaintiff-patient can establish (i.e., prove) that he or she would not have consented to the treatment intervention in issue had full disclosure been made

The court in *Canterbury*[20] clearly spells out the requirement for a causal connection between the negligent omission on the part of a health care clinician to make legally sufficient disclosure to a patient and resultant patient injury:

> *No more than breach of any other legal duty does nonfulfillment of the physician's obligation to disclose alone establish liability to the patient. An unrevealed risk that should have been made known must materialize, for otherwise the omission, however unpardonable, is legally without consequence.* Occurrence of the risk must be harmful to the patient, for unrelated injury *is nonactionable [emphasis added]. And, as in malpractice actions generally, there must be a causal relationship between the physician's failure to adequately divulge (information) and damage to the patient.*
>
> A causal connection exists when, but only when, disclosure of significant risks incidental to treatment would have resulted in a decision against it *[emphasis added]. The patient obviously has no complaint if he would have submitted to the therapy notwithstanding awareness that the risk was one of its perils. On the other hand, the very purpose of the disclosure rule is to protect the patient against the consequences which, if known, he would have avoided by foregoing the treatment.*

Litigation over informed consent to treatment should never occur if primary health care professionals remember that disclosure of treatment-related information is a requisite element of the provider-patient communication process. The disclosure elements (discussed subsequently) are relatively straightforward, and the process, if made a routine part of provider-patient communications, is neither unduly burdensome nor time-consuming.

> Disclosure of information to patients is relatively straightforward, and the process, if made a routine part of provider-patient communications, is neither unduly burdensome nor time-consuming.

Obviously, open and thorough communication between health care providers and patients is key to minimizing health care malpractice liability exposure. The word *consent* literally means that the provider and patient jointly should agree on a recommended treatment intervention before it is implemented.[21] Decades of medical research have shown that patients achieve optimal intervention outcomes when they are informed partners in their own care.[22]

One confounding factor to the health care provider-patient communication process is the fact that some patients may wish not to participate in the treatment decision-making process with their providers. Rather, some patients—even though they have full mental capacity—prefer to leave treatment decision making to family members or trusted others. Regarding revelation of terminal illnesses, this impediment to provider-patient communications may be race- or ethnicity-related. One study revealed that, whereas black and white geriatric patients generally believe that it is appropriate for providers to discuss terminal illnesses with their patients, those of Korean descent and Hispanics often do not.[23] In complicated fact scenarios like those presented in this exemplar, health care clinicians are strongly encouraged to consult with facility and/or personal legal advisors for advice on how to proceed and to document their actions carefully.

Hoffman[24] reported that patients face a "superabundance" of medical information to sort through in making care-related decisions and that many patients do not want to make difficult treatment decisions on their own. Hoffman also cited a 2005 New York Times–CBS poll that revealed the following:

- Physicians only reveal to patients their diagnoses in 38% of cases.
- Physicians offer their patients only one treatment option 55% of the time.
- Physicians do help patients make medical decisions 65% of the time.

Disclosure Elements for Legally Sufficient Disclosure of Information to Patients

Although legal requirements differ from state to state for what constitutes legally sufficient information disclosure in the provider-patient informed consent communication process, the following elements are commonly included in most or all states. For specific advice on what information must be imparted to patients under specific state laws, consult with legal counsel.

For patient consent to treatment to be legally "informed," the following items of disclosure information should be addressed:

Diagnosis and Pertinent Evaluative Findings. Health care clinicians should always discuss with patients the patients' diagnoses and pertinent evaluative findings (unless the patient effectively waives disclosure or another exception applies). Although it may be particularly difficult for health care professionals to avoid the use of health care professional jargon in communications because of their training, communication with other providers, and continuing education, they must remember to speak to patients using layperson's language, in a language understandable by the patient, and at the level of understanding appropriate for the patient.

Nature of the Treatment Intervention Recommended. After patient evaluation is completed and a diagnosis is made, a clinician formulates a proposed intervention plan designed to optimize function or achieve some other therapeutic result. This recommended intervention must be disclosed to the patient before its implementation, and the patient must agree to it. If specific treatment has been prescribed by a physician or other provider legally privileged to make referrals, then the prescribed treatment must likewise be described to the patient. In either case the patient must consent to treatment.

Recommended treatment intervention must be described to the patient before its implementation, and the patient must agree to the treatment.

Material (Decisional) Risks of Serious Harm or Complications. Any credible risk of possible serious harm or complication associated with a proposed treatment intervention must be disclosed to a patient before treatment commences. The term *material* refers to a risk of harm that would cause an ordinary reasonable patient to think seriously about whether he or she would accept or reject a proposed treatment intervention. (In some cases the term *material* has been construed by courts to mean the risk of harm that a particular patient would subjectively consider to be serious, even if that particular patient is not an ordinary reasonable person.) For every health discipline, a number of material risks must be disclosed to patients.

One nonobvious material risk associated with physical therapy involves axillary crutch gait instruction. Unless a physical therapist warns a patient about the material risk of possible axillary nerve and vessel injury associated with leaning on the soft axillary pads on the top portions of the crutches, a patient might reasonably believe that the soft pads are designed to be leaned upon. By disclosing this potential risk, a physical therapist may prevent patient injury and malpractice litigation. A material risk of harm that must be disclosed by prosthetists providing artificial limbs to clients is the risk of harm associated with skin breakdown around a prosthesis. A patient must be informed by his or her prosthetist that the signs and symptoms of pain, redness, and skin breakdown in the vicinity of a prosthesis are not normal and may result in serious adverse consequences and must immediately be made known by the patient to his or her providers.

The law generally recognizes that the only material risks that need to be disclosed to patients are those that are nonobvious to ordinary reasonable persons. Obvious risks, such as the risk of being cut by a sharp needle or of being burned by an extremely hot thermal treatment modality, are generally understood by adult lay patients and are not required to be discussed. However, patients may not fully comprehend the gravity of the risk of harm associated with seemingly obvious risk scenarios. Consider the following hypothetical example:

> A 68-year-old male patient with a medical diagnosis of diabetes mellitus and a left lateral malleolar diabetic ulcer on his ankle is referred to physical therapy for "evaluation and hydrotherapy, as appropriate." After evaluation and initial treatment, the physical therapist advises the patient to soak his left foot in very warm water at home for 20 minutes, twice a day. The patient asks, "How warm should the water be?" The therapist replies, "As warm as you can tolerate on the unaffected part of your left foot." Unfortunately, the physical therapist had neglected to evaluate the patient's whole foot, which was severely desensitized as a result of peripheral neuropathy. The next day, the patient returns to the clinic with third-degree thermal burns to his left foot. The patient had boiled water, poured it into a basin, and placed his left foot into the scalding water, resulting in serious injury. The patient's left foot was amputated several weeks later.

Out of concern for patient welfare and as a matter of prudent risk management, the health care provider should always discuss even seemingly obvious risks of serious harm or complications of treatment with patients to prevent needless patient injury and liability exposure. If patients understand the treatment goals established on their behalf and take an "ownership" interest in the treatment goals, they will be more motivated to achieve better functional outcomes.

Expected Benefits of Treatment. It is incumbent upon health care clinicians to establish functionally relevant, measurable, short- and long-term treatment goals for patients under their care. As an integral part of the informed consent process, health care clinicians must also reveal and discuss with patients the goals established for them. If patients understand the treatment goals established on their behalf and take an "ownership" interest in the treatment goals, they will be more motivated to achieve better functional outcomes.

Reasonable Alternatives to the Proposed Intervention. If there are reasonable alternatives to a proposed treatment or intervention, these must be disclosed to and discussed with the patient. In addition to describing reasonable alternatives to proposed treatments, clinicians must also discuss with patients the attendant material risks (if any) and expected benefits of such reasonable alternatives. This disclosure element may pose a problem under managed care, in that alternative treatments or interventions, even if more efficacious than a recommended treatment, may not be available or funded under the patient's health insurance plan. This fact does not, however, obviate the need for discussion of all reasonable alternative treatments or interventions.

After disclosing all informed consent parameters to a patient—diagnostic and evaluative findings, nature of recommended treatment, material risks, expected benefits, and reasonable alternatives (Box 8-1)—a health care clinician is obliged to take one further step. The provider must ensure that the patient understands all the information conveyed by asking for and by satisfactorily answering patient questions related to treatment. If the patient's primary language is one other than English, the provider must provide translation, as needed, to ensure that the patient understands all information conveyed.

Occasionally, a patient refuses treatment recommended by a health care provider or ordered by a physician or other referring entity, even after informed consent disclosure has been made. Certain additional steps must be taken by a health care provider whenever a patient refuses care. The clinician must first ensure that the patient understands the disclosure information conveyed and must solicit further questions or comments about the proposed treatment or intervention that the patient may have to offer. If this reiteration and summarization of the informed consent process does not resolve the problem, the clinician should explain, in an empathetic and objective manner, the expected consequences of refusal of treatment or intervention to the patient's health status, as applicable. Discussion with the patient should be interactive and participative rather than directive, and the clinician should display sincere concern for the patient's best health interests (beneficence) and respect for patient autonomy over decision making.

If the patient persists in his or her refusal to allow recommended treatment, this fact and a summarization of the "informed refusal" prevention measures used on the patient's behalf should be well documented in the patient's health record. In addition, the clinician is legally and ethically responsible to coordinate expeditiously with the referring entity, if any, and other key health care professionals having a need to know about the patient's refusal of care.

BOX **8-1** ▪ **Informed Consent to Treatment**

Disclosure of relevant treatment-related information includes the following:
- Patient diagnosis or evaluative findings
- Nature of treatment or intervention recommended or ordered
- Material (decisional) risks of serious harm or complication associated with the proposed treatment or intervention
- Expected benefits or goals associated with the proposed treatment or intervention
- Reasonable alternatives, if any, to the proposed treatment or intervention

If a patient refuses treatment, this fact and a summarization of the "informed refusal" prevention measures used on the patient's behalf should be well documented. The clinician is legally and ethically responsible to coordinate with any referring health care professional about the patient's refusal of care.

Even after a patient agrees to accept a recommended medical intervention, noncompliance may ensue. According to Brody,[25] the reasons for nonadherence to medical prescriptions are many and complex. The most common reasons for patient noncompliance are poor communication by health care providers and forgetfulness on the part of patients. The remedies to minimize the occurrence of noncompliance, then, are as follows: better communication with patients during informed consent disclosure and care processes; the issuance of clear, written instructions; and follow-on consultation with patients about their progress.

Health care clinical professionals and managers need to develop innovative ways to improve patient understanding about their practices and procedures. Rogers[26] reported on an innovative, interactive patient waiting room at the Jay Monahan Center for Gastrointestinal Health in Manhattan, New York City. According to the director, Dr. Mark Pochapin, the process of waiting for care by patients should be active, not passive. The waiting room has two walls of video screens playing patient education videos. An outreach director circulates among patients to answer general questions. (Caution, though. Remember the Health Insurance Portability and Accountability Act and the Privacy Rule, Chapter 6!) Similarly, Hutson and Blaha[27] use video questionnaires to assess patients' understanding of what is communicated to them by providers about their procedures after informed consent disclosure.

Brody[28] offered several important tips for better patient communication for primary health care professionals. Of key importance is to gauge patients' baseline understanding before delving into complex medical terminology. Her article offers a Health Literacy Test that patients can take as a self-assessment in the waiting room before seeing their providers.

Patients, too, bear responsibility for their own care and well-being. Patients should bring a copy of their medication list to medical appointments for primary health care providers to review and should alert their providers to any allergies they have.[29] According to Franklin,[30] patients might also consider creating a comprehensive medical problem list for their primary providers and tell providers which problems have the highest priority for them. Patients should consider conducting preliminary research about their medical problems on the Internet before medical visits, recognizing that, even though they might have access to similar medical information as their health care providers, they probably lack the expertise to evaluate it fully. Finally, reticent patients should consider bringing a trusted friend or family member with them to medical appointments so that important questions about their care are asked and answered.

Legal Standards for Adequacy of Informed Consent

Two possible legal standards are used to determine whether a health care professional made sufficient disclosure of treatment-related information in order to permit a patient to make an informed decision about care. The states are nearly equally divided in their use of each available standard; however, a slight majority of jurisdictions use a **professional standard** for disclosure.[31] In states using this legal disclosure standard, a health care professional is required to impart to a patient only that information that another health care professional from the same discipline, who would be acting under the same or similar circumstances, would see fit to disclose. Health care malpractice litigation involving informed consent issues in states using the professional standard requires the introduction of expert testimony concerning (1) the propriety of the disclosure information actually conveyed by a defendant–health care provider to a plaintiff-patient and (2) the expert's professional opinion about what information is generally appropriate for disclosure to patients under the same or similar circumstances.

A number of states use a **layperson's standard** for disclosure. In these jurisdictions a health care professional is required to disclose all relevant information that an ordinary reasonable patient, acting under the same or similar circumstances as the patient in issue, would consider material to make an informed decision about treatment. Obviously, the lay standard imposes greater responsibility on health care providers, who must carefully contemplate what information an ordinary reasonable lay patient would deem to be material for every possible treatment or intervention.

The court in *Canterbury* enunciated in a reasoned manner the rationale for and the parameters of the ordinary reasonable layperson's standard for the first time as follows:

> We do not agree that the patient's cause of action is dependent upon the existence and nonperformance of a relevant professional tradition. There are, in our view, formidable obstacles to acceptance of the notion that [a health care professional's] obligation to disclose is either germinated or limited by medical practice. To begin with, the reality of any discernible custom reflecting a professional consensus on communication of option and risk information to patients is open to serious doubt. We sense the danger that what in fact is no custom at all may be taken as an affirmative custom to maintain silence, and that [health professional-witnesses] to the so-called custom may state merely their personal opinions as to what they or others would do under given conditions.
>
> The decision to unveil the patient's condition and the chances for as to remediation is ofttimes a non-medical judgment and, if so, is a decision outside the ambit of the special standard. Prevailing medical practice does not define the standard. In our view, the patient's right of self-decision shapes the boundaries of the duty to reveal. That right can be effectively exercised only if the patient possesses enough information to enable an intelligent choice. The scope of the [provider's] communication to the patient, then, must be measured by the patient's need, and that need is the information material [emphasis added] to the decision. Thus the test for determining whether a particular peril must be divulged is its materiality to the [ordinary reasonable] patient's decision: all risks potentially affecting the decision must be unmasked.

One advantage to both parties to an informed consent–based health care malpractice lawsuit of the application by the court of the layperson standard for assessing disclosure is that, under most circumstances, expert testimony about health care professional discipline-specific disclosure standards is not required, for lay jurors are responsible to decide what information an ordinary reasonable patient would need to hear in order to make an informed decision about accepting or rejecting treatment. This fact saves money at trial that otherwise would be paid to expert witnesses, which benefits both parties to the lawsuit. Additionally, when expert witnesses are not used in a case, substantial time is usually saved in litigating the material issues in the case.

Exceptions to the Requirement to Obtain Patient Informed Consent

Several well-established exceptions exist to the requirement otherwise universally to obtain patient informed consent before carrying out health care treatment interventions. The two most important ones are the **emergency doctrine** and **therapeutic privilege**.[32]

Under the emergency doctrine, whenever a patient seeks evaluation and treatment in a life-threatening emergency situation and is unable to communicate his or her wishes regarding treatment (such as when the patient is unconscious), it is generally presumed that the patient would consent to reasonable, lifesaving medical intervention. Consider the following hypothetical case scenario:

> *A student nurse on a clinical rotation is evaluating a 65-year-old male rehabilitation patient, who is recovering from a left cerebrovascular accident. Suddenly, the patient suffers a myocardial infarction and grasps his chest. The patient is initially unable to speak because of pain and shortness of breath; he then becomes unconscious. What action should the student take? (At the time of the incident, there is no one, including the student's supervisory clinical preceptor, in the clinic area.)*

This scenario presents an example of a situation in which the emergency doctrine exception to the law of patient informed consent is applicable. In such a situation, it is generally presumed, as a matter of law, that an ordinary reasonable person would wish to avail himself or herself of lifesaving treatment intervention. Absent clear evidence of contrary patient desires, the student should immediately commence cardiopulmonary resuscitation and activate the emergency medical response system.

Of course, there are exceptions to the exception of a presumption favoring rendition of care in life-threatening emergencies. For example, if a patient's desire not to receive lifesaving care in the event of an emergency has been memorialized in a valid patient advance directive (discussed in Chapter 6), health care professionals and supportive personnel are obligated to respect the patient's autonomy and not initiate lifesaving treatment. A similar exception applies when a valid "do not resuscitate" order (discussed later in this chapter) appears in a patient's medical record.

> If a patient's desire not to receive lifesaving care in the event of an emergency has been memorialized in a valid patient advance directive, health care professionals and supportive personnel are obligated to respect the patient's autonomy and not initiate lifesaving treatment.

Therapeutic privilege is rarely invoked and even less often sanctioned by the courts as legally acceptable because the exercise of the privilege derogates from the foundational biomedical ethical principle of respect for patient autonomy and self-determination.

What course of action can a nonphysician health care professional team member treating a patient take when he or she disagrees with a physician's invocation of therapeutic privilege? Consider the following hypothetical case example:

An occupational therapist treating a 32-year-old female patient (who is diagnosed with terminal, end-stage metastatic breast cancer) meets with the other rehabilitation team members for a weekly team conference. At the meeting the patient's attending physician advises the team members that he is discharging the patient to home to allow her to die in peace with her family. The attending physician tells the team treating the patient that he is invoking therapeutic privilege concerning the patient's prognosis. (The patient already knows her diagnosis.) The occupational therapist knows, from her recent conversations with the patient, that the patient wishes to know about her prognosis and apprises the rest of the team of this fact. The physician becomes angry and reminds the occupational therapist that he is the patient's physician and the leader of the rehabilitation team. The physician ends the discussion by imposing a "gag order" on the entire treatment team, ordering all of them to remain silent if asked by the patient about her prognosis.

Is this the end of the matter? Not necessarily. In this case the occupational therapist is unable to abide by the physician's decision as a matter of personal ethics. What can she do? Several acceptable options are open to the occupational therapist. First, the occupational therapist should consider requesting a private meeting with the physician to express her concerns about the gag order. Assume that she does this and poignantly states her position. Assume further that her resistance to his edict enrages the physician, who summarily ejects the occupational therapist from his office stating, "Just do what I ordered!"

At this point, there are three options open to the occupational therapist. She may resign herself to acceptance of the physician's order. However, in this case the patient, who has become accustomed to confiding in the occupational therapist, begins to pressure her for information about her prognosis. Additionally, the occupational therapist's personal code of ethics does not allow her to be untruthful to the patient.

The occupational therapist, at this point, may be justified in removing herself from the patient's treatment team—because she cannot abide by the physician's order—and allowing another occupational therapist who can accept the "gag order" to continue to care for the patient. However, in this case, the occupational therapist believes that this option is unethical and therefore an unacceptable "cop-out."

> Therapeutic privilege is rarely invoked and even less often sanctioned by the courts as legally acceptable because the privilege derogates from the foundational biomedical ethical principle of respect for patient autonomy and self-determination.

The last available option to the occupational therapist is perhaps the best one, after exercising all reasonable efforts to discuss the situation civilly with the physician. This option is formally to request an ethics consultation from the **institutional ethics committee** in the facility. The institutional ethics committee is a multidisciplinary committee of health care professionals and other related professionals that offers consultative services and convenes to hear and make recommendations about cases involving ethical dilemmas. Any health care organization should always have in place a mechanism for licensed and certified health care professionals and others to avail themselves of the advice and intervention of the institutional ethics committee. No stigma should ever be associated with requesting consultation from the institutional ethics committee. Similarly, the fact that the occupational therapist acted reasonably in requesting an ethics consultation should not cause her to suffer retribution from the physician whose judgment is challenged. It may be necessary for facility administrators to educate physicians and other health care professionals about the role(s) of the institutional ethics committee regularly so that misunderstandings and anger over its intervention do not occur.

Two other scenarios (involving the treatment of incompetent or minor patients) may seem to be possible exceptions to the requirement to obtain patient informed consent to treatment; however, such is not the case. When a patient lacks legal capacity to consent to treatment—because the patient cannot understand information conveyed and is legally adjudicated as incapacitated or because the patient is a minor and cannot consent to a particular intervention as a matter of law—a health care professional must obtain informed consent from a **surrogate decision maker** (or substitute).

The disclosure of information made to a surrogate decision maker is exactly the same as would be made to a competent patient. The surrogate decision maker, appointed by the patient or by law, acts on the patient's behalf and has the same right to have key information disclosed and to have questions answered to the surrogate's satisfaction before treatment commences.

One exception to the general rule that parents or guardians normally consent on behalf of their minor children is that minors, especially when they are nearing the age of majority (age 18), may have the right under applicable state law to exercise autonomy personally to consent (usually without revelation to their parents) to treatment in cases involving elective abortion, treatment of drug (including alcohol) abuse, and the treatment of sexually transmitted diseases. These exceptions to the general rule of substituted consent for minors vary from state to state, and providers must consult proactively with legal counsel to remain current on the state of the law so as to protect the rights of all parties.

Another difficult dilemma involving incapacitated patients centers around informed consent involving patients who, practically but not legally, lack the mental capacity to make knowing, intelligent, voluntary, and unequivocal decisions about their care. Although the determination of patient capacity to make decisions about health care interventions is a question for physicians and jurists, other health care professionals involved in the care of particular patients can offer important input into competency determinations based on their observations and interactions with patients.

Little guidance is available in the health care professional literature for physicians and other health care professionals on mental capacity assessment. An excellent article that presents a framework for patient competency assessment (including dimensions of competence and a series of questions to assess mental capacity) is "Assessing Patient Competence for Medical Decision Making."[33] Another by Spremulli[34] offers a screening assessment for capacity developed by the author.

In cases of questionable patient competency to make treatment-related decisions, health care professionals are urged to raise the issue expeditiously with physicians, facility administrators, legal counsel, and institutional ethics committees so that a competency determination can be undertaken, if appropriate. When a question of patient competency exists, a competency assessment is required to comply with legal require-ments concerning consent to care and to meet foundational ethical standards, includ-ing respect for patient autonomy and dignity, beneficence, and nonmaleficence.

Patient Informed Consent in an Era of Managed Care

The managed care model of health care delivery has spawned at least two informed consent–related ethical dilemmas for health care professionals. First, compliance by pro-viders with "gag clauses" in health care professional employment contracts with man-aged care organizations may result in situations in which clinicians do not make full disclosure of treatment-related information to patients. Second, nondisclosure by health care professionals to patients of financial incentives paid to them for providing less care to patients fails to respect patient autonomy over treatment-related decision making.

Gag clauses are provisions in health care professional–managed care organization employment contracts that obstruct a provider's ability to make full disclosure to patients of treatment-related information.[35] When a health care professional chooses to comply with a managed care gag clause provision and thereby places his or her own employment interests above patient welfare considerations, nondisclosure of key treatment-related information during informed consent processes may result. In particular, compliance by health care professionals with managed care gag clauses may prevent patients from receiv-ing information about reasonable alternatives to proposed interventions not funded by patients' insurance plans. Managed care plans have severely limited their use of gag clauses in employment contracts with primary health care providers because of public pressure,[36] legislative initiatives,[37] and professional association action.[38]

Failure on the part of health care professionals to disclose to a patient any provider contractual financial incentives tied to providing less care evidences a lack of respect for patient autonomy. Patients have the right to receive all pertinent disclosure infor-mation related to their care. Is there any person who would not want to know that his or her health care provider is paid, in whole or in part, for saving money for the provider's employer by providing less care to the patient? The same kind of pressure by the general public, the press, professional associations, and legislatures is urgently needed to provide definitive guidance in this area.

> Compliance by providers with gag clauses in health care professional employment contracts with managed care organizations and failure by providers to disclose actual and potential conflicts of interest to patients may result in situations in which clinicians do not make full disclosure of treatment-related information to their patients.

LIFE AND DEATH DECISION MAKING

Health care professionals work intensively with patients who are at or may be near the end of their lives. Twenty-seven percent of Medicare expenditures occur in the last 6 months of patients' lives.[39]

As patient care team members, primary and support health care professionals ac-tively participate in conferences in which life and death issues involving their patients are addressed. All health care professional codes of ethics address professional responsibilities related to patient life and death decision making, at least indirectly, through provisions requiring professionals to respect patient autonomy, maintain patient confidentiality, and act in patients' best interests while providing care services, among numerous other issues.

Life and death decisions are largely made by patients (or their surrogate decision makers) and their primary physicians and surgeons. Other health care professionals have the opportunity to offer unique insight about patients under their care to surrogate and physician decision makers, as members of institutional ethics committees, as primary and supportive team members, and in other important capacities.

Euthanasia

The Greek word *euthanasia* signifies "good" or "easy death." No area of health care professional service delivery has generated greater confusion, controversy, or judicial oversight than the area of euthanasia. Euthanasia seemingly involves conflicts among, and inconsistent compliance on the part of health care providers with, the four biomedical ethical principles of autonomy, beneficence, nonmaleficence, and justice. Is any form of euthanasia ethically, legally, and/or morally acceptable?

Euthanasia issues most often center around patients who are terminally ill or in a persistent vegetative state. A terminally ill patient is one with an incurable disease that is expected to result in the patient's death.[40] A patient who is in a persistent vegetative state is one who may exhibit "motor reflexes, but evinces no indication of significant cognitive function."[41] Classifying a patient as terminally ill or in a persistent vegetative state not only has medical significance but also has legal, ethical, economic, and sociocultural implications.[42]

Processes such as the withdrawal or withholding of ordinary or extraordinary life-sustaining support devices or measures or of sustenance represent means of passive euthanasia. Active euthanasia, however, involves deliberate intervention by health care providers or others that facilitate or cause patients' death in order to relieve patient pain and suffering.[43] Although the U.S. Supreme Court in essence legitimized passive euthanasia in its 1990 *Cruzan*[44] decision, neither the states (with one exception) nor the federal government have sanctioned active euthanasia as legally and ethically acceptable medical practice.

On November 8, 1994, the voters in Oregon passed the Oregon Death with Dignity Act (ODDA), the nation's first physician-assisted suicide law. ODDA authorizes physicians to write prescriptions for competent, terminally ill adult patients who are expected to die within 6 months, when such patients meet statutory requirements, including the making of three separate requests for suicide, obtaining a second medical opinion concerning their prognosis, and complying with the requisite 15-day waiting period.[45]

The law excludes from coverage (1) those competent adult patients physically unable to take the lethal medication on their own; (2) patients with nonterminal diagnoses, including chronic, debilitating conditions; (3) execution of patient requests for suicide made through advance directives or surrogate decision makers; and (4) non-Oregonians. The ODDA does not compel physicians and other health care professionals to take part in assisting patients to die.

The federal government, through its then-Attorney General John Ashcroft and successor Albert Gonzales, challenged the ODDA on the grounds that Oregon physicians violated the Controlled Substances Act of 1970[46] by prescribing euthanasia medications. On January 17, 2006, the U.S. Supreme Court upheld the ODDA, rejecting federal interference with a matter of pure state jurisdiction.[47]

An April 2005, Harris Interactive poll found that 70 percent of Americans believe that physicians should be allowed actively to assist terminally ill patients to end their lives and suffering, In 1982, only 53 percent of Americans agreed with physician-assisted patient suicide.[48]

Do Not Resuscitate Orders

Do not resuscitate (DNR) orders in patient medical records are written physician directives to staff health care professionals that preclude the otherwise automatic initiation of cardiopulmonary resuscitation efforts in the event of patient cardiorespiratory arrest. DNR orders do not affect other life-sustaining interventions.

Four principal circumstances may justify the writing of a DNR order:

- At the request of a competent patient
- Pursuant to a valid patient request under a living will or similar legal instrument
- At the request of a properly designated third-party surrogate decision maker empowered under a durable power of attorney for health care decision making
- When, in the judgment of a patient's primary physician (and another, or other, physicians as required by law or institutional policy), resuscitative efforts would be futile[49]

Health care providers must learn (and take the time) to communicate more effectively with patients regarding patients' desires on end-of-life care. A Robert Wood Johnson Foundation study revealed that in 47 percent of cases, physicians were unaware that patients under their care did not want cardiopulmonary resuscitation in the event of cardiac arrest.[50] Because managed care has limited the amount of time that primary health care providers can spend with individual patients, all health care providers on teams treating patients must expeditiously communicate patient expressions of desires concerning treatment options to the patients' primary physicians and to others on the patient care team.

Primary physicians must carefully document specific information concerning DNRs in patients' medical records. Although the requisite information varies from state to state, the following information is commonly required to be annotated:

- Justification and supporting rationale for the DNR order
- Information on a DNR: patient's condition, mental capacity, and advance directives
- Summary of physician communications with the patient and/or the patient's significant others, guardian, or surrogate decision maker
- Summary of input from an institutional ethics committee or other ethics consultants[51]

Clinical managers should involve legal counsel and bioethicists and applied ethicists in in-service educational experiences with clinical staff caring for patients for whom DNR orders are or might be written.

Is There a "Constitutional Right to Die"?

The mixed legal-ethical issue of whether there is a legal right to die under the federal Constitution has baffled jurists, attorneys, politicians, and health care professionals and policy makers for some time. The U.S. Supreme Court has confronted this issue in three cases: *Cruzan* v. *Director, Missouri Department of Health*[52] and, decided on the same day, *Washington* v. *Glucksberg*[53] and *Vacco* v. *Quill*.[54] In all three cases the Supreme Court declined to interpret the existence of a federal constitutional right to die.

On January 11, 1983, Nancy Beth Cruzan was involved in a rollover motor vehicle accident, in which she suffered anoxia for up to 14 minutes, eventually leaving her in a persistent vegetative state. After 4 years, her parents sought judicial permission of the Missouri state courts to remove Nancy's artificial feeding and hydration tubes so that she could die naturally. Nancy, like most Americans, had not executed any advance directives. The Missouri Supreme Court overturned the ruling of the trial-level court granting the Cruzans permission to remove Nancy's nutritional apparatus, finding that such action could only take place if there was clear and convincing evidence that this action comported with Nancy's wishes.

The U.S. Supreme Court affirmed the decision of the Missouri Supreme Court and held that (1) there is a federal constitutional (privacy) right to refuse medical treatment, which survives a patient's subsequent incapacity and (2) it is the states' prerogative to determine the legal standard for establishing an incompetent patient's wishes concerning life-sustaining treatment. States establish such procedural safeguards on behalf of incapacitated patients under their inherent ***parens patriae*** **power**.

In June 1997, in *Washington* v. *Glucksberg* and *Vacco* v. *Quill,* the U.S. Supreme Court upheld two state statutes (Washington and New York) banning physician-assisted suicide, a form of active euthanasia. The court found that there is no fundamental federal constitutional privacy right to unregulated assisted suicide. Five of the nine Supreme Court justices left open, in their separate concurring opinions, the possibility of revisiting the issue of assisted suicide at some later time.

The case of Terri Schiavo (1963-2005) involved the legal issue of withdrawal of nutrition from a woman in a 15-year persistent vegetative state. Her husband petitioned the courts for removal of her feeding tube, while her parents opposed the petition on the grounds that they believed that their daughter was conscious. After court cases in Florida state and the federal courts, including interim removal, reinsertion, and reremoval of Mrs. Schiavo's feeding tube, she died March 31, 2005.[55] An autopsy confirmed that Mrs. Schiavo was not conscious, but was in a persistent vegetative state, having suffered severe, irreversible brain damage. She also was blind.[56]

Cloning

Another salient bioethics issue involves cloning. Cloning is the process of reproducing a genetically identical duplicate of an organism. This issue became critical early in 1997 when Scottish researchers cloned a sheep and sought a patent for their cloning process. (The U.S. Supreme Court had previously ruled that living organisms are potentially patentable.)

Significant ethical and legal impediments to cloning exist. On August 9, 2001, President Bush signed into law a provision allowing limited human embryonic stem cell research under strict criteria. Under federal guidelines, informed consent for donation of a research embryo is required. The derivation process must have been initiated before the enactment of the federal law in 2001, and the embryo must have been created for reproductive purposes and must be no longer needed. Currently, some 71 lines of embryonic stem cells are being investigated by scientists in 14 laboratories around the world under these criteria.[57]

NONDISCRIMINATION IN HEALTH CARE DELIVERY

Managed care—the private sector analog to public sector health care reform initiatives of the early 1990s—has refocused health care delivery from a unitary quality patient care focus to one that is coprimarily focused on systemic cost containment and quality patient care. Under any system of health care delivery, ethical questions of distributive (macrolevel) and comparative (microlevel) justice arise. Policy makers, politicians, providers, and (most importantly) patients have for some time sought solutions to balance national interests in containing health care costs and optimizing the quality of patient care services under managed care.

According to the National Coalition on Health Care, total health care expenditures in 2005 were $2 trillion, or $6,700 per person, in the United States. This figure is expected to double to $4 trillion by 2015, making up 20 percent of the nation's gross domestic product.[58]

Despite such levels of spending, a study by Families USA revealed that hospitalized pediatric patients without health insurance were twice as likely to die from their injuries as those with medical insurance. For traumatic brain injury patients, 8.2% of insured inpatients suffered mortality, whereas 13.8% of uninsured patients died in hospitals.[59]

According to Dr. Michael Ozer of Physicians for a National Health Program, the only solution to the health care crisis is an effective national health care system. Dr. Ozer pointed out that insurance companies in the United States spend more than one third of health care dollars on administration and marketing, enrolling healthier, more profitable patients to boost profits. Forty-seven million Americans are insured for health care, and health care premiums and costs for those covered continue to wax compared with ever-waning coverage.[60]

In April 2006, Massachusetts became the first state to enact comprehensive health care reform at the state level. The legislation is designed to broaden coverage to include all Massachusetts residents and places financial responsibilities or "mandates" on all parties to make the new system work. Through a state-chartered health insurance broker or "connector," individuals and small businesses are enabled to purchase lower-cost health insurance.[61]

A study in *Pediatrics*[62] revealed substantial variance in state-to-state participation in Medicaid by primary care pediatricians. State-administered Medicaid programs are required by law to provide equal access to health care for children whose parents or guardians lack the ability to pay for services. Yet this study of 3773 primary care pediatricians revealed that Medicaid participation rates were significantly lower where reimbursement was lower, where capitated (fixed fee) programs were in place, and where the administrative paperwork burden associated with care was relatively higher.

EMTALA, the Emergency Treatment and Active Labor Act,[63] mandates that health care providers and organizations that receive federal funds examine and not transfer indigent patients in need of emergency medical services until they are stable. EMTALA was enacted to create a uniform national standard for caring for indigent emergent patients and patients in active labor, and to supplement the scant number of inconsistent state laws addressing patient "dumping."

The mandate of EMTALA ends, however, once a patient stabilizes. A disturbing series of articles in the *Los Angeles Times* chronicled how indigent patients may be literally being dumped onto city sidewalks by hospitals and medical centers because of inability to pay for continued services. California State Senator Gil Cedillo (D-Los Angeles) has labeled such practices reverse false imprisonment and has introduced legislation to ban homeless patient dumping.[64] As of May 16, 2007, Kaiser Permanente, the nation's largest health maintenance organization, agreed to a settlement in order to have criminal charges dismissed against it by the Los Angeles city attorney's office that requires Kaiser quickly to establish new protocols to prevent further homeless patient dumping and to have its progress monitored by an independent former U.S. attorney.[65]

EXERCISE

Most persons, including health care professionals, are shocked when they become aware of the cruel practice of homeless patient dumping. Yet, allegedly, health care professionals and administrators are the perpetrators of this conduct. Draft a concise paragraph that restates your position on the basic dignity and rights of all patients, including the right to comprehensive care services. Start it off, "The United States is the most affluent and compassionate nation on Earth."

AIDS and Other Life-Threatening Illnesses

Worldwide in 2006, 39.5 million persons were infected with the human immunodeficiency virus (HIV), with 1.4 million in North America.[66] HIV and the resultant acquired immunodeficiency syndrome (AIDS) are among the most serious health problems facing providers, patients, and policy makers. Health care professionals unquestionably are under legal and professional ethical duties to treat patients who are HIV-positive and those with AIDS. The Americans with Disabilities Act and case law interpreting the act clearly recognize HIV and AIDS as physical disabilities protected under its provisions (i.e., employment [Title I] and access to public and private health care services [Titles II and III]).

Health care professionals are obligated by legal and professional ethical standards to sublimate any negative biases they may have toward patients with HIV and AIDS. The law and standards of professional ethics disallow the manifestation of negative attitudinal biases against patients. The Association of Nurses in AIDS Care has multiple position statements on widely variegated aspects of AIDS care that make excellent starting points for health care professional associations, organizations, and systems to review.[67]

EXERCISE

How do the professional ethics code, policies, and standards of your discipline specifically address HIV and AIDS? Compare the provisions of your discipline to those of one other health care profession.

Ethical concerns related to treatment of patients with HIV or AIDS include confronting one's own prejudices (attitudinal biases), safe-guarding patient confidentiality, and protecting third parties who might be at risk of harm because of exposure to the patient's infected bodily fluids.[68] Patient confidentiality principles remain the same, whether health care professionals are treating patients who have AIDS, back pain, or any other condition. (The *Tarasoff* exception to privacy, under which breach of confidentiality may be justified to protect identified third parties threatened with serious bodily harm, would apply with equal force to a patient threatening intentionally to infect identified third parties with HIV.) Finally, concerning risk of infection from bodily fluids, the principle of universal precautions requires any health care provider exposed to patient bodily fluids to treat all such patients as potentially infectious and take appropriate self-protective precautions, irrespective of the patient's pathological condition.

Is there a professional ethical duty to disclose to patients the fact that a health care provider is HIV-positive? Clearly, the incidence of occupational HIV transmission among health care workers is on the increase[69] The Centers for Disease Control and Prevention recommend that health care professionals who perform invasive or other exposure-prone procedures on patients be aware of their own HIV status and that those who are HIV-positive refrain from performing such procedures without patient consent.[70] Absent a state or federal law requiring otherwise, there is no general legal duty to reveal one's HIV status to patients, colleagues, or others. One's HIV status, like one's cancer status, is a private matter—even for clinical health care professionals.

> Health care professionals have no legal duty to reveal their HIV status to patients, colleagues, or others.

Provider Access to Health Care Services Delivery

Patients are not the only participants in the managed care arena who face denial of access to health care service delivery systems. Health care professionals, too, may face exclusion from participation in health care service delivery systems for a variety of reasons—some ethically and legally acceptable and some not.

Any willing provider laws and regulations exist at federal and state levels designed to safeguard the rights of licensed and certified health care professionals freely to practice their professions and to participate in health care delivery services under managed care. Generally, under these laws, all qualified providers who are willing to participate in managed care health delivery services and who are able to meet the reasonable inclusion standards of managed care organizations, insurers, or other payers must be included in provider networks. Absent the existence of "any willing provider" laws in a state, managed care organizations may contract exclusively with select health care providers and groups for service delivery and exclude all others from participation. According to the National Council on State Legislatures, in May 2007, 21 states had in place "any willing provider" laws, most of which apply to pharmacists, who are deemed most likely to be adversely affected by exclusive provider arrangements under managed care.[71] On April 8, 2003, the U.S. Supreme Court validated the any willing provider legislation of Kentucky in the case of *Kentucky Association of Health Plans, Inc. v. Miller.*[72]

NAFTA, the North Atlantic Free Trade Agreement, an international treaty signed by the United States, Canada, and Mexico, was enacted on December 17, 1992. NAFTA provides for ease of entry into and between member nations for 63 classes of temporary nonimmigrant alien business professionals desiring to work in member nations, including many health care professionals.[73] The Department of Homeland security issued 65,000 6-year H-1B visas to foreign specialty workers (including health care professionals) in 2006, with the same quota allotted for 2007.[74]

Pro Bono Health Care Service Delivery

When professional service is provided *pro bono publico* (Latin for "for the public good"), it is provided at a reduced fee or for no fee, depending on the ability of the service recipient to pay. For primary health care professionals who participate in *pro bono* activities, the benefits are tangible and intangible.

The public image of an individual provider, his or her business organization, and his or her profession are enhanced through a strong commitment to public service. Personal and collective satisfaction result when professionals respond to a compelling need for the services of the profession. In addition, improvement in the goodwill of an organization enhances revenue and/or profit; a network is created among colleagues performing similar services; and professional associations and public entities provide technical and administrative support that ensures overall success of *pro bono* efforts.[75]

> Personal and collective satisfaction result when professionals respond to a compelling need for the services of a profession.

In Search of a Model for Pro Bono *Service*

Of all the professions, the legal profession may have the most extensive documented history of *pro bono* service and expectations. *Pro bono* professional service in the United States has traditionally focused on the legal profession. Many of the *pro bono* concepts used by the legal profession may be directly transferable to the health care professions.

The legal profession has a centuries-old commitment to provide legal services to persons who cannot afford them. In the twentieth century, this altruistic goal was formalized into a canon of ethical conduct by the American Bar Association in its *Canons of Professional Ethics* (1908),[76] the **Model Code of Professional Responsibility** (1969),[77] and the *Model Rules of Professional Conduct* (1983).[78] Although the original

Canons of Professional Ethics made *pro bono* service mandatory for attorneys, the *Model Code* and *Model Rules*—adopted by the state bars of all 50 states—label attorneys' *pro bono* service obligation as an "ethical," rather than a "legal," obligation.

In Rule 6.1 of the *Model Rules of Professional Conduct,* the American Bar Association established the following professional ethical standard for attorneys regarding *pro bono* service:

> *A lawyer* should *[emphasis added] render public interest legal service. A lawyer may discharge this responsibility by providing professional services at no fee or at a reduced fee to persons of limited means or to public service or charitable groups or organizations, by services in activities for improving the law, the legal system or the legal profession, and by financial support for organizations that provide legal services to persons of limited means.*

The nonbinding "Comment" to Rule 6.1 of the *Model Rules of Professional Conduct* expounds on this ethical principle by stating the following:

> *Every lawyer, regardless of professional prominence or professional work load, should find time to participate in or otherwise support the provision of legal services to the disadvantaged. The provision of free legal services to those unable to pay reasonable fees continues to be an obligation of each lawyer, as well as the profession generally.*

Health Care Professions and Pro Bono *Service*

With 47 million Americans uninsured or underinsured for health care and a quarter of the population over 65 years of age living below the poverty line,[79] there is obviously a tremendous need for *pro bono* health care in the United States. Some of this need is currently being met by individuals and groups.

Legislators and health care policy makers have created, or have attempted to create, various incentives to encourage health care professionals to engage in *pro bono* activities. As of January 2005, 42 states and the District of Columbia offered some form of charitable immunity from malpractice liability to volunteer health care professionals.[80] Such statutory immunity typically protects physicians and other health care providers from liability so long as the providers' conduct does not constitute gross negligence, recklessness, or willful misconduct.

Fear of Health Care Malpractice Liability as a Barrier to Greater *Pro Bono* Service

Fear of liability exposure prevents many health care professionals engaged in clinical service delivery from providing or expanding *pro bono* services. Part of the fear stems from the belief that because patients with low incomes may be more prone to adverse care outcomes because of relatively poor baseline health, they will more likely file claims against, or sue, their health care providers. A Maryland study concluded that obstetric Medicaid patients showed no greater likelihood than women in general to file medical malpractice claims against their obstetricians.[81] Simple initiatives—including effective communication with patients and their significant others; empathy; good rapport; and accurate, timely documentation of patient evaluation and care—go a long way in protecting providers from liability.

One way to dampen a provider's fear of malpractice liability exposure incident to *pro bono* service activities would be the creation of a legislative exception by Congress to the mandatory reporting requirements of the National Practitioner Data Bank. Designed in part to serve as a resource for verifying the accuracy of information provided by licensed health care professional job applicants to employers, the National Practitioner Data Bank also requires health care organizations and systems, licensing entities, professional associations and malpractice payment entities to report malpractice payments.[82]

Pro Bono Publico Service: A Social Responsibility

All health care professionals and professional associations, clinical entities, and academic health centers should carefully examine the model for *pro bono* service established by the legal profession and consider implementing minimally intrusive *pro bono* service expectations of members, employees, faculty, and staff, as applicable. State agencies, which license primary health care providers, should consider codifying *pro bono* expectations into law in the form of rules and regulations in state practice acts.

In addition to establishing *pro bono* policies, professional associations, clinical sites and universities, and state and federal agencies must continue to assume responsibility for integrating *pro bono* efforts across all health care disciplines, providing continuing education, networking, and administrative and other support for volunteers who give their time to help socioeconomically disadvantaged clients. Professional corporations, practice groups, and individual providers also may consider incorporating *pro bono* policies into their practices and publicizing their *pro bono* efforts to encourage and provide guidance to others.

The following are just a few recent examples of innovative health-related and other professional *pro bono* activities. The Occupational Therapy Program at Samuel Merritt College in Oakland, California, offers a free rehabilitation clinic for indigent patients.[83] Nursing students at the University of Texas Medical Branch in Galveston assist Texas probate courts and guardians of wards of the state as volunteer consultants.[84] A drug partnership between international health agencies and the world's fourth largest drug manufacturer, Sanofi-Aventis, sells antimalarial medicines at cost to poor patients in Africa, Indonesia, and the Philippines.[85] Companies such as Deloitte and Touche, among many others, encourage and give incentives to their employees to "give back" to charitable causes.[86]

Pro bono service should be an expectation—never a requirement—of all professionals to whom the states have granted the exclusive right to practice professions for profit. The tangible and intangible benefits to patients served, volunteer providers, practice groups, professional associations and professions, and society at large are limitless.

PROFESSIONAL PRACTICE ISSUES

Financial Responsibility: Ethical Duties of Patients and Providers

Although health care is not just an ordinary business, there obviously are business and financial implications associated with its delivery. Most, if not all, health care providers and organizations require monetary compensation from patients or third-party payers in order to survive and thrive. These entities must price their services according to ethical and legal standards.

Patient Duty to Pay Fair Value for Professional Services

Patients are not bound by a formal code of ethical conduct in their relations with health care professionals, as are the latter. However, certain legal duties are incumbent upon patients receiving treatment in health care delivery settings. The principle duty of patients (absent legal excuse or release by the provider) is to pay market or fair value for professional services rendered. This legal obligation is the primary duty of patients cited by authorities as creating legal consideration under the implied health care professional–patient contractual relationship. (The principle legal duty incumbent upon the provider is, of course, to exercise his or her best clinical judgment to effect an optimal therapeutic result for the patient.)

> Patients are not bound by a formal code of ethical conduct in their relations with health care professionals. The principle legal duty incumbent upon the provider is to exercise his or her best clinical judgment to effect an optimal therapeutic result for the patient.

Health Care Professionals' Duties

Pricing of Services

Health care organizations—whether operated for-profit or not-for-profit—are businesses and must normally generate sufficient operating revenue (absent receipt of subsidies, donations, or investment or other nonoperating revenue) to cover the direct and indirect costs of patient care. Direct costs include salaries for professional and support staff and supplies and equipment used in patient care activities. Indirect costs include employee benefits, administrative and maintenance expenses, depreciation on equipment, and housekeeping and laundry expenses.[87]

The processes associated with pricing of health care services and products give rise to potential ethical problems, issues, and dilemmas for health care providers and administrators. Managed care and prospective payment systems have given rise to discounted and fixed reimbursement for inpatient and outpatient health care services.

EXERCISE

How do the code of ethics and related standards of your discipline address the pricing of professional services?

The common thread of "reasonableness" among the health care professional ethics codes in setting fees is augmented by the implied principle that fees for professional services must also be "realistic"; that is, fees for professional services must be set high enough to generate sufficient net income for the professional to enjoy a fair living standard commensurate with his or her labor efforts and level of education and experience.

Under managed care, many health care providers deliver care under contractual capitation arrangements. Under **capitation**, providers agree to provide all necessary professional services to program subscribers (patients) for a fixed fee, often expressed as "per member per month."[88] Before entering into capitation arrangements, providers must consult with their legal counsel and financial advisor; conduct a relevant market analysis; and ensure that projected revenues under the contract will exceed projected expenses, so that established fees are reasonable and realistic.

Gifts

The word *gift* in German means poison. Because the areas of patient, referral entity, business associate, vendor, and other sources of gifts to health care providers raise such serious conflict of interest ethical concerns, health care providers would do well to remember the German meaning of "gift" when dealing with this issue in most cases.

In her excellent overview article, "Gift-giving or Influence Peddling: Can You Tell the Difference,"[89] Finley suggested that patient gifts of *de minimis* monetary value, directed toward an organization, rather than a specific health care provider, are acceptable. Consider the following example:

> *A neuromuscular rehabilitation patient being discharged after 6 weeks of intensive inpatient care delivers to her occupational therapist a 2-lb box of Godiva chocolates and expresses her thanks for excellent care rendered. How should the therapist respond?*

The occupational therapist should respond by expressing gratitude for the gift on behalf of the entire rehabilitation team, informing the patient that it will be shared with all professional, support, and administrative services team members. In this case, it would probably be unnecessary and might be seen as imprudent to decline the gift altogether.

EXERCISE

Review the ethics code of your discipline for guidance about gifts. How do formal ethics guidelines compare with actual customary practice concerning acceptance of gifts from patients and third parties?

Impaired Providers

Health care providers impaired by drugs (including alcohol), mental distress, or other causes pose a serious risk of substantial harm to patients under their care and research subjects; to colleagues, visitors, and others; and to themselves. For that reason, professional ethical standards and licensure and certification regulations and other state and federal laws make mandatory the reporting of suspected impairment by peers.

Ethics codes of representative health care professions make clear that health care professionals have the personal ethical responsibility to recognize the signs and symptoms of possible abuse affecting themselves and to refrain from carrying out interventions that might harm patients or others. Because a primary purpose of health care professional codes of ethics is patient and public protection, it is expected that ethics codes will require peer reporting of unethical, illegal conduct or suspected incompetence.

EXERCISE

Review the ethics code and licensure/certification provisions of your discipline regarding impaired providers. Are the provisions adequate to protect the public from harm by impaired providers? If not, what changes need to be made to them?

Professional Relations

Professional relations within and among health care disciplines generally have been consistently positive over time. However, some professional ethical issues involving intradisciplinary and interdisciplinary health care professional relations bear mentioning.

In recent times, millions of dollars in legal fees have been spent prosecuting or defending intradisciplinary and interdisciplinary encroachment or "turf" or jurisdictional battles within, between, and among health care professional disciplines and organizations. Issues addressed in these legal battles range from jurisdiction to domains of practice to credentialing to antitrust. In perhaps the most prominent of these legal cases in recent times, *Wilk* v. *American Medical Association,*[90] a federal appellate court ruled that the medical community had carried out an illegal boycott of the chiropractic profession in violation of Section One of the Sherman Antitrust Act of 1890.[91]

Health care professionals, individually and collectively, and health care professional organizations should consider resolving such disputes in a more amicable manner than through civil litigation. These groups should consider using alternative dispute resolution methods, including conciliation between the parties to disputes, as well as third-party mediation and arbitration.

In mediation, a neutral third-party intermediary facilitates a mutually agreeable solution to a dispute by the parties themselves. In arbitration, a neutral third party conducts the administrative equivalent of a private civil legal proceeding and renders a decision to which the parties to the dispute contractually agree to be bound. Under either method of alternative dispute resolution, a public record of proceedings is avoided, the cost of dispute resolution in terms of time and money is reduced, and professional goodwill may be enhanced.

EXERCISE

How does your ethics code address professional relations? Compare the provisions of your discipline to those of two other complementary health disciplines.

Research Considerations

Ethical issues in research settings center largely on two issues: the protection of human research subjects and the integrity of research processes.[92] Federal regulations governing the use of human subjects in research promulgated by the Department of Health and Human Services[93] are derived in part from U.S. law and in part from customary international law and multinational human rights treaties. Responsibility for the protection of human research subjects rests with institutional review boards (IRBs), which are multidisciplinary committees that establish research protocol guidelines; review and approve research proposals for their institutions that involve human research subjects; and enforce compliance with federal, state, and institutional requirements and standards.

The integrity of research scientists is a paramount concern to the research community, for obvious reasons. From the funding of research projects to public trust, research—especially involving human subjects—must have the respect of the scientific community, government, and public at large.

Researchers, similar to health care clinicians, academicians, and students, have ethical responsibilities. Scientists have the same core values that others have within a given profession[94] and are obligated to comply with the professional codes of ethics governing their respective disciplines.

Researchers are ethically bound to protect the well-being of research subjects and to ensure that each individual is provided detailed disclosure of information regarding the research, ensuring that informed consent is given to participate. Researchers must also maintain appropriate confidentiality of the personal identities of research subjects. Researchers must avoid conflicts of interest that might bias their research findings. Researchers are similarly obliged to avoid distorting or misrepresenting results, and they must appropriately credit others for their source materials and contributions to research projects.[95]

Altman and Broad[96] reported on the disturbing series of recent cases involving scientific fraud, including the case of Dr. Hwang Woo Suk of Seoul National University and his human cloning studies, which results published in *Science* were subsequently retracted. The authors highlight that the integrity of scientific research is protected by a triple safety net: peer review, the scientific journal referee system, and replication of reported results by other scientists. To help combat fraud in science, in 2004, major scientific journals banded together to require registration of studies in public databases as a precondition to later publication of results.[97]

Health Care Professional Student and Faculty Ethical Concerns

In professional education settings, academicians (including guest lecturers), clinical faculty, and students have ethical responsibilities. The same fundamental duties of competency, confidentiality, fidelity, respect, and truth that apply to professional-patient relationships apply with equal force to relationships between students and faculty. Many of these professional ethical duties are codified into case law and statutes, making them legal duties as well. For example, the legal duty of confidentiality of student records incumbent on academicians and educational program administrators is governed by the Family Education Rights and Privacy Act of 1974 (the Buckley Amendment).[98]

Students, as well as faculty, have fundamental professional ethical duties governing their conduct. For example, relative to truth, students have the ethical duties not to cheat on examinations and not to plagiarize or fail to credit, as appropriate, the work product of others when paraphrasing them. Health care professional students also have the ethical duty not to intentionally defraud prospective employers by signing preemployment contracts solely to receive current financial incentives.

Sanctions for violations of ethical duties in professional education exist along a progressive continuum, just as they do along the disciplinary continuum in employment settings. Students who violate ethical obligations may face the award of a failing grade or suspension or expulsion from their educational programs for serious breaches of ethics. Faculty who breach professional ethical standards may incur the loss of a chance for tenure or even the loss of employment for serious breaches of their ethical responsibilities.

Faculty and student ethical responsibilities are commonly spelled out with varying degrees of clarity in faculty and student handbooks, respectively. Although standards may appear vague, sanctions for violations of standards cannot be stated in a vague fashion because of the constitutional procedural due process considerations of notice and substantive fairness, which are prerequisites to adverse action—at least in public institutions of higher learning.

Among other ethical duties of academic and clinical faculty are the duty to certify that health care professional students participating in clinical affiliations are competent to perform the tasks expected of them and the duty to supervise students in laboratory and clinical settings, as appropriate. Students bear the special ethical duties to follow reasonable instructions issued to them by their professors and clinical instructors and to act only within the scope of their personal and legal competence.

Ethics Committees and Consultations

Institutional ethics committees (IECs) are multidisciplinary committees within health care organizations that include health care and related professionals (i.e., clergy, social workers, and attorneys) and occasionally lay members. In addition to their educative and policy-making roles, IECs offer consultative services to physicians and other health care providers and administrations on cases involving ethical problems, issues, and dilemmas.

A primary goal of an IEC ethics consultation is to provide collective advice to physicians and other clinical health care decision makers about patient care issues. As the adage goes, "Two (or six, or twelve) heads are always better than one." The consultative role of the IEC to physicians and others is advisory, not directive. It remains, as it always has been, the primary responsibility of a patient's attending or primary physician or surgeon (or other primary care professional) to execute patient care decisions. Through IEC intervention, however, it is often easier for physicians and other health care providers and their patients and families to reach ethical consensus concerning optimal patient care decisions.

What is the role of an attorney in the ethics consultative process? A health care organization attorney should act as a legal consultant to an IEC, offering advice on the legal implications of alternative decisions to decision makers. An attorney should neither dictate a solution to the IEC nor be permitted to dominate discussion with risk management concerns.[99] Attorneys are educated by law schools to be legal advisors, not surrogate decision makers (although they are too often misused as such). An IEC (or any decision maker) should never have to say, "We're just doing what the lawyer told us to do."

Ethics consultations can be obtained from sources other than IECs as well. Private ethics consultants and professional associations are other sources for ethics consultation. By way of example, ETHICSearch is a service of the Standing Committee on Ethical and Professional Responsibility of the American Bar Association for member attorneys, at no cost for routine matters or at nominal cost for complicated inquiries requiring consultant research.[100]

EXERCISE

Investigate whether the professional association and/or state licensing agency of your discipline has in place a no-fee ethics consultation service for members.

Informed Consent Issues in Research Settings

The informed consent of human research subjects is a fundamental requirement of and prerequisite to carrying out clinical research involving human beings. The process of obtaining research subject informed consent is more complex than for obtaining patient informed consent to routine health care interventions. In part, this is because research-related consent is subject to greater institutional, administrative, and legal oversight than treatment-related informed consent and in part because research-related subject consent normally must be documented in long-form, according to strict, rather than flexible, standards. (Documentation standards for patient informed consent to treatment or related intervention are more varied; individual documentation in patient health records of treatment-related informed consent may not even be ethically and legally required.)[101]

The intense regulation of human subject research resulted in large part from the Nuremberg trials that followed World War II. In those trials, approximately 20 prominent German physicians were tried for human rights violations involving cruel and inhumane medical experimentation of prisoners of war. Most were convicted, and several were hanged.

Subsequent to the Nuremberg trials, the Nuremberg Code of 1947 was drafted and adopted. This code, in part, established as codified international law that "the voluntary consent of the human subject is absolutely essential" (to legally and ethically carry out permissible medical research).[102] The Nuremberg Code was augmented in 1975 by the Helsinki Declarations of 1964 (I) and 1975 (II), which established the international law requirement of independent review of research proposals involving human subjects as follows: "The design and performance of each experimental procedure involving human subjects should be clearly formulated in an experimental protocol which should be transmitted to a specially appointed independent committee for consideration, comment, and guidance."[103]

Based in large part on these international treaties and on human rights abuses in the American Tuskegee Syphilis Study, the Department of Health and Human Services (then the Department of Health, Education, and Welfare) adopted human subject research guidelines in the late 1970s that delineated the permissible scope of and procedures for human subject research activities that use federal funding. These guidelines also established the requirement for independent review of human subject research protocols by IRBs. The federal guidelines were amended in 1981 to delete the requirement for IRB approval of a limited class of very-low-risk human subject research protocols.[104]

Special federal guidelines dictate required elements that must be included in human subject research informed consent forms. These guidelines include the following parameters:

- The consent form must impart sufficient information about a proposed study, its procedures, expected benefits, material risks, and reasonable alternatives to enable a potential subject to make a knowing, intelligent, and voluntary decision about whether to agree to participate.
- The investigator (or approved designee) must personally explain the parameters to the potential subject.
- The consent form must be written in the first person and must be in layperson's language, without significant technical medical "jargon." If the potential subject's language of comprehension is other than English, a translation of the consent form is required.
- In general, consent forms from other institutions may not be used to obtain human subject research consent.
- The consequences of subject injury must be clearly spelled out, including therapeutic measures to be taken in the event of subject injury and who bears the cost of such care.
- Any compensation or benefit that the subject will receive for participation in a research study must be clearly stated in the informed consent form.
- A copy of the signed form must be given to the subject. If the subject is also a patient, a copy of the research consent form must be filed in the patient's medical treatment record. The original copy of the consent form must be retained for at least 5 years after completion of the study.
- The consent form must be witnessed. The witness or witnesses attest only to a subject's signature, not to the subject's comprehension of disclosure elements or comprehension of them.
- The informed consent form must state contact telephone numbers for the principal investigator, where the subject can personally reach the investigator 24 hours a day.

Additional safeguards for research subject protection include the following:

- No person may be excluded from consideration as a research subject because of race, ethnicity, or language. The equitable inclusion of women and minorities in research is strongly encouraged.
- The subject's confidentiality and autonomy enjoy absolute respect and protection. The subject has the right to review all data collected from and about him or her and to withhold permission for their use by the researcher.

- The subject may withdraw consent at any time, without prejudice.
- The subject may not be prejudiced in receiving necessary and equitable care based on a decision not to participate in a research study.

Judicial activism is strong in protecting the rights of medical research subjects. In the case of *T.D.* v. *New York Office of Mental Health,*[105] the court ruled that nontherapeutic research involving greater than minimal risk of harm to minors and adult subjects lacking mental capacity is illegal under New York state law based on the fact that these subjects cannot give informed consent to participate. In so ruling, New York joined a growing number of states in banning such research. The same rule of law applies in the United Kingdom.[106]

SUMMARY

Informed patient consent to health care evaluation and treatment intervention is a legal and ethical prerequisite to care. Health care clinicians responsible for patient evaluation and treatment and intervention—especially rehabilitation professionals— bear primary responsibility for obtaining patient informed consent. Informed consent to rehabilitation intervention by nonphysician health care professionals is not the responsibility of referring physicians at one end of the continuum, nor of assistants or other supportive personnel carrying out the professionals' directives at the other end of the continuum.

Although the elements of legally sufficient patient informed consent vary from state to state (according to state or federal law, as applicable), the following disclosure elements must normally be imparted to patients (or their surrogate decision makers) before health care commences:

- Diagnosis and pertinent evaluative findings
- Nature of the intervention(s) recommended or ordered
- Risk of potential harm or complications material to the patient's decision whether to accept or reject treatment
- Expected benefits (i.e., goals) of treatment
- Reasonable alternatives to the proposed treatment or intervention

In addition to the disclosure elements, a health care professional must also solicit and satisfactorily answer any patient questions before the informed consent process is consummated. A variety of legally acceptable ways exist to document patient informed consent to treatment.

Two principal exceptions to the requirement to obtain patient informed consent are the emergency doctrine and therapeutic privilege. In life-threatening emergency situations, it is generally presumed that patients grant implied consent to medical interventions designed to save their lives. (Exceptions to the exception may also apply, such as when a specific patient's prior contrary wishes are known.) Therapeutic privilege allows a physician to withhold diagnostic and/or prognostic information from a patient who is deemed to be psychologically incapable of dealing with the information. Rarely is therapeutic privilege allowed because the exception derogates from respect for patient autonomy and patient control over treatment-related decision making.

Human subject research informed consent is normally more formal and complex than patient informed consent, in part because of the substantial federal, state, and institutional oversight over human subject research activities and in part because of the (recent) history of horrific abuse of human subjects in medical research. The details of the processes of human research subject informed consent are governed at the operative level by independent IRBs. A judicial trend is to disallow nontherapeutic research posing greater than minimal health risks involving minors and incompetent subjects.

Managed care has given rise to informed consent practice issues, most involving actual or perceived provider conflicts of interest. The fundamental biomedical ethical principles of beneficence and respect for patient autonomy are in direct conflict with managed care contractual gag clauses, which may prevent providers from making full disclosure of treatment-related information to patients and nondisclosure about provider financial incentives to provide less care to patients. The courts have yet to rule definitively on these issues but will likely declare these managed care initiatives unconscionable and unenforceable.

CASES AND QUESTIONS

1. A nurse practitioner in private practice asks you for advice on the propriety of placing a rubber-stamped informed consent summary in each patient's treatment record to demonstrate that the patients have been provided with appropriate disclosure information and in fact have given informed consent to intervention. How do you advise the client?
2. As a facility risk manager, what steps can you take to ensure that health care professionals universally make appropriate disclosure of treatment-related information and obtain patient informed consent to intervention?
3. A 54-year-old terminally ill cancer patient expresses during an evaluation by an orthotist her desire to "die with dignity." What action(s), if any, should the orthotist take based on the patient's assertion?

SUGGESTED ANSWERS TO CASES AND QUESTIONS

1. Informed consent is a communicative process and not a stamp or patient signature on a form. A rubber-stamped summary of the information imparted to a patient might constitute some evidence of what was said to the patient but is normally unnecessary for routine interventions. Under managed care—where time is at a premium—the optimal method of documenting patient informed consent to intervention may be in a document such as a clinic policies and procedures manual or quality management manual, instead of placing individual documentation in patient treatment records for routine interventions. Health care providers will be expected by clinic managers, insurers, and the courts universally to comply with the institutional informed consent standards enunciated in such manuals.
2. Steps to ensure that providers carry out their legal and ethical duties related to disclosure of treatment-related information and the obtaining of patient informed consent include the following:
   • Ensuring that newly employed providers read and verify in writing their understanding of the clinic policy regarding patient informed consent
   • Monitoring selected patients for comprehension of disclosure information and consent to intervention

- Providing periodic in-service education, involving clinical professionals, ethicists, and legal counsel, on legal and ethical issues related to patient informed consent.

3. Analyze this problem under the systems approach to health care professional ethical decision making.

Step 1: Identify the ethical problem. The patient has made a statement during orthotic evaluation, which possibly affects end-of-life medical interventions. The patient has the inherent right to self-determination over health care interventions affecting her person and body. What action(s), if any, should the orthotist take, based on the patient's assertion?

Step 2: Identify relevant facts and unknowns; formulate reasonable assumptions. *Facts*: The patient is terminally ill with cancer; she is undergoing orthotic evaluation; she has expressed a desire to "die with dignity." *Unknowns*: Family situation, advance directives in force, other considerations? *Assumptions*: The patient appears competent and sincere and in need of professional consultation regarding her statement.

Step 3: Assess viable courses of action. (1) Take no action, because the patient's statement is confidential. (2) Document the patient's statement, but take no further action. (3) Alert the patient's physician and nurse about her statement.

Step 4: Implement a course of action. Execute option 3—alert the patient's physician and nurse.

Step 5: Obtain feedback on the chosen course of action; modify or change, as necessary. The orthotist should follow up the next day with the physician or nurse regarding action taken based on the patient's reported statement.

SUGGESTED READINGS

Banaji MR, Bazerman MH, Chugh D: How (un)ethical are you? *Harvard Business Review* 81(12):56-64, 2003.

Begley S: Racism studies find rational part of brain can override prejudice, *Wall Street Journal* p B1, Nov 19, 2004.

Dewan S: Waiting list for AIDS drugs causes dismay in South Carolina, *New York Times* p A14, Dec 29, 2006 (longest waiting list in the United States for free lifesaving drugs).

Foy N: Texas law gives hospitals right to end life support, *San Antonio Express News* p 1A, March 27, 2005.

Friedman A: Beyond medicine, a doctor's urge to save a patient from herself, *New York Times* p D5, Dec 12, 2006 (autonomy versus paternalism).

Gazella K: End-of-life wishes vary among racial and ethnic groups, genders, *Senior News*, 18(3):1, 2006.

Hoffman J: The last word on the last breath, *New York Times* p D1, Oct 10, 2006.

Klitzman R: The quest for privacy can make us thieves, *New York Times* p D1, May 9, 2006.

Kuhl BA, Radensky PW: Legal issues involving genetic databases, *Health Lawyers News* pp 11-12, Sep 2001.

Kurtz SM, Silverman J, Draper J, Silverman J: *Teaching and learning communication skills in medicine*, ed 2, Oxford, United Kingdom, 2005, Radcliffe Publishing.

Rozovsky FA: *Consent to treatment*, ed 2, Gaithersburg, Md, 1990, Aspen.

Scott RW: Medical Spanish: a new approach, Sudbury, Mass, 2008, Jones and Bartlett.

Somerville MA: Therapeutic privilege: variation on the theme of informed consent, *Law Med Health Care* 12(1):4, 1984.

Timm K: Informed consent in clinical research, *Orthopaedic Practice* 7(3):14, 1995.

University of California, San Francisco: Human research protection program. Retrieved Sept. 22, 2007, from www.ucsf.edu.

Usmar C: A new beginning: caring for coma-emergent patients, *Today in PT* pp 30-33, April 30, 2007 (includes the revised Rancho Los Amigos Cognitive Scale).

Washington D: *Medical apartheid: the dark history of medical experimentation on black Americans from colonial times to the present,* New York, 2007, Doubleday. (On May 17, 1997, President Bill Clinton apologized to eight Tuskegee survivors and families on behalf of the United States.)

Winslow R: Videos, questionnaires aim to expand role of patients in treatment decisions, *Wall Street Journal* p B1, 1992.

Zezima K: The Muslim patient will see you now, doctor, *New York Times* p A16, Sep 1, 2004 (cultural sensitivity).

REFERENCES

1. Beauchamp TL, Childress JF: *Principles of biomedical ethics,* ed 5, New York, 2001, Oxford University Press.

2. In an early leading case on informed consent, *Schloendorf* v. *Society of New York Hospital,* 105 NE 2nd 92 (NY, 1914), Justice Benjamin Cardozo wrote, "Every human being of adult years and sound mind has a right to determine what shall be done with his [or her] own body, and a surgeon who performs an operation without [a] patient's consent commits an assault for which he [or she] is liable in money damages."

3. Katz J: *The silent world of doctor and patient,* New York, 1984, Free Press. "[D]isclosure and consent, except in the most rudimentary fashion, are obligations alien to medical thinking and practice."

4. Furrow BR, Johnson SH, Jost TS, Schwartz RL: *Health law: cases, materials and problems,* ed 2, St Paul, Minn, 1991, West Publishing (p 322).

5. *Schloendorf* v. *Society of New York Hospital.* See reference 2.

6. *Natanson* v. *Kline,* 350 P.2d 1093 (Kansas, 1965).

7. *Canterbury* v. *Spence,* 464 F.2d 772 (Washington, DC, 1972), cert. [US Supreme Court appeal] denied, 409 US 1064, 1974.

8. *Schloendorf* v. *Society of New York Hospital.* See reference 2.

9. "The fundamental distinction between assault and battery on one hand, and [professional] negligence such as would constitute malpractice, on the other, is that the former is intentional and the latter unintentional. ... "*Natanson* v. *Kline.* See reference 2.

10. *Spence* v. *Todaro,* No 94-3757 (ED Pa, 1994).

11. *Friter and Friter* v. *Iolab Corp.,* 607 A.2d 1111 (Pennsylvania Supreme Court, 1992).

12. *Flores* v. *Center for Spinal Evaluation and Rehabilitation,* 865 SW 2nd 261 (Tex App, 1993).

13. In re *Quinlan,* 355 A.2d 647 (NJ, 1976).

14. *Bouvia* v. *Superior Court,* 179 Calif App 3d 1127, 225 Calif Rptr 297 (Calif App, 1986).

15. *Cruzan* v. *Director, Missouri Department of Health,* 497 US 261 (1990).

16. Patient Self-Determination Act, 42 United States Code Sections 1395, 1396.

17. 42 United States Code Section 1395cc(f)(1)(A)(i).

18. The author is grateful to Brooke Army Medical center for use of its Patient Bill of Rights and Responsibilities. Kudos to U.S. military medical professionals caring for wounded service members returning from Afghanistan and Iraq.

19. The Joint Commission: *2007 Comprehensive accreditation manual for hospitals,* Chicago, 2007, The Commission.

20. *Canterbury* v. *Spence*. See reference 7.
21. Curtin LL: Ethics in management: informed consent: cautious, calculated candor, *Nurs Manage* 24(4):18, 1995.
22. How is your doctor treating you? *Consumer Reports* p 81, 1995.
23. Tanner L: Study asks how much patients want to know, *Senior News* p 15, Oct 1995.
24. Hoffman J: Awash in information: patients face lonely, uncertain road, *New York Times* p A1, Aug 14, 2005.
25. Brody JE: Just what the doctor ordered? Not exactly, *New York Times,* p D8, May 9, 2006.
26. Rogers TK: It's a busy waiting room that keeps patients busy, *New York Times* p 22, Nov 20, 2005.
27. Hutson MM, Blaha JD: Patients' recall of preoperative instruction for informed consent for an operation, *J Bone Joint Surg Am* 73:160, 1991.
28. Brody JE: The importance of knowing what the doctor is talking about, *New York Times* p D7, Jan 30, 2007.
29. Brody JE: To protect against drug errors, ask questions, *New York Times* p D7, Jan 2, 2007.
30. Franklin D: Patient power: making sure your doctor really hears you, *New York Times* p D5, Aug 15, 2006.
31. Furrow BR, Johnson SH, Jost TS, Schwartz RL: *Health law: cases, materials and problems,* ed 2, St Paul, Minn, 1991, West Publishing (p 336).
32. *Canterbury* v. *Spence*. See reference 7.
33. Searight HR: Assessing patient competence for medical decision making, *Am Fam Physician* 45:751, 1992.
34. Spremulli M: Decision-making in health care: competence to consent to treatment, *Advance for Physical Therapists & PT Assistants,* p 33, July 15, 2005.
35. O'Brien C: *Memo: background and supporting documentation on gag clauses,* Chicago, 1995, American Medical Association.
36. Bursztajn HJ, Saunders LS, Brodsky A: Medical negligence and informed consent in the managed care era, *Health Lawyer* 9(5):14, 1997.
37. Liang BA: The practical utility of gag clause legislation, *J Gen Intern Medicine* 13(6):419-421, 1998.
38. American Medical Association, Council on Ethical and Judicial Affairs: Ethical issues in managed care, *JAMA* 273:330, 1995.
39. Emanuel EJ: Cost savings at the end of life: what do the data show? *JAMA* 275(6):1907-1914, 1996.
40. Audie L: *Murphy Memorial Veterans Hospital: policy memorandum No. 119617—withholding or withdrawal of life-sustaining treatment,* San Antonio, Texas, 1996, Murphy Memorial Veterans Hospital.
41. *Cruzan.* See reference 15.
42. Furrow BR, Johnson SH, Jost TS, Schwartz RL: *Health law: cases, materials and problems,* ed 2, St Paul, Minn, 1991, West Publishing (p 1056).
43. Deepak G, Sushma B, Seema M: Euthanasia: issues implied within. Part 1, *Journal of Pain, Symptom Control and Palliative Care* vol 4, No. 2, 2006. Retrieved May 14, 2007, from www.ispub.com.
44. *Cruzan.* See reference 15.
45. ORS 127.800.-995, Oct 27, 1997. Between 1998 and 2006, 292 patients were served by the law. See Oregon Department of Human Services: *Death with Dignity Act annual reports.* Retrieved May 14, 2007, from http://egov.oregon.gov/DHS/ph/pas/ar-index.shtml.
46. The Controlled Substances Act of 1970, 21 United States Code Section 829(a).

47. *Gonzales* v. *Oregon,* 546 U.S. 243 (2006).
48. Jacoby S: The right to die, *AARP Bulletin* pp 8-9, Nov 2005.
49. American Medical Association: Guidelines for the appropriate use of do not resuscitate orders: Council on Ethical and Judicial Affairs, *JAMA* 265:1868, 1991.
50. Patient's wishes on "end-of-life care" should be discussed with health professionals, *PT Bulletin* p 19, Dec 22, 1995.
51. Woodruff WA: Letting life run its course: do-not-resuscitate orders and withdrawal of life-sustaining treatment, *Army Lawyer* pp 6-18, April 1989.
52. Cruzan. See reference 15.
53. 521 U.S. 702 (1997).
54. 521 U.S. 793 (1997).
55. Eisenberg D: Lessons from the Schiavo battle, *Time* pp 22-30, April 4, 2005.
56. Stacy M: Autopsy: Schiavo in vegetative state, *San Antonio Express News* p 1A, June 16, 2005.
57. Stem Cell Information (National Institutes of Health): *Federal policy.* Retrieved May 15, 2007, from http://stemcells.nih.gov/policy.
58. National Coalition on Health Care: *Health insurance cost.* Retrieved May 18, 2007, from www.nchc.org/facts/cost.shtml.
59. Wolf R: Study: uninsured kids fare worse at hospitals, *USA Today* p 2A, March 2, 2007.
60. Ozer M: National health system would fix health care crisis, *San Antonio Express News* p 4H, April 18, 2007.
61. Moffit, R.E. The Massachusetts Health Plan: An Update and Lessons for Other States. Heritage Foundation, Retrieved May 18, 2007, from www.heritage.org.
62. Berman S, Dolins J, Tang S, Yudkowsky B: Factors that influence willingness of private primary care pediatricians to accept more Medicaid patients, *Pediatrics* 110:239-248, 2002.
63. The Emergency Treatment and Active Labor Act, 42 United States Code Section 1395dd.
64. Winton R: Patient dumping may seem criminal but ... , *Los Angeles Times* p B1, Feb 25, 2007.
65. Winton R, DiMassa CM: Kaiser accepts patient dumping settlement, *Latimes.com* May 16, 2007. Retrieved May 19, 2007. Kudos to reporters.
66. 2006 AIDS epidemic update. Retrieved May 20, 2007, from www.unaids.org.
67. Association of Nurses in AIDS Care. Retrieved May 20, 2007, from www.anacnet.org.
68. Deacon H, Boulle A: Factors affecting HIV/AIDS-related stigma and discrimination by medical professionals, *Int J Epidemiol* 36(10):185-186, 2007.
69. Worker Health Chartbook 2004. Surveillance of Health Care Workers with AIDS. NIOSH Pub. 2004-146. Retrieved Sept. 26, 2007, from www.cdc.gov.
70. Recommendations for Prevention of Transmission of HIV in Health Care Settings. Retrieved Sept. 26, 2007, from www. cdc.gov.
71. National Council on State Legislatures: Managed Care State Laws, retrieved May 20, 2007, from www.ncsl.org
72. *Kentucky Association of Health Plans, Inc.* v. *Miller,* 538 U.S. 329 (2003).
73. 8 C.F.R. Part 214, Department of Homeland Security (2007).
74. US Citizenship and Immigration Services: H1B annual report 2006, retrieved May 20, 2007, from www.uscis.gov.
75. Lardent EF: Recruitment and retention of volunteer attorneys. In *The resource: a* pro bono *manual,* Chicago, 1983, American Bar Association.
76. American Bar Association: *Canons of professional ethics,* Chicago, 1908, The Association.
77. American Bar Association: *Model code of professional responsibility,* Chicago, 1969, The Association.

78. American Bar Association: *Model rules of professional conduct,* Chicago, 1983, The Association.

79. Russell LH, Bruce EA: *The elder economic security standard background,* Feb 1, 2007. Elder economic security project, retrieved May 21, 2007, from www.geront.umb.edu.

80. American Medical Association: *State licensing and liability laws for volunteer physicians,* Jan 31, 2005. Retrieved May 21, 2007, from www.ama-assn.org.

81. Mussman MG, Zawistowich I, Weisman CS: Medical malpractice claims filed by Medicaid and non-Medicaid recipients in Maryland, *JAMA* 265:2992, 1991.

82. National Practitioner Data Bank, Health care integrity and protection, retrieved May 21, 2007, from www.npdb-hipdb.hrsa.gov.

83. Hayner K: Samuel Merritt College seeks adults for free adult rehabilitation clinic, *Reporter* p 3, Winter 2005.

84. UTMB nursing students assist probate court, *Texas Bar Journal* 66(11):860, 2003.

85. Drug partnership introduces cheap antimalarial pill, *New York Times* 2007, March 1, 2007.

86. Knight D: Giving back: companies becoming advocates for workers volunteering time to causes, *Indianapolis Star* p D1, April 30, 2006.

87. Cleverley WO: *Essentials of health care finance,* ed 4, Gaithersburg, Md, 1997, Aspen.

88. Ibid. pp 53, 61.

89. Finley C: Gift-giving or influence peddling: can you tell the difference? *J Am Phys Ther Assoc* 74:143, 1994.

90. *Wilk v. American Medical Association,* 895 F 2d 352, cert. denied, 498 US 982 (1990).

91. The Sherman Act of 1890, 15 United States Code Section 1.

92. Portney LG, Watkins MP: *Foundations of clinical research: applications to practice,* Norwalk, Conn, 1993, Appleton & Lange.

93. Title 45 Code of Federal Regulations, Part 46: Protection of human subjects, Washington, DC, June 23, 2005, Department of Health and Human Services.

94. *On being a scientist: responsible conduct in research,* ed 2, 1995, Washington, DC, National Academy Press (pp 6-8).

95. Ibid, pp 8-18.

96. Altman LK, Broad WJ: Global trend: more science, more fraud, *New York Times* p D1, Dec 20, 2005.

97. Meier B: Major medical journals will require registration of trials, *New York Times* p C9, Sep 9, 2004.

98. The Family Educational Rights and Privacy Act of 1974, 20 United States Code Section 1232 et seq.

99. Mathis RD: The roles of the law and the lawyer in clinical ethics. In *Health care ethics short course,* San Antonio, Texas, 1993, Brooke Army Medical Center.

100. Stein RA: Just call the ethics experts, *ABA Journal* p 98, March 1997.

101. Scott RW: *Legal aspects of documenting patient care,* ed 3, Sudbury, Mass, 2006, Jones and Bartlett.

102. Principle 1, Nuremberg Code of 1947. In *Trials of war criminals before the Nuremberg military tribunals under control council law No. 10,* vol 2, Washington, DC, 1949, US Government Printing Office.

103. World Medical Association Declaration of Helsinki: Principle 2 (Adopted by the 18th World Medical Assembly, Helsinki, Finland, 1964, and amended by the 29th World Medical Assembly, Tokyo, Japan, 1975), 35th World Medical Assembly, Venice, Italy, 1983 and 41st World Medical Assembly, Hong Kong, 1989.

104. Code of Federal Regulations: *Protection of human subjects,* Title 45, Part 46, Washington, DC, 2005, US Government Printing Office.

105. *TD v. New York State Office of Mental Health,* WL 695417 (N. App, 1996).

106. Barnes PG: Beyond Nuremberg, *ABA Journal* 83(3):24, 1997.

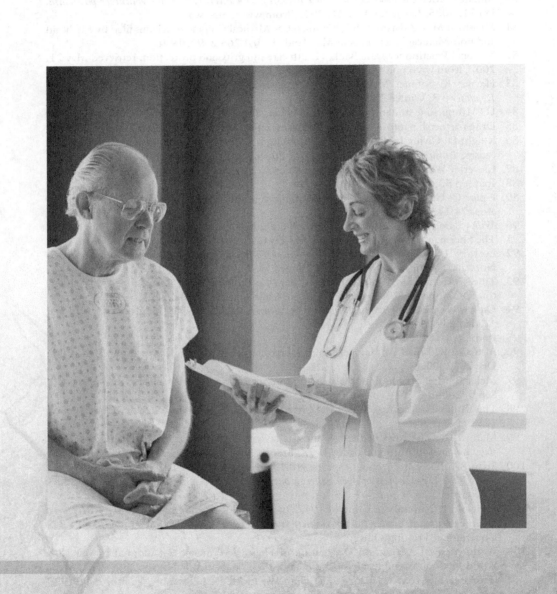

Epilogue

Although the legal and ethical obligations incumbent upon health care professionals are many and complex, they can be better understood through education, and, as a result, providers can have greater peace of mind while they carry out their formidable duties.

Those are the principle purposes of this book: to educate health care professionals about key legal concepts and make them aware of their rights and duties under law; to give them a framework to assess their official conduct for compliance with ethical standards; to provide them with a systems model for ethical decision making; and to help ensure that health care professionals do not fear the legal system nor practice defensively in response to it.

Because the law is ever changing, readers are urged to involve organizational attorneys and legal and ethical consultants in their practices and continuing education experiences. Through better understanding of the legal system, health care professionals will simultaneously protect the vital interests of their patients and themselves.

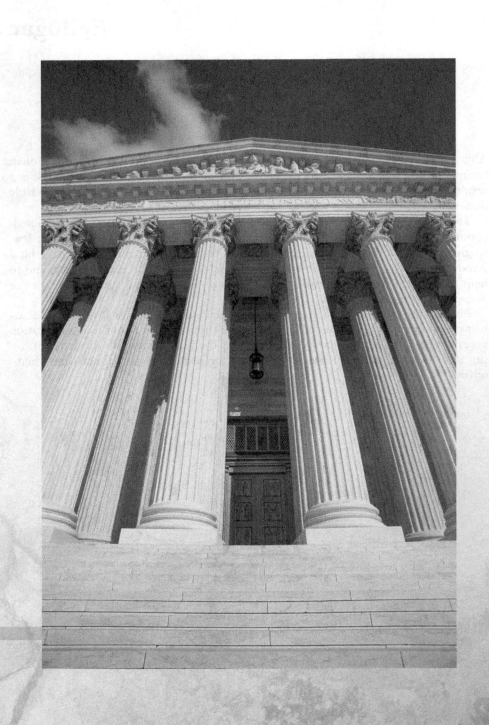

Index

401(k) plans, 136-137

A

Ab initio, 148
Abandonment, 56-59, 93, 241
Absolute liability. *See* Strict liability
Absolute privileges, 96
Abuse, 97-99, 107-108
Access, nondiscrimination and, 242-243
Accommodation, 129-130
Acquittals, 110
Active euthanasia, 117, 239
Actors, ethics and, 26
Acts, intentional torts and, 92-93
Actual cause, 63
Actus reus, 90, 108, 120
Administrative law, 8-9, 162-163
Administrative Procedures Act of 1946, 163
Adoption, 137-138
Advance directives, 194
Advertising professional services, 165
Aetna Health Inc. v. Davila, 53
Affiliation, 179
Affirmative defenses, 71
Against medical advice, 76
Agape concern, 33
Age Discrimination in Employment Act, 128
Agency by estoppel, 70
Agency for Healthcare Research and Quality, 63
Aggravated burglary, 118
Agreement, contracts and, 172-173, 175
Agreements, oral and written, 175-176
AIDS, 241-242
Alibis, 111
Alteration of records, 81
Alternatives, informed consent and, 230
American Board of Certification, 31
American Hand Society, 62
American Medical Association, Wilk v., 164, 248
Americans with Disabilities Act, 8, 128-132, 207, 241-242
Analytical principalism, 35
Answers, 71, 114
Anticipatory deadly force, 112

Antidumping law, 38
Antitrust law, 163-164
Antonio, Wards Cove Packing Co. v., 134
"Any willing provider" laws, 243
Apparent agency, 70
Appeals, 16, 114
Arbitration, 248
Arizona State Bar, Bates and Van O'Steen v., 165
Arraignments, 114
Arrests, 113
Ashcroft, John, 238
Assault, 93-94, 105-106, 116
Assisted suicide, 117, 237-239
Assumption of risk, 74-75
At will employment, 126
Attorneys
  conflicts of interest and, 190-191
  contingent fees and, 13
  institutional ethics committees and, 250-251
  pretrial depositions and, 167-168
  pro bono services and, 244
  when to seek legal advice from, 166-167
Attractive nuisances, 68
Authorized disclosure, 185
Auto theft, 118
Automatism, 111
Autonomy, 29, 38-39, 41, 222

B

Bail, 7
Barnett case, 131
Barondess, Jeremiah, 36
Bates and Van O'Steen v. State Bar of Arizona, 165
Battery, 94-95, 116, 214, 223, 224
Belmont Report, 37
Beneficence, 34-35
BFOQ. *See* Bona fide occupational qualifications
Bilateral contracts, 170, 171, 175
Bill of Rights, 5-6, 7
Bioethics, defined, 30
Biomedical ethical principles, 34-38
Bisexuality, 130
Boadle, Byrne v., 15

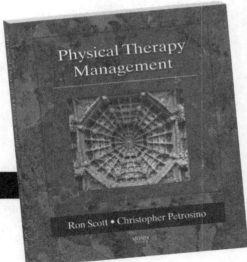

Printed in the United States
By Bookmasters